Recent Results in Cancer Research 52

Fortschritte der Krebsforschung
Progrès dans les recherches sur le cancer

The Ambivalence of Cytostatic Therapy

Edited by

E. Grundmann and R. Gross

With 58 Figures

Springer-Verlag
Berlin · Heidelberg · New York 1975

Gesellschaft zur Bekämpfung der Krebskrankheiten, Nordrhein-Westfalen e. V. and European Organization for Research on Treatment of Cancer, V. Symposium in Düsseldorf, November 8/9, 1973

Prof. Dr. EKKEHARD GRUNDMANN, Pathologisches Institut, 4400 Münster, Westring 17

Prof. Dr. RUDOLF W. J. GROSS, Medizinische Universitätsklinik, 5000 Köln 41, Joseph-Stelzmannstr. 9

Sponsored by the Swiss League against Cancer

ISBN-13 : 978-3-642-80942-2 e-ISBN-13 : 978-3-642-80940-8
DOI : 10.1007 / 978-3-642-80940-8

Library of Congress Cataloging in Publication Data. Gesellschaft zur Bekämpfung der Krebskrankheiten Nordrhein-Westfalen. The Ambivalence of Cytostatic Therapy (Recent results in cancer research; 52) Proceedings of the society's 5th symposium, held in Düsseldorf Nov. 8—9, 1973, and sponsored by the Swiss League against Cancer. Includes bibliographies and index. 1. Cancer — Chemotherapy — Congresses. 2. Antineoplastic agents — Congresses. I. Grundmann, Ekkehard. II. Gross, Rudolf, 1917—. III. Schweizerische Nationalliga für Krebsbekämpfung und Krebsforschung. IV. Title. V. Series. [DNLM: 1. Antineoplastic agents — Adverse effects. 2. Cell division — Drug effects. 3. Neoplasms — Drug therapy. Wl RE106P v. 52 / QZ267 C997] RC261.R35 vol. 52 [RC271.C5] 616.9'94'008s [616.9'94'061] 75-6742.

Softcover reprint of the hardcover 1st edition 1975

Typesetting, printing and binding:
Konrad Triltsch, Graphischer Betrieb, 87 Würzburg, Germany.

Contents

I. Tumor Induction by Cytostatics?

II. Tumor Induction by Immunodeficiency?

III. Cell Synchronization in Tumor Therapy

List of Delegates

R. Baserga, Temple University of Medicine, Dept. of Pathology, 3400 North Broad St., Philadelphia/PA. 19140, USA.

N. Brock, ASTA-Werke AG, Pharmakologische Abteilung, D-4812 Brackwede, Germany.

A. Caputo, Istituto Regina Elena, I-00161 Roma, viale Regina Elena 291, Italy.

F. Ehring, Fachklinik Haus Hornheide, D-4401 Handorf/Münster, Germany.

R. Fritzsche, Universitäts-Frauenklinik, D-4400 Münster, Westring 11, Germany.

R. Gross, Medizinische Universitätsklinik, D-5000 Köln 41, Joseph-Stelzmann-Str. 9, Germany.

E. Grundmann, Pathologisches Institut der Universität, D-4400 Münster, Westring 17, Germany.

M. G. Hanna, Frederick Cancer Research Center, P.O. Box B Frederick, MD 21701 and Oak Ridge National Laboratories, Biology Division, P.O. Box Y, Oak Ridge, TN 37830, USA.

W. Hunstein, Medizinische Universitätsklinik, D-6900 Heidelberg 1, Hospitalstr. 3, Germany.

N. S. Irey, Armed Forces Institute of Pathology, Registry of Tissue Reactions to Drugs, Washington/DC. 20306, USA.

H. O. Klein, Medizinische Universitätsklinik, D-5000 Köln 41, Joseph-Stelzmann-Str. 9, Germany.

R. Kroes, Rijksinstituut voor de Volksgezondheid, Bilthoven, Antoni Leeuwenhoeklaan 9, Netherlands.

G. Krueger, Pathologisches Institut der Universität, D-5000 Köln 41, Joseph-Stelzmann-Str. 9, Germany.

K. J. Lennartz, Pathologisches Institut d. Universität, D-5000 Köln 41, Joseph-Stelzmann-Str. 9, Germany.

I. Penn, University of Colorado, Medical Center, 4200 East Ninth Avenue, Denver/CO. 80220, USA.

F. S. Philips, Sloan-Kettering-Institute for Cancer Research, Trafalgar 9-3000, New York/NY. 11021, USA.

P. POUILLART, Groupe Hospitalier Paul Brousse, Institut de Cancérologie et d'Immunogénétique, 14/16 Ave. P. Vaillant-Couturier, F-94 Villejuif, France.

M. F. RAJEWSKY, Max-Planck-Institut f. Virusforschung, D-7400 Tübingen, Spemannstr. 35, Germany.

H. R. SCHERF, Deutsches Krebsforschungszentrum, Inst. f. Toxikologie u. Chemotherapie, D-6900 Heidelberg, Im Neuenheimer Feld 280, Germany.

D. SCHMÄHL, Deutsches Krebsforschungszentrum, Inst. f. Toxikologie u. Chemotherapie, D-6900 Heidelberg, Im Neuenheimer Feld 280, Germany.

B. SCHNEIDER, Medizinische Hochschule, Inst. f. Biometrie, D-3000 Hannover-Kleefeld, Karl-Wiechert-Allee 9, Germany

J. SCHUMANN, Fachklinik Haus Hornheide, D-4401 Handorf/Münster, Germany.

H. L. STEWART, N.I.H., National Cancer Institute, Registry of Experimental Cancers, Bldg. 37 (ERF), R. 202, Bethesda/MD. 20014, USA.

M. TUBIANA, Institut Gustave Roussy, 16bis, Ave. P. Vaillant-Couturier, F-94 Villejuif, France.

M. C. VANDEPUTTE, Katholieke Universiteit te Leuven, Rega Instituut, B-3000 Leuven, Minderbroederstraat 10, Belgium.

L. M. VAN PUTTEN, Radiobiological Institute, Rijswijk, Lange Kleiweg 151, Netherlands.

J. H. WEISBURGER, Naylor Dana Institute for Disease Prevention, American Health Foundation, Valhalla, NY. 10595.

M. WINNEWISSER, Max-Planck-Institut für Psychiatrie, D-8000 München 40, Kraepelinstraße 10, Germany.

The Carcinogenic Properties of Some of the Principal Drugs Used in Clinical Cancer Chemotherapy

J. H. WEISBURGER, D. P. GRISWOLD, J. D. PREJEAN, A. E. CASEY, H. B. WOOD, and E. K. WEISBURGER

INTRODUCTION

Years ago, a team at the Chester Beatty Research Institute in London made the important observation that active cancer chemotherapeutic agents might also be carcinogenic (6). Thus, they discovered the potent carcinogenicity of 4-aminostilbene and derivatives. This concept, however, was not universally recognized and applied. In fact, it was rediscovered with one of the drugs developed at the Chester Beatty Research Institute, namely chlornaphazine. This drug was successful in leading to remissions of Hodgkins' disease and related neoplastic conditions, but the patients so treated developed cancer in the urinary bladder some years later (1).

Subsequently, attention was drawn to the potential carcinogenic risk attached to certain cancer chemotherapeutic agents (25). When lung tumor induction in the A strain mouse was used as indicator, it was shown that some of these drugs did indeed possess carcinogenic potential. Later the carcinogenic risk of a larger series of drugs used in cancer chemotherapy was investigated at a number of dose levels in the same test system (26). The authors found quite varied carcinogenic potential. Moreover, they concluded that there was no correlation between the carcinogenicity of a given drug and its potential chemotherapeutic effect in an L1210 leukemia assay.

In the intervening years, others have also questioned the carcinogenicity of certain drugs, as evidenced by a number of symposia on this subject (1, 28). The extensive data collected by Professor SCHMÄHL, with whom we have exchanged information over the years, are reported in this volume. In addition, there has been progress in the mechanistic understanding of the carcinogenic process. It became clear that chemicals with alkylating properties may well have carcinogenic potency, depending on structure, reactivity, and the test system. Biochemical conversion by the host of precursors to such alkylating agents likewise entailed carcinogenic risk, often at a higher level because the reactive entity was produced within the cell. Exogenously given alkylating agents were often less active, because they could undergo competitive deactivating

* We are indebted for advice to Dr. C. G. ZUBROD, Dr. S. CARTER, Dr. E. FREIREICH, and Dr. H. L. FALK, and for editorial assistance to Mrs. F. WILLIAMS and Mrs. M. MERVIS.

This work was performed at Southern Research Institute under contract no. NIH-NCI-E-73-3214 from the National Cancer Institute.

reactions before reaching the key intracellular targets for the expression of carcinogenicity (2, 5, 9, 12, 14, 15, 17, 29, 30, 31, 32).

On the other hand, it was thought that drugs used in cancer chemotherapy, because of their specific antimetabolite functions, might not be carcinogenic if (1) they were not converted to alkylating agents, and (2) they did not otherwise affect the host in a general way, such as through an alteration in the immune response.

As a follow-up on studies which developed data on carcinogenic risk in the strain-A mouse system with the induction of pulmonary tumors as an indicator (26), it was felt that a more general investigation of the carcinogenic potential of drugs used clinically in the United States at present would be desirable.

Thus, plans were formulated by the staff of the National Cancer Institute and their advisors to conduct a detailed study in mice and rats on the carcinogenicity of drugs commonly used in the clinic, including certain key mixtures used concurrently or in a sequential protocol in patients. Since the drugs were used only for a portion of a lifespan, the protocols realistically reflected this. Hence, the drugs were injected for 6 months to mice and rats, followed by a holding period for one additional year to reveal delayed toxic effects and to allow the expression of carcinogenicity. These protocols are different from those generally used for the assessment of carcinogenicity of other environmental agents, such as food additives, where the risk extends over the whole lifetime (33).

The current report is preliminary, for not all of the data obtained with the 43 drugs and mixtures studied have been fully analyzed. Other data have also been presented in preliminary reports (20).

MATERIALS AND METHODS

Animals

Sprague Dawley-derived Charles River CD rats were procured at weaning, from the Charles River Laboratories, Wilmington, Massachusetts 01887. Swiss Webster-derived mice were purchased from Manor Farms, Inc., Staatsburg, New York. The animals were maintained in quarantine until they were 6 weeks of age, then randomly distributed into experimental and control groups. The animal facilities, constructed to maintain directional flow of all materials and personnel, were maintained at 60% humidity and a temperature of 24°C. The animals were housed in stainless steel cages with no more than 5 rats or 7 mice per cage. Later in the study, the number of animals was reduced to 2 to 3 per cage. The diet was Purina Laboratory Chow 5010C, a fortified pelleted food, which was sterilized by autoclaving prior to feeding. Feed, bedding, cages, and water bottles were periodically checked to insure freedom from bacterial and mold contamination.

Preliminary Toxicology

The maximally tolerated dose (MTD) under our experimental conditions was determined in preliminary experiments (33). Existing data expressing doses in terms of wt/m^2 body surface were used as initial guidelines. Groups of 5 animals each were given 5 preselected dose levels of each compound, formulated in an appropriate vehicle, by i. p. injection 3 times per week for a total of 45 days (20 injections). The animals were held an additional 45 days to detect delayed toxicity. The MTD was taken as that dose which assured survival of the animals for the trial period and gave a distinct depression of weight gain during the treatment period, but no more than 20%. The animals at the highest tolerated dose levels were killed and examined thoroughly, and the key tissues were processed for histopathologic study.

Carcinogenicity Tests

Groups of 25 male and 25 female animals, rats and mice, were given 3 i. p. injections per week of the MTD level, as determined above, of each drug for a 6-month period. Other identical groups of animals received 0.5 MTD. Thus, each test involved 50 male and 50 female mice, and the same number of rats. Where excessive mortality was seen, whether due to treatment with the recommended dose levels or (as was found with the male mice) due to fighting, additional groups of animals, including controls, were started at appropriate dose levels to assure adequate numbers of animals for evaluation at the end of the study.

There were untreated control rats and mice as well as groups of animals given the vehicle only, where a vehicle was used to formulate the drug for injection.

The animals were carefully observed during treatment and a further 12-month holding period. Their weight gains and general appearance were monitored. Animals in poor condition were isolated and killed when survival appeared in jeopardy. All animals were killed at the end of the 18-month test period. They were necropsied and examined for grossly apparent lesions, which were recorded. The following tissues were preserved in fixative (4% buffered formalin solution) for subsequent histopathologic examination: pituitary, brain, thyroid, thymus, heart, lungs, stomach, duodenum, jejunum, ileum, caecum, colon, liver, pancreas, spleen, adrenal, kidney, urinary bladder, mammary, marrow, ovary and Fallopian tubes, uterus, seminal vesicle, prostate, testicle, skin, and peripheral blood (smear) and any tumor masses.

The data were evaluated in most instances by the Fischer exact method with a 2 x 2 probability table, comparing the experimental groups with the corresponding control groups of untreated mice or rats.

In this preliminary report, the results obtained at both dose levels are combined to facilitate the presentation.

RESULTS

Untreated Control Animals

Since the control animals necessarily serve as a reference point for an evaluation of the results obtained with the drug-injected experimental mice or rats, we are first presenting data on survival and tumor incidence with the untreated control groups (21) (Tables 1 through 4). Most of the tumors in the control

Table 1. Mortality and tumor incidence in 179 male and 181 female Sprague-Dawley rats observed for 540 days

Weeks of observation	No. dying with tumors/ No. dead Male	Female
13	0/0	0/0
26	0/0	0/1
39	0/0	1/1
52	0/5	3/7
65	2/10	5/9
77	3/9	9/12
>77[a]	55/155	57/151
Total	60/179	105/181

[a]77-week survivors were sacrificed at day 540.

Table 2. Location of 219 spontaneous tumors occurring in 165 (60 males and 105 females) of 360 Sprague-Dawley rats observed for 540 days

Site and tumor	Male	Female
Skin and subcutaneous tissues:		
Fibroma	1	
Fibrosarcoma		1
Hemangioma		1
Sebaceous gland adenoma	1	
Squamous papilloma		1
Myxolipoma		1
Mammary gland:		
Fibroadenoma	2	43
Lobular adenoma		2
Lobular adenocarcinoma	1	13
Columnar cell carcinoma	1	
Hematopoietic and lymphatic tissues:		
Disseminated myelocytic sarcoma	2	
Disseminated lymphosarcoma		1
Hemangioma (lymph node)		1
Lung:		
Alveolar cell adenoma	1	
Bronchogenic carcinoma	2	1
Stomach:		
Squamous papilloma	1	
Squamous cell carcinoma	1	
Peritoneum:		
Lipoma		1

Table 2 (Continued)

Site and tumor	Male	Female
Pancreas:		
Acinar adenoma		1
Uterus:		
Leiomyosarcoma		1
Fibrovascular polyps		2
Vagina:		
Stromal polyp		1
Testis:		
Interstitial cell adenoma	4	
Interstitial cell adenocarcinoma	2	
Prostate:		
Adenocarcinoma	1	
Pituitary:		
Adenoma	12	25
Adenocarcinoma	16	28
Fibrosarcoma	1	
Adrenal:		
Cortical adenoma	11	16
Cortical adenocarcinoma	1	
Pheochromocytoma	2	2
Thyroid:		
Adenoma	4	1
Adenocarcinoma	3	2
Parathyroid:		
Adenoma	2	
Brain:		
Astrocytoma	2	
Total	74	145

mice were noted in the last 6 months of the observation period. In mice lung tumors were most prevalent, followed in decreasing order of frequency by tumors in the hematopoietic and lymphatic tissues, the skin and subcutaneous tissues, the endocrine-related organs such as breast, ovary, uterus, testis, pituitary, adrenal, thyroid, and scattered other lesions.

In the Charles River (CD) male rats there were no tumors in the first 65 weeks, and most neoplastic lesions were seen at the 18-month necropsy point. Female rats exhibited some early mammary tumors but these were detected most frequently at necropsy. In addition, male and female rats had an appreciable number of pituitary and somewhat fewer adrenal tumors. A small number of tumors occurred in other tissues.

Table 3. Mortality and tumor incidence in 101 male and 153 female Swiss-Webster mice observed for 540 days

Weeks of observation	No. dying with tumors/ No. dead Male	Female
13	0/0	0/0
26	1/7	0/0
39	2/8	0/6
52	1/10	3/17
65	5/11	1/13
77	9/23	9/30
>77[a]	10/42	25/97
Total	28/101	38/153

[a]77-week survivors were sacrificed at day 540.

Table 4. Location of 79 spontaneous tumors occurring in 66 (28 males and 38 females) of 254 Swiss-Webster mice observed for 540 days

Site and tumor	Male	Female
Skin and subcutaneous tissues:		
Fibrosarcoma	2	
Leiomyosarcoma		1
Sebaceous gland adenoma	3	
Fibroepithelial polyp	1	
Cavernous hemangioma	1	
Mammary gland:		
Lobular adenocarcinoma		3
Cystadenoma	1	
Hematopoietic and lymphatic tissues:		
Disseminated lymphosarcoma		1
Disseminated reticulum cell sarcoma	1	1
Plasmacytoma (Thymus)	1	
Lymphosarcoma (Thymus)	1	1
Cavernous hemangioma (Spleen)		1
Lung:		
Alveolar cell adenoma	4	7
Alveolar cell adenocarcinoma	6	14
Metastatic carcinoma from mammary gland		1
Thoracic Cavity:		
Osteosarcoma		1

Table 4 (Continued)

Site and tumor	Male	Female
Liver:		
Hepatocytic adenoma	1	
Hemangioendothelial sarcoma	1	
Kidney:		
Nephroblastoma	1	
Adenocarcinoma	1	
Urinary Bladder:		
Papilloma	1	
Carcinoma	2	
Ovary:		
Adenocarcinoma		2
Adenoleiomyoma		1
Granulosa cell tumor		3
Uterus:		
Hemangiosarcoma		1
Fibrous polyp		2
Testis:		
Interstitial cell adenoma	2	
Interstitial cell adenocarcinoma	1	
Pituitary:		
Chromophobe adenoma		1
Chromophobe adenocarcinoma		2
Adrenal:		
Fibrosarcoma	1	
Thyroid:		
Light cell adenoma	1	1
Cystadenoma		1
Brain:		
Astroblastoma		1
Muscle:		
Fibrosarcoma	1	
Total	34	45

Tumors Induced by Drugs

Actinomycin D (NSC-3053) induced sarcomas in the peritoneal cavity, the site of injection, in male and female rats. Thus, it had a typical local action. However, no tumors due to the drug were seen in mice (Table 5).

Table 5. Main tumors induced by cancer chemotherapeutic drugs

		Mice			
		Males		Females	
Drug and NSC no.	Dose range (mg/kg/dose)	Tumors[a]	p^b	Tumors[a]	p^b
Actinomycin D 3053	0.18-0.37	-	-	-	-
Chlorambucil 3088	1.5-3.0	Lung tumors 22/35	<0.001	Lung tumors 20/28	<0.001
		Lymphosarcomas 6/35	0.004	Lymphosarcomas 4/28	0.012
				Ovarian tumors 10/28	<0.001
Melphalan 8806	0.75-1.5	Lung tumors 11/44	0.012	Lung tumors 10/23	0.001
		Lymphosarcomas 13/44	<0.001	-	
Cytoxan 26271	12-25	Lung tumors 7/30	0.031	Lung tumors 10/35	0.027
		Bladder papillomas - 4/30	0.048	-	
Mitomycin C 26980	0.25-0.5	-	-	-	-
Uracil mustard 34462	0.12-0.5	Lung tumors 7/37	0.095	Lung tumors 23/40	<0.001
		Liver tumors 4/37	0.018	Ovarian tumors 10/40	<0.001
				Lymphomas 20/40	<0.001
DIC 45388	25-50	Lung tumors 21/41	<0.001	Lung tumors 16/19	<0.001
		Lymphomas 15/41	<0.001	Uterine tumors 5/19	<0.001
		Splenic tumors 10/41	<0.001		
Phosphorodiamidic acid, cyclohexyl-amine, salt 52695	50-100	Lung tumors 14/39	0.004	Lung tumors 21/39	<0.001
				Lymphomas 10/39	<0.001
				Esophageal papillomas 3/39	<0.001
				Uterine tumors 5/39	0.004
1-Acetyl-2-pico-linolhydrazine 68626	125-250	Lung tumors 13/27	<0.001	Lung tumors 19/25	<0.001
				Ovarian and uterine tumors 9/25	<0.001
Natulan 77213	12-25	Lung tumors 15/33	<0.001	Lung tumors 23/34	<0.001
				Lymphomas 9/34	<0.001
				Renal tumors 3/34	0.006
				Uterine tumors 8/34	<0.001

Streptozotocin 85999	6-12	Lung tumors 18/30	<0.001	Lung tumors 33/39	<0.001
		Renal tumors 18/30	0.007	Renal tumors 7/39	<0.001
				Uterine tumors 6/39	0.001
Streptozotocin plus nicotinamide (250 mg)	6-12	Lung tumors 25/46	<0.001	Lung tumors 34/45	<0.001
		Renal tumors 2/46	0.371	Renal tumors 1/45	0.227
		Pancreatic tumors 1/46	0.313	Pancreatic tumors 1/45	0.227
Dibromomannitol 94100	90-180	Lung tumors 8/25	0.006	Lung tumors 19/40	<0.001
				Lymphomas 9/40	<0.001
Dibromodulcitol 104800	45-90	Lung tumors 8/41	0.073	Lung tumors 14/30	<0.001
		Lymphomas 10/41	<0.001	Lymphomas 8/30	<0.001
Diethylnitrosamine 132 (positive control)	6	Lung tumors 26/32	0.001	Lung tumors 25/31	<0.001
		Liver tumors 3/32	0.043	Liver tumors 5/31	<0.001

[a]Number of animals with specific tumor/number of animals examined.

[b]Significance of difference in occurrence of tumors in treated and untreated groups.

Table 5 (continued)

		Rats			
		Males		Females	
Drug and NSC no.	Dose range (mg/kg/dose)	Tumors[a]	p[b]	Tumors[a]	p[b]
Actinomycin D 3053	0.022-0.045	Peritoneal sarcomas 32/38	<0.001	Peritoneal sarcomas 25/36	<0.001
Chlorambucil 3088	2.2-4.5	Lymphomas 8/33	<0.001	-	-
Melphalan 8806	0.9-1.8	Peritoneal sarcomas 11/20	<0.001	Peritoneal sarcomas 10/23	<0.001
Cytoxan 26271	5-10	Breast carcinoma 1/50	0.530	Breast carcinoma 9/53	0.035
				Breast adenoma 24/53	0.028
Mitomycin C 26980	0.038-0.15	Peritoneal sarcomas 27/29	<0.001	Peritoneal sarcomas 30/31	<0.001
Uracil mustard 34462	0.15-0.3	Peritoneal sarcomas 10/38	<0.001	Peritoneal sarcomas 8/39	<0.001
		Lymphomas 6/38	<0.001	Lymphomas 4/39	0.004
		Pancreatic tumors 3/38	0.005	Ovarian tumors 4/39	<0.001
				Breast carcinomas 8/39	0.03
DIC 45388	50-100	Lymphomas 18/34	<0.001	Lymphomas 12/22	<0.001
		Renal tumors 4/34	<0.001	Breast carcinomas 16/22	0.001
		Heart tumors 8/34	<0.001	Heart tumors 2/22	0.011
Phosphorodiamidic acid, cyclohexylamine, salt 52695	37-75	Bladder tumors 4/26	<0.001	Bladder tumors 4/28	<0.001
		Prostate tumors 2/26	0.043	Breast carcinomas 10/28	<0.001
		Subcutaneous tumors 4/26	0.003		
1-Acetyl-2-picolinolhydrazine 68626	125-250	Pancreatic tumors 2/44	0.038	-	-
Natulan 77213	30-60	Breast carcinomas 18/47	<0.001	Breast carcinomas 20/37	<0.001
		Lymphomas 11/47	<0.001	Lymphomas 4/37	0.003
		Leukemia 14/47	<0.001	Leukemia 13/37	<0.001

Streptozotocin 85999	6-12	Renal tumors 19/42	<0.001	Renal tumors 16/46	<0.001
		Peritoneal sarcomas 4/42	0.001	Liver Tumors 19/46	<0.001
		Pancreatic tumors 3/42	0.006	Pancreatic tumors 4/46	<0.005
		Muscle tumors 3/42	0.006		
Streptozotocin plus nicotinamide (250 mg)	6-12	Renal tumors 21/40	0.001	Renal tumors 22/49	<0.001
		Liver tumors 7/40	<0.001	Liver tumors 5/49	<0.001
		Pancreatic tumors 7/40	<0.001	Pancreatic tumors 4/49	0.008
		Peritoneal sarcomas 3/40	0.006	Peritoneal sarcomas 2/49	0.045
Dibromomannitol 94100	125-250	Peritoneal sarcomas 6/37	<0.001	Peritoneal sarcomas 2/40	0.032
		Subcutaneous tumors 6/37	<0.001	-	-
Dibromodulcitol 104800	75-150	Subcutaneous tumors 18/34	<0.001	-	-
Diethylnitrosamine 132 (positive control	5	Liver tumors 11/32	<0.001	Liver tumors 18/18	<0.001
				Renal tumors 6/18	<0.001

[a]Number of animals with specific tumor/number of animals examined.

[b]Significance of difference in occurrence of tumors in treated and untreated groups.

Chlorambucil (NSC-3088) induced mainly lung tumors in both male and female mice, and a smaller number of lymphosarcomas. Females had ovarian tumors. Chlorambucil appeared to have no carcinogenicity in female rats, but males had a few lymphosarcomas, myelogenous leukemias, and reticulum cell sarcomas.

Melphalan (NSC-8806) led to lung tumors in male and female mice and lymphosarcomas in males. Sarcomas of the peritoneal cavity appeared in about 50% of the surviving rats.

Cytoxan (NSC-26271) induced lung tumors in male and female mice and some papillomas of the urinary bladder in male mice. With female rats tumor formation in the mammary gland was increased above the control incidence. An effect of cytoxan on the bladder has already been reported in rats (10).

Mitomycin (NSC-26980) was active in inducing peritoneal sarcoma in a considerable number of male and female rats, but no real effect was noted in mice.

Uracil Mustard (NSC-34462), the most active of the drugs studied by Shimkin's team in strain-A mice (26), induced mainly lung tumors in male and female mice. In addition, there were malignant lymphomas in females, and liver tumors in males only. Females also had a higher incidence of ovarian tumors than did the untreated controls. At a dose of 0.5 mg/kg there were only 4 male and 5 female mice surviving from each group of 25, with a median date of death at day 281 and day 240 respectively. Of the 5 females, 4 had malignant lymphomas. At a dose of 0.25 mg/kg males had a median day of death of 315 (range 200-283) and females 483 (163-550). With a dose of 0.12 mg/kg the median date of death was day 426 (109-551) for males and day 407 (208-551) for females.

Uracil mustard led to lymphomas and peritoneal tumors in male and female rats, and breast as well as ovarian tumors in female rats. Only 4 males and 4 females survived more than 100 days at 0.6 mg/kg; median day 156 (range 122-332) for males, 151 (127-285) for females. With 0.3 mg/kg uracil mustard, the median day was 350 (241-548) for males, and 394 (292-548) for females, while with 0.15 mg/kg it was 456 (280-547) for males and 493 (141-547) for females.

4(5)-(3,3-Dimethyl-1-triazeno)imidazole-5(4)-carboxamide (DIC; NSC-45388) was also a carcinogen. It induced lung tumors, lymphomas, and hemangiomas (spleen) in male mice. In test females lung tumors and uterine tumors were more frequent than in female controls. With a dose of 50 mg/kg the median survival was 177 days (range 163-270) for males and 128 (116-179) for females. With 25 mg/kg/dose it was 331 days (104-549) for males and 306 (275-429) for females. In rats, this drug was an active carcinogen causing lymphomas, renal and breast tumors. In both males and females tumors in the heart, which are rarely seen, were obtained. Very few animals survived with a dose of 200 mg/kg (male 108, females 105 days). Even with 100 mg/kg/dose, the median survival was only 141 days (118-191) for males and 126 (118-135) for females. With 50 mg/kg the survival was 202 (132-302) and 195 (106-304) days, respectively. Other authors have also reported on the carcinogenicity of this drug (27).

N,N-Bis(2-chloroethyl)-N'-3-hydroxypropyl phosphorodiamidic acid as the cyclohexylamine salt (NSC-52695) led to lung tumors in male and female mice. In test females lymphomas were more frequent than in female controls, and some esophageal and uterine tumors occurred. At the dose of 100 mg/kg survival was relatively poor, an average of 147 days (116-263) for males, and 231 (152-289) for females. Males, therefore, had relatively few tumors. Most tumors were obtained at the lower dose of 50 mg/kg with a longer median survival of 302 days (116-545) for males and 389 days (229-475) for females.

In rats the phosphorodiamidic acid salt caused an increased frequency of tumors of the urinary bladder in both males and females. In females the incidence of breast tumors was elevated compared to that in controls. In males other tumors were rather more frequent. As in mice, survival and tumor yield were poor at the higher dose of 75 mg/kg, with a median day of death of 159 (116-494) for males and 180 (110-337) for females. At a dose of 37 mg/kg survival was 349 days (207-545) in male rats and 444 (150-545) for females.

1-Acetyl-2-picolinolhydrazine (NSC-68626) induced lung tumors in male and female mice and, in addition, an appreciable number of ovarian and uterine tumors. The mean survival was over 500 days for males and females at 125 mg/kg, but at 250 mg/kg, survival was poor. No outstanding tumor incidence was seen in rats given this drug.

Natulan, or procarbazine (NSC-77213), which had already been demonstrated to be carcinogenic (4, 7, 18) caused lung tumors in male and female mice. In addition, females had lymphomas and some kidney and uterine tumors. In the rat it induced lymphomas and leukemias in both sexes and breast cancer in both female and male rats.

The important drug streptozotocin (NSC-85998) led to tumors at a variety of sites, mainly in the lung but also in the kidney of both male and female mice. The incidence of uterine tumors was elevated in the females. When it was administered together with nicotinamide, the same tumor spectrum was obtained, but in addition a small number of mice had pancreatic tumors. At a dose of 12 mg/kg, survival was better in female mice (mean 318 days, range 150-376) than in males (mean 257, range 158-459). At the lower dose of 6 mg/kg survival was 467 days (100-505) in males and 477 days (296-549) in females.

Streptozotocin was quite carcinogenic for the liver and kidney in female rats; and for the kidney alone in male rats. Similar effects have been reported elsewhere (13). In addition, this drug induced local cancer in the peritoneal cavity and some pancreatic tumors in male and female rats. When it was administered together with nicotinamide, with the intention of preventing the onset of diabetic conditions (24), a similar tumor distribution was seen, again with emphasis on tumors in the kidney, liver, pancreas, and peritoneal cavity, in decreasing order of frequency. At the dose of 12 mg/kg survival was shorter in females (mean 283 days, range 167-339) than in males (mean 320 days, range 103-547). At a dose level of 6 mg/kg it was longer, with a mean of 448 days for males (270-547) and 447 days (374-547) for females. Other authors also found pancreatic tumors in this system (22).

Dibromomannitol (NSC-94100) had a borderline effect in the lung. However, this drug induced a sizeable number of lymphomas in female mice. In males survival was poor with the high dose of 180 mg/kg, but females did better, with a mean of 502 days (214-549). At the lower dose of 90 mg/kg, males with a mean survival of 520 days (116-545), were in the same range as females (mean 529 days, range 456-549).

In rats, the dose of 250 mg/kg gave virtually no tumors in males or females because of poor survival for only 188 days (142-369) and 117 days (115-362), respectively. At the lower dose of 125 mg/kg, skin tumors and peritoneal sarcomas were seen more frequently in males than in females, mean days of death being 547 and 541, respectively.

Dibromodulcitol (NSC-104800) was instrumental in the development of lymphomas in male and female mice, and there was a small yield of lung tumors, especially in female mice. Survival was much shorter at the dose of 90 mg/kg, with 241 days (120-446) for males and 285 (180-550) for females, than with 45 mg/kg, where it was 345 (100-550) and 513 (152-550) days, respectively. In male rats this drug led to a significant increase in the incidence of subcutaneous tumors. Females were not affected in this way.

Diethylnitrosamine was used as a positive control. It induced many lung tumors in male and female mice, and hemangiomas in a smaller proportion of animals. In addition, male and female rats exhibited a high yield of liver tumors and some cases of pulmonary carcinoma, while females exhibited kidney adenomas and carcinomas.

DISCUSSION

The main aim of the studies reported is to forecast potential carcinogenic risks with drugs currently used effectively in the clinic in securing increased survival of cancer patients. Data of this type will prevent a recurrence of unexpected episodes where cancer has been seen for the second time in patients previously "cured" of another neoplastic condition (1, 8, 11, 28, 31). It will help emphasize the need for continued observation of such patients. In an earlier study, we concluded that the carcinogenic effect did not necessarily parallel the antineoplastic action (26). If the current series of tests yields further documentation of trends along these lines, it will enable clinicians to select the most effective drug with the lowest long-term risk to the patient, on the basis of sound, rational data.

At this time, a complete evaluation of our massive effort to produce reliable information on the oncogenicity of 43 drugs and mixtures currently in use is not possible. Numerous tissues from over 5000 rats and 5000 mice have to be studied histologically and the data must be analyzed with reference to the tumor incidence in simultaneous or contemporary controls.

The action of some of the drugs, such as actinomycin D, melphalan, mitomycin, uracil mustard, dibromomannitol and dibromodulcitol, was similar to that of the so-called direct alkylating agents, in that they induced cancer in the peritoneal cavity, the site of injection. The rat appeared to be more susceptible in this respect than the mouse. With some agents this seemed to be the only lesion produced.

Some other drugs had a broad spectrum of carcinogenicity affecting a variety of organs. These included the cyclohexylamine salt of a phosphorodiamidic acid derivative, Natulan, DIC and streptozotocin. The last compound affected target organs in rats and mice, including the kidneys and the pancreas. In addition, virtually all active agents characteristically induced pulmonary tumors in mice, a fact already utilized in earlier studies (26) with the strain-A mouse, which is more sensitive than the Swiss strain employed here.

Several of the agents led to tumors in the hematopoietic and lymphatic system in one or both of the species utilized. This finding appears to parallel the related clinical finding where patients treated with this type of drug appeared to develop secondary neoplastic lesions in the hematopoietic system (8, 11). It is not clear whether these tumors are indirect evidence for an oncogenic effect of the drug or whether this could reflect a specific or general immunosuppressive action (3, 16, 19, 23). Preliminary information indicates that in our test series, 6-mercatopurine (NSC-755) may have induced lymphosarcomas in mice, a species in which it is a known immunosuppressant. On the other hand, methotrexate (NSC-740) appears to be free of this adverse effect, even though it also exerts an immunosuppressive effect. A similar statement can be made for prednisone, although not all data have been completely analyzed.

It was useful to perform the final studies on carcinogenicity at two dose levels, the maximally tolerated dose, and one-half of this dose. Despite the careful preliminary toxicology, several drugs gave rise to delayed toxicity with mortality of animals prior to the planned end of the tests. Such groups with high mortality often showed few tumors, despite the carcinogenicity apparent at the lower dose. Had this lower dose not been programmed, a year or more would have been lost.

The data presented do not necessarily reflect the full carcinogenic potential of the drugs studied. As noted, the protocols utilized attempted to mimic, in part, a clinical pattern of administration for a portion of the lifespan of the animal. For a complete assessment of carcinogenicity, the exposure period would need to be longer (33). Nonetheless, a number of substances were found to be carcinogenic. It is hoped that patients in whom remission of the disease is satisfactorily achieved following treatment with these drugs are carefully followed so as to detect any adverse effects as early as possible.

REFERENCES

1. CLAYSON, D. B.: Carcinogenic hazards due to drugs. In: Drug-Induced Diseases, Vol. 4, p. 91. Eds.: L. LEYLER, H. M. PECK. Amsterdam: Excerpta Medica 1972.
2. DRUCKREY, H.: Chemical structure and action in transplacental carcinogenesis and teratogensis. In: Transplacental Carcinogenesis, p.45. Eds.: L. TOMATIS, U. MOHR, W. DAVIS. Lyons: IARC (Scientific Publication No. 4) 1973.
3. GATTI, R. A., GOOD, R. A.: Occurrence of malignancy in immuno-deficiency diseases. A literature review. Cancer 28, 89 (1971).
4. GRISWOLD, D. P., JR., CASEY, A. E., WEISBURGER, E. K., WEISBURGER, J. H.: The carcinogenicity of multiple intragastric doses of aromatic and heterocyclic nitro or amino derivatives in young female Sprague Dawley rats. Cancer Res. 28, 924 (1968).
5. HADDOW, A.: On the biological alkylating agents. Persp. Biol. Med. 16, 503 (1973).
6. HADDOW, A., HARRIS, R. J. C., KON, G. A. R., ROE, E. M. F.: The growth inhibitory and carcinogenic properties of 4 aminostilbene and derivatives. Phil. Trans. A. 241 (1948).
7. HEUSON, J. C., HEIMANN, R.: Ibenzmethyzin (Natulan), a highly effective mammary carcinogen in the Huggins System. Europ. J. Cancer 2, 385 (1966).
8. HOLLAND, J. F.: Epidemic acute leukemia. New Engl. J. Med. 283, 1165 (1970).
9. IRVING, C. C.: Interaction of chemical carcinogens with DNA. In: Methods in Cancer Research, Vol. 7, p. 189. Ed.: H. BUSCH. New York: Academic Press 1973.
10. KOSS, L. G., LAVIN, P.: Effects of a single dose of cyclophosphamide on various organs of the rat. II. Response of urinary bladder epithelium according to strain and sex. J. nat. Cancer Inst. 44, 1195 (1970).

11. KYLE, R. A., PIERRE, R. V., BAYRD, E. D.: Multiple myeloma and acute myelomonocytic leukemia. New Engl. J. Med. 283, 1121 (1970).
12. MAGEE, P.: Toxicity of nitrosamines: Their possible human health hazards. Food Cosmet. Toxicol. 9, 207 (1971).
13. MAUER, S. M., LEE, C. S., NAJARIAN, J. S., BROWN, D. M.: Induction of malignant kidney tumors in rats with streptozotocin. Cancer Res. 34, 158 (1974).
14. MILLER, E. C., MILLER, J. A.: Approaches to the mechanisms and control of chemical carcinogenesis. In: Environment and Cancer, p. 5. Baltimore: Williams and Wilkins 1972.
15. MILLER, J. A., MILLER, E. C.: Chemical carcinogenesis: Mechanisms and approaches to its control. J. nat. Cancer Inst. 47, V (1971).
16. MOORE, M., NISBET, N. W., HAIGH, M. V., Eds.: Immunology of Malignancy. Brit. J. Cancer 28, Suppl. I (1973).
17. NAKAHARA, S., TAKAYAMA, S., SUGIMARA, T., ODASHIMA, S., Eds.: Topics in Chemical Carcinogenesis. Tokyo: University of Tokyo Press 1972.
18. OLIVERIO, V. T.: Derivatives of triazenes and hydrazines. In: Cancer Medicine, p. 806. Eds.: J. F. HOLLAND, E. FREI. Philadelphia: Lea and Febiger 1973.
19. PREHN, R. T.: Immune involvement in oncogenesis. In: Proceedings of the Seventh National Cancer Conference, p. 401. Philadelphia: J. B. Lippincott 1972.
20. PREJEAN, J. D., GRISWOLD, S. P., PECKHAM, J. C. CASEY, A. E., WEISBURGER, E. K., WEISBURGER, J. H.: Carcinogenicity of clinically used anticancer agents. (Abstract). Proc. Amer. Ass. Cancer Res. 14, 79 (1973a).
21. PREJEAN, J. D., PECKHAM, J. C., CASEY, A. E., GRISWOLD, D. P., WEISBURGER, E. K., WEISBURGER, J. H.: Spontaneous tumors in Sprague Dawley rats and Swiss mice. Cancer Res. 33, 2768 (1973b).
22. RAKIETEN, N., GORDON, B. S., BEATY, A., COONEY, D. A., DAVIS, R. D., SCHEIN, P. S.: Pancreatic islet cell tumors produced by the combined action of streptozotocin and nicotinamide. Pros. Soc. exp. Biol. (N. Y.) 137, 280 (1971).
23. RAPP, H. J., HANNA, M. G., JR.: Chairmen, Conference on Immunology of Carcinogenesis. Nat. Cancer Inst. Monogr. No. 35 (1972).
24. SCHEIN, P. S., COONEY, D. A., VERNON, M. L.: The use of nicotinamide to modify the toxicity of streptozotocin diabetes without loss of antitumor activity. Cancer Res.27, 2324 (1967).
25. SHIMKIN, M. B.: Pulmonary-tumor induction in mice with chemical agents used in the clinical management of lymphomas, Cancer 7, 410 (1954).
26. SHIMKIN, M. B., WEISBURGER, J. H., WEISBURGER, E. K., GUBAREFF, N., SUNTZEFF, V.: Bioassay of 29 alkylating chemicals by the pulmonary tumor response in Strain-A mice. J. nat. Cancer Inst. 36, 915 (1966).
27. SKIBBA, J. L., ERTURK, E., BRYAN, G. T., Induction of thymic lymphosarcoma and mammary adenocarcinoma in rats by oral administration of the antitumor agent, 4 (5)-(3,3-dimethyl-1-triazeno)-imidazole-5(4) carboxamide. Cancer 26, 1000 (1970).
28. TRUHAUT, R.: Potential carcinogenic hazards from drugs. UICC Monograph Series, Vol. 7. Berlin, Heidelberg, New York: Springer 1967.
29. UEHLEKE, H.: Stoffwechsel von Arzneimitteln als Ursache von Wirkungen, Nebenwirkungen und Toxizität. Fortschr. Arzneim.-Forsch. 15, 147 (1971).
30. VAN DUUREN, B. L., Ed.: Biological Effects of Alkylating Agents. Ann. N. Y. Acad. Sci. 163, 589 (1969).
31. WEISBURGER, J. H.: Chemical carcinogenesis. In: Cancer Medicine, p. 45. Eds.: J. F. HOLLAND, E. FREI. Philadelphia: Lea and Febiger 1973.
32. WEISBURGER, J. H.: Chemical carcinogenesis. In: Toxicology: The Basic Science of Poisons. Eds.: L. CASARETT, J. H. DOULL. New York: McMillan 1975.

33. WEISBURGER, J. H., WEISBURGER, E. K.: Tests for chemical carcinogens. In: Methods in Cancer Research, Vol. 1, p. 307. Eds.: H. BUSCH. New York: Academic Press 1967.

Experimental Investigations with Anti-Cancer Drugs for Carcinogenicity with Special Reference to Immunedepression

D. Schmähl

INTRODUCTION

In previous studies (1962, 1963) we found that transplantation of tumors to pretreated recipient animals (X-rays (1) or alkylating cytostatic compounds (2)) hastens the growth of the transplanted tumor and increases the frequency of metastases. Since at the time of pretreatment no tumor cells were present in the animals the phenomena observed later must have been an effect on the host system and not on the tumor cells. It was suggested that the pretreatment with X-rays or alkylating agents disturbs the immune system and thus causes the more malignant tumor growth (2).

Our findings, which have been reproduced and verified by several authors (3, 4), caused us to re-examine cytostatic substances, this time for potential carcinogenic effects, and particularly to investigate whether there is a correlation between carcinogenic and immunodepressive activity. This question appeared especially important since cytostatic compounds were and are being used increasingly not only in the treatment of malignant tumors, but also in the therapy of autoaggressive diseases and benign hyperproliferations, sometimes without a vital indication. Alkylating cytostatic substances have even been recommended and used in the therapy of the contracture of DUPUYTREN (5) and multiple sclerosis (6). Since it is known that cytostatic compounds are rather aggressive drugs the question arises as to whether or not their use without vital indication is justified in view of possible carcinogenic effects. In addition, there have been a few clinical reports describing carcinogenic effects observed in patients subjected to long-term cytostatic treatment after tumor operations (3).

EXPERIMENTS

In an initial communication (7) we reported that after administration of cyclophosphamide and triazichone to rats, malignant tumors appeared in 54% (cyclophosphamide) and 41% (triazichone) of the animals respectively, when these substances were given in dosages (calculated to kg bodyweight) proportional to those used in human therapy. No tumors were observed in the control series.

On the basis of these observations we made a comparative study of 16 of the most common carcino-chemotherapeutic agents (as commercial preparations), including alkylating agents, antimetabolites, antibiotics and natural substances paying particular attention to carcinogenic effects (8). In these experiments we used more than 1200 rats of the BR 46 strain. The substances were administered intravenously in equitoxic dosages in two different experimental schemes. In the first one, 7% of the LD_{50} was given once weekly for 52 weeks. The total doses (again calculated to kg bodyweight) corresponded with those given clinically (9). In a second scheme, 17% of the LD_{50} of three compounds was given only five times at intervals of 14 days in order to simulate postoperative chemoprophylaxis.

We did not determine dose-response relationships in this study because we consider this to be an essential task of the drug-producing firms. The aim of our experiments, however, was to examine comparatively whether the cytostatics currently in use differ from each other in their carcinogenic and immunodepressive activity.

The results of these studies are shown in Tables 1-3. From Table 1 it can be seen that carcinogenic effects were produced almost exclusively by the alkylating cytostatics, whereas the antimetabolites and natural substances tested did not have carcinogenic effects. The observed tumor frequencies were significantly above the control values (9). We did not observe a special organotropy of the carcinogenic effect of the alkylating cytostatics; tumors developed in various organs and organ systems, as Table 2 shows. Hemangioendotheliomas, leukemias, and subcutaneously or intraperitoneally formed sarcomas had a certain predominance, accounting for about 40% of all tumors produced. These tumor types were not seen in the control animals.

It was particularly striking and surprising that a relatively strong carcinogenic effect was also seen when the drugs were administered only five times at intervals of 14 days (see Table 3). Here again, only the alkylating substances showed carcinogenic effects. The distribution pattern of the tumors was similar to that seen in the previous study, except that the predominance of malignant hemangioendotheliomas was even more significant than in the earlier study.

Table 1. Survey of experiments in male BR-46 rats, testing the carcinogenicity of anticancer drugs. Dose: 7% of LD_{50} weekly for 52 weeks i.v. Drugs tested: a) Myleran, Degranol, Dichloren, Mitomen, Endoxana, Thiotepa, Trenimon, Natulan b) 6-Mercaptopurin, 5-Fluoruracil, Methotrexat, c) Colcemid, A-Blastomase, Proresid, vinblastin, d) Whole-body irradiation. N_0 = Number of animals in the beginning. $N_{1.Tu}$ = Effective number of animals living when the first tumor appeared

Experiment	Number of animals		Malignomas %		Induction time t_{50} months
	N_0	$N_{1.Tu}$	N_0	$N_{1.Tu}$	
Controls	89	65	5	6	23 ± 5
Alkylating agents[a]	391	271	19	24	15 ± 4
Antimetabolites[b]	148	73	2	4	16 ± 5
Natural compounds[c]	200	121	2	3	16 ± 4
X-rays[d]	120	114	20	22	14 ± 4

Table 2. Types of malignomas in male BR-46 rats after administration of anticancer drugs and X-rays (Dosage see Table 1)

Kind of malignoma →	Pheochromocytoma	Leukemias	Lymphosarcomas	Hemangioendotheliomas	Skin Carcinoma	Testis Carcinoma	Lung Carcinoma	Liver Carcinoma	Kidney Carcinoma	Ear-duct Carcinoma	Intestinal Carcinoma	Liposarcomas	Fibrosarcomas i. p.	Fibrosarcomas s. c.	Sternum sarcoma	Osteosarcoma	Meningeosarcoma	Kidney sarcoma	Neurilemmoma	Mamma sarcoma
Experiment																				
Controls	1																			3
Alkylating agents	5	8	2	11	1	2	1	1	1	3	3	3	8	6	1	1	2	3	1	1
X-rays		18		1			1		1	1						1	1			1

Table 3. Survey of experiments in male BR-46 rats after 5 x i.v. administration of anticancer drugs fortnightly with 17% of LD_{50} each. a) mammary sarcomas, 1 pheochromocytoma, b) 10 hemangioendotheliomas, 3 leukemias, 2 pheochromoblastomas, 1 osteochondrosarcoma, c) 2 hemangioendotheliomas, 8 sc./i.p. fibrosarcomas, 5 mammary sarcomas, 3 lymphosarcomas, 1 pheochromocytoma, 3 lung carcinomas, 2 bladder carcinomas, 1 gastric carcinoma, 1 esophageal carcinoma, 1 saliva-gland carcinoma

Experiment	Number of animals N_0	$N_{1.Tu}$	Malignomas % N_0	$N_{1.Tu}$	Induction time t_{50} months
Controls	89	65	5[a]	6	23 ± 5
Vinblastine	96	31	1	3	24
Endoxan	96	66	16[b]	24	18 ± 4
Mitomycin C	96	79	28[c]	34	18 ± 4

Table 4. Incidence of malignomas in female NMRI mice after i.v. administration of 7% of LD_{50} of Endoxan weekly for 1 year

Experiment	Number of animals N_0	$N_{1.Tu}$	Malignomas % N_0	$N_{1.Tu}$	Induction time t_{50} months
Controls	50	46	6	7	14 ± 4
Endoxana	50	46	58	61	9 ± 5

Table 4 shows that the carcinogenicity, e.g. of cyclophosphamide, was proved not only in rats, but also in mice. In mice the carcinogenic effect was even more marked than in rats since in the test animals malignant tumors developed ten times more frequently than in the control series.

Besides the series treated with cytostatic substances a positive comparative group was formed which was treated with whole-body irradiation in equitoxic dosages (52 sessions with 7% of LD_{50} each time). As can be seen from Table 1, the tumor yield corresponded with that observed in the series treated with alkylating substances, except that in the X-ray series leukemias were the predominant tumor type (see Table 2). In this series the "radiomimetic effect" of the alkylating substances with regard to carcinogenesis was again significantly visible.

Besides the carcinogenesis experiments, we performed the hemagglutination test and Jerne's plaque test to examine to what extent the substances tested have immunodepressive properties. The results of these investigations are listed in Table 5. There did not appear to be any close correlation between carcinogenic and immunodepressive action. While some antimetabolites, e.g. Methotrexate, showed a significant immunodepressive activity, they did not show carcinogenic effects. On the other hand, some potently carcinogenic compounds, e.g. mitomycin, had only a weak immunodepressive action.

Table 5. Relationship between immunodepression and carcinogenicity of some anticancer drugs in male BR-46 rats. HA = Hemagglutination-test, APT = Agar-Plaque test

Compound	Immunodepression				Carcinogenicity
	1 x 40% of LD_{50}		14 x 7% of LD_{50}/weekly		
	HA	APT	HA	APT	
Methotrexate	++	++	-	+	-
5-Fluoruracil	-	++	+	-	-
6-Mercaptopurin	++	++	-	+	-
Vinblastin	-	-	+	-	-
Proresid	-	-	+	-	-
Colcemid	-	-	+	-	-
Endoxana	++	++	++	++	++
Dichloren	-	++	++	+	++
Trenimon	-	-	+	++	++
Thiotepa	-	-	++	-	++
Natulan	-	-	++	-	+++
Myleran	-	-	-	+	+
Degranol	-	-	++	+	+
Mitomycin C	-	+	-	+	+++
X-rays	-	-	++	-	++

Table 6. Survey of experiments in male Sprague-Dawley rats on the carcinogenicity of cyclophosphamide combined with hydrocortisone given once weekly i.v. or p.o. d = single dose; D = total dose; MIT = medium induction time of the tumors; MLE = mean life expectation

Experiment	No. of animals N	d mg/kg/week	D mg/kg	Malignant tumors N	Malignant tumors %	MIT days	MLE days
Control	52	-	-	6	12	671 ± 150	745 ± 105
Cyclophosphamide + Hydrocortisone	32	13 50	676 2600	14	44	500 ± 140	500 ± 190
Cyclophosphamide	32	13	676	13	40	510 ± 90	500 ± 175
Hydrocortisone	32[a]	50	2600				

[a]No evaluation yet possible; 12 animals still alive.

Table 7. Influence of immunodepression with hydrocortisone (HC) or cyclophosphamide (CP) on the local carcinogenic action of 3,4 - benzpyrene (BP) after s.c. injection in male Sprague-Dawley rats

Experiment	No. of animals	Single dose mg/kg	Total dose mg/kg	Local sarcomas N	Local sarcomas %	Induction time t_{50} months
BP	45	30	30	44	97	5 ± 1
BP + HC	20	30 50	30 1050	19	95	5 ± 1
BP + CP	49	30 13	30 325	45	92	6 ± 1
BP	32	3	3	25	78	10 ± 4
BP + HC	32	3 50	3 2600	26	81	8 ± 3
BP + CP	32	3 13	3 676	14 7	44 22[a]	8 ± 3 14 ± 6

[a]Malignomas not arising locally; produced by carcinogenicity of CP.

The absence of any correlation between immunodepression and carcinogenesis in the formation of tumors by chemical substances has also been established in other experiments (11). Table 6 shows the results of unpublished investigations that were carried out to test whether the carcinogenic effect of cyclophosphamide can be intensified when the animals are simultaneously treated with hydrocortisone. This substance is also known to have an immunodepressive action. We observed, however, that in the series which received cyclophosphamide alone, tumor yield, induction time and tumor types (again predominantly hemangioendotheliomas) were practically the same as in the series where cyclophosphamide had been given together with hydrocortisone. The results of these experiments on the carcinogenic effect of cyclophosphamide are consistent in our previous findings (7, 8), though in the earlier tests we used Sprague-Dawley rats instead of BR 46 rats. In the plaque test according to Jerne the dosage of hydrocortisone (50 mg/kg/week) leads the immune response to fall to 25% of the normal value.

In former experiments we had already observed (11) that the formation of malignant hepatomas after the administration of diethylnitrosamine cannot be influenced by simultaneous immunodepressive treatment with cyclophosphamide or hydrocortisone. In Table 7 more recent results, with 3,4 benzpyrene, are demonstrated. Rats received single doses, by injection, of benzpyrene (30 mg/kg and 3 mg/kg single dose respectively) that are sufficient to lead to local sarcomas after induction periods of various lengths. While the control group was given benzpyrene alone, in the other groups hydrocortisone and cyclophosphamide were administered weekly in dosages of 50 mg/kg and 13 mg/kg respectively. The formation of local sarcomas at the site of injection and the induction period of these tumors were used as a decisive parameter. It was not possible to alter the tumor yield or the induction periods significantly by the treatment with hydrocortisone and cyclophosphamide. It was, however, observed that when benzpyrene was given in a small dose of 3 mg/kg together with cyclophosphamide in a dose of 13 mg/kg for 52 weeks, after an average induction period of 14 ± 6 months not only local sarcomas but also systemic carcinomas occurred, which could not be related to the influence of benzpyrene and had to be attributed to the carcinogenic effect of cyclophosphamide (Fig. 1). This experiment made it clear that after a longer induction period each carcinogen developed its own typical effects. At least the resorptive carcinogenic effect of cyclophosphamide became manifest.

COMMENTS

Our results, obtained with a large animal sample (about 3000 rats),led us to recommend that alkylating cytostatics be used in the case of vital indications only. This, of course, includes cancer diseases with poor prognosis as well as autoaggressive diseases that cannot be influenced by other therapeutic means. But the use of cytostatic drugs in postoperative chemoprophylaxis appears questionable to us in certain circumstances. Formerly it was often recommended as a general rule that every cancer operation be linked with a chemotherapeutic follow-up treatment. We now feel we have to dissociate ourselves distinctly from this recommendation. We have also warned particularly against the treatment of juvenile patients with alkylating drugs if there is no vital indication for their use. If a patient is still young and common clinical experience suggests that he or she has a good chance of being cured by operation and/or radiation (e.g. mamma carcinoma Steinthal I), chemotherapeutic follow-up treatment should be omitted, especially as its therapeutic benefit must be considered doubtful.

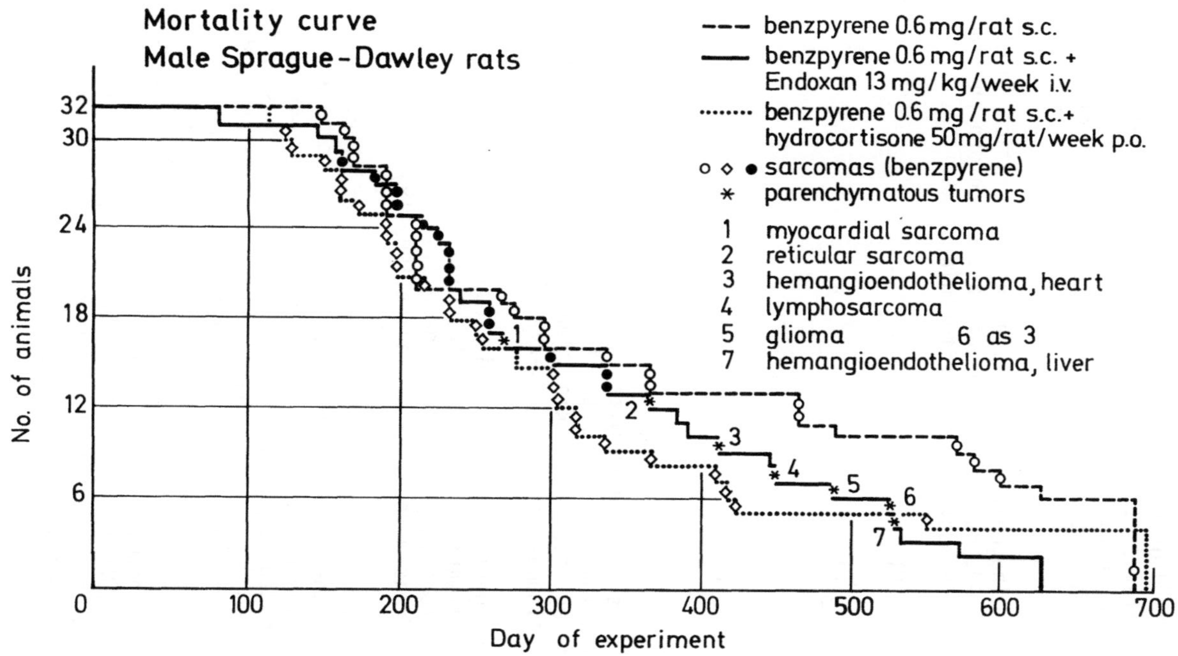

Fig. 1. Local sarcomas at the site of injection after topical application of benzpyrene and malignomas of internal organs after additional administration of cyclophosphamide

Our warning has been correctly understood by most clinicians and research workers. We have no wish to encourage therapeutic nihilism, but we do wish to insist on strict indications for the use of such dangerous substances. Our admonition seems to us the more justified because the carcinogenic effect of alkylating compounds in man has been unquestionably proved. In this connection I wish to mention especially the occurrence of tumors, particularly of the respiratory tract, in people formerly employed as mustard-gas workers (12-14). The proof of the carcinogenic effect of alkylating mustard compounds is more conclusive in healthy humans than in patients because tumors following mustard exposure have an average induction period of 18-22 years (13 , 14). After this length of time cancer patients are normally not accessible to observation . But what has been proved in healthy humans is naturally also valid for sick ones, especially since we have to realize that in therapy with alkylating compounds of the mustard or ethylenimine type permanent mustard poisoning is therapeutically achieved. If noncancer patients are treated with alkylating agents when there is no vital indication, the possibility must be faced that iatrogenic carcinomas may occur after an induction period of about 20 years.

Substantial evidence for the carcinogenicity of alkylating cytostatics in cancer patients has also been obtained, especially in the case of chlornaphazine (15-17), which is a β-naphthylamine mustard, as the formula shows.

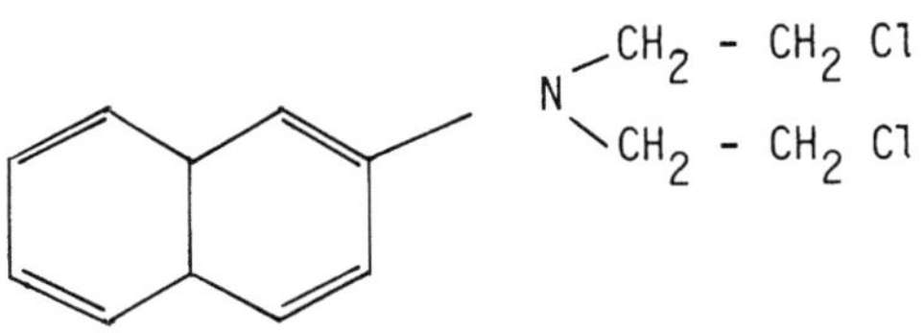

chlornaphazine (formula I)

After treatment of erythroblastosis patients with chlornaphazine carcinomas of the bladder that must be attributed to this treatment occurred in a high percentage. These tumors occurred after a strikingly short induction period of only 3-5 years. Bladder carcinomas were not observed in control subjects.

There have also been reports suggesting that in individual cases malignomas have been induced in man by treatment with cytostatic drugs other than chlornaphazine (3, 18-21, 31). Therefore many clinicians have also given warnings against the use of alkylating drugs without vital indication (19).

It is still not fully clear whether the carcinogenic activity of alkylating cytostatic compounds depends on their alkylating properties or must be attributed to their immunodepressive action. This question has become particularly important since it was noted (22) that recipients of organ transplants showed a significantly higher tumor frequency than control populations, and that malignant lymphomas in particular developed after uncommonly short induction periods. Many authors have attributed this to the immunodepression that is necessary in the case of organ transplantation and leads to a loss of the surveillance function of the immune system (23). This view, however, has not remained uncontradicted (23). Nevertheless it is still thought possible that a cytostatic long-term treatment carries a carcinogenic risk to the patient because of its immunodepressive effects (24, 25).

Our experimental results have led us to the view that the alkylating properties of a cytostatic compound are probably a more essential factor in its carcinogenic effect than its immunodepressive activity, because in our studies we failed to potentiate the chemically-induced carcinogenesis obtained with nitroso compounds, hydrocarbons and alkylating substances by additional immunodepressive measures. Other authors have described different results, particularly those working with mice (23, 30). Therefore it must of course be considered that immunodepression, too, may play a role in the phenomenon of carcinogenesis due to alkylating cytostatics. However, it should be realized that for the afflicted patient it is not so important whether his malignoma following a cytostatic drug has been caused via alkylating properties or via immunodepression.

There is now no doubt that there are drugs possessing carcinogenic properties (17, 26, 27). These include alkylating anticancer drugs that have proved significantly carcinogenic in animal experiments (7, 8, 9, 28, 29) as well as in clinical observations. Since nil nocere is still the prime precept of each component of any therapy, every pharmacotherapist is obliged to protect patients against potential risks; in this particular case, this means to use alkylating cytostatic drugs for vital indications only.

REFERENCES

1. SCHMÄHL, D., STUTZ, E.: Abhängigkeit der Tumorentwicklung bei Ratten nach i.v. Injektion des Yoshida-Acites-Sarcoms von vorausgegangener Röntgenganzkörperbestrahlung. Naturwissenschaften 49, 424 (1962).
2. SCMÄHL, D.: Wert und Gefahr der Krebschemotherapie. Dtsch. med. Wschr. 88, 1463 (1963).
3. SCHMÄHL, D.: Entstehung, Wachstum und Chemotherapie maligner Tumoren. 2nd ed. Aulendorf:Cantor 1970.
4. NOWAK, C., ELBE, S., ARNOLD, W., BENDER, E.: Untersuchungen über den Einfluß einer Vorbehandlung mit Cyclophosphamide, Ribo-Azauracil und Mercaleukin auf die experimentelle Metastasierung im syngenen Tumor-Wirts-System. Arch. Geschwulstforsch. 41, 1, 137 (1973).
5. AROU, E.: Le traitement médical de la maladie de Dupuytren par un agent cytostatique (méthyl-hydrazine). Presse méd. 76, 1956 (1968).
6. DANIELCZYK, W.: Erfahrungen mit Cytostatica bei der multiplen Sklerose. Wien. klin. Wschr. 82, 697 (1970).
7. SCHMÄHL, D.: Cancerogene Wirkung von Cyclophosphamid und Triazichon bei Ratten. Dtsch. med. Wschr. 92, 1150 (1967).
8. SCHMÄHL, D., OSSWALD, H.: Experimentelle Untersuchungen über carcinogene Wirkungen von Krebs-Chemotherapeutika. Arzneimittel-Forsch. 20, 1461 (1970).
9. SCHMÄHL, D., OSSWALD, H., IMMICH, H.: Zur Frage der carcinogenen Wirkung von Krebs-Chemotherapeutika und Immunsuppressiva. Arzneimittel-Forsch. 21, 435 (1971).
10. SCHERF, R. H., KRÜGER, C., KARSTEN, C.: Untersuchungen an Ratten über immunosuppressive Eigenschaften von Cytostatica unter besonderer Berücksichtigung der carcinogenen Wirkung. Arzneimittel-Forsch. 20, 1467 (1970).
11. SCHMÄHL, D., WAGNER, R., SCHERF, H. R.: Der Einfluß von Immunosuppressiva auf die Cancerisierung der Rattenleber durch Diäthylnitrosamin und die Fibrosarkomentstehung durch 3,4-Benzpyren. Arzneimittel-Forsch. 21, 403 (1971).

12. WADA, S., MIYANISHI, M., NISHIMOTO, Y., KAMBE, S.: Mustard gas as a cause of respiratory neoplasia in man. Lancet 1968, 1161.
13. SATO, T., UTSUMI, S., KAJIKARA, K., IKEDA, H.: A case of cancer of the larynx found in mustard gas poisoning. Jap. J. Otolog. 70, 1773 (1967).
14. HELLMANN, U.: Katamnestische Studien an kampstoffgeschädigten Personen unter besonderer Berücksichtigung psychiatrischer Spät- und Dauerschäden. Inaugural dissertation, Marburg, 1970 .
15. THIEDE, T., CHIEVITZ, E., CHRISTENSEN, B. C.: Chlornaphazine as a bladder carcinogen. Acta med. scand. 175, 721 (1964).
16. LAURSEN, B.: Cancer of the bladder in patients treated with chlornaphazine. Brit. med. J. 1970, 684.
17. CLAYSON, W.: Carcinogenic hazards due to drugs. Drug-induced diseases 4, 91, (1972).
18. RIECHE, K.: Zur Frage der Cancerogenität von Cytostatica. Arch. Geschwulstforsch. 34, 240 (1969).
19. HARTWICH, G.: Nebenwirkungen cytostatischer und immunosuppressiver Therapie. Fortschr. Med. 91, 357 (1973).
20. STERNBERG, S. S., PHILIPS, F. S., Cronin, A. P.: Renal tumors and other lesions in rats following a single intravenous injection of Daunomycin. Cancer Res. 32, 1029 (1972).
21. SCHEIDEGGER, S.: Lungenfibrose, rezidivierende Vasculitis und multizentrisches Lungencarcinom nach cytostatischer Therapie mit Alkeran. Verh. dtsch. Ges. Path. 56, 364 (1972).
22. PENN, I.: Malignant tumors in organ transplant recipients. Berlin, Heidelberg, New York: Springer 1970.
23. GLEICHMANN, H., GLEICHMANN, E.: Immunosuppression and neoplasia. Klin. Wschr. 51, 255, 260 (1973).
24. MICHLMAYR, G., GÜNTHER, R., LEDERER, B., HUBER, H.:Malignes Lymphom nach zweijähriger immunosuppressiver Therapie einer Periarteriitis nodosa. Med. Klin. 68, 180 (1973).
25. TRESKE, U.: Iatrogene Leukämogenese als potentielle Gefahr der immunosuppressiven Cytostaticatherapie. Paper presented at the 73rd Meeting of the Nordwestdtsch. Ges. inn. Med., Bremen (1969).
26. FRAUMENI, J. F., MILLER, R. W.: Drug induced cancer. J. nat. Cancer Inst. 48, 1268 (1972).
27. SCHMÄHL, D.: Toxikologische Probleme der iatrogenen Carcinogenese. Verh. dtsch. Ges. Path. 56, 133 (1972).
28. PREJEAN, J. D., CASEY, A. E., GRISWOLD, D. P., PECKHAM, J. C., WEISBURGER, E. K., WEISBURGER, J. H.: Carcinogenicity of clinically used anticancer agents. Abstr. Amer. Ass. Cancer Res. 79, (1973), 112, (1972).
29. SHIMKIN, J. B., WEISBURGER, J. H., WEISBURGER, E. K., GUBAREFF, N., SUNTZEFF, V.: Bioassay of 29 alkylating agents by the pulmonary-tumor response in strain A mice. J. nat. Cancer Inst. 36, 915 (1969).
30. GRUNDMANN, E., HOBIK, H. P.: Lymphoretikuläre Sarkome bei immunologisch geschädigten Mäusen. Z. Krebsforsch. 79, 298 (1973).
31. RUPPRECHT, L., BLESSING, M. M.: Fibrosarkom der Harnblase nach siebenjähriger Chemotherapie einer Lymphogranulomatose im Kindesalter. Dtsch. med. Wschr. 98, 1663 (1973).

Tests for Tumor Induction by Antitumor Agents*

F. S. Philips and S. S. Sternberg

We have a long-standing interest in studies of the cytotoxic effects of antitumor agents *in vivo* and we have been struck by their high capacity to induce selective lesions in cell-renewal systems. In this respect antitumor agents have appeared to be unique among various classes of pharmacologically active substances. For this reason we were greatly interested in the reports by HUGGINS (6) and other workers (8) that the potent carcinogen 7,12-dimethylbenz(a)anthracene, (DMBA), has toxic effects on hematopoietic cells in bone marrow, thymus, and spleen, on spermatogenesis, and on intestinal crypt epithelium. It seemed appropriate to ask whether antitumor agents which have similar cytotoxic effects might also have carcinogenic activity like DMBA. We chose to study this possibility by testing for tumor induction in mammary epithelium of virgin, female rats. As shown by HUGGINS and others this system is highly susceptible to polycyclic aromatic hydrocarbon carcinogens. It is also susceptible to the carcinogenic effects of X-irradiation (3).

We gave our rats a number of representative chemotherapeutic agents in doses that were in the lethal or near-lethal range and sufficient to induce lesions in normal proliferating tissues. Surviving animals were observed for 5 months, a period during which large numbers of mammary tumors appear in DMBA-treated rats. Table 1 describes the induction of tumors by DMBA in the rats we used. The data show that the median lethal dose (MLD) of DMBA was about 250 mg/kg. Most animals receiving doses near the MLD succumbed in less than 30 days, probably as the result of severe atrophy of hematopoietic tissues (8). An abundance of mammary tumors appeared in the animals that survived doses in the lethal range. Significant numbers also arose in rats given lower doses. For example, the non lethal dose of 50 mg/kg (about 1/5 of the MLD) induced tumors in about 50% of animals and each rat so affected had an average of two or more tumors. Even doses as low as 12.5 mg/kg (1/20 of the MLD) induced single tumors in a few animals.

Quite opposite results were obtained in rats receiving high doses of the antitumor agents listed in Table 2. With the exception of hydroxyurea and ethylcarbamate, the substances were given in lethal or near-lethal doses. Again with the exception of hydroxyurea and urethan there were no mammary tumors in any of the surviving rats. None had grossly observable tumors at any other sites. The two tumors in the urethan-treated rats were histologically found to be mammary neoplasms. The single tumor in the hydroxyurea group was small and detected only at necropsy. Regrettably it was lost during preparation for histological study.

* Supported in part by Grant CA 08748 from the National Cancer Institute and by the Elsa U. Pardee Foundation.

Table 1. Toxicity and mammary tumors in female rats receiving single doses of 7,12-dimethylbenz(a)anthracene[a]

Dose	No.	No.dead		At 150 days		
(mg/kg)	tested	0-30 days	30-150 days	No. surviving	No. with tumors	Tumors per survivor
600	10	10		0	0	
400	15	15		0	0	
300	48	31	4	13	12	5.3
200	50	17	5	28	20	2.8
133	50	1	2	47	39	3.2
100	26	0	2	24	19	2.3
50	24	0	0	24	14	1.1
25	29	0	0	29	8	0.3
12.5	20	0	2	18	2	0.1

[a]CD rats (pathogen-free line of Sprague-Dawley), 5 weeks old, were given single doses in peanut oil by intragastric intubation.

Table 2. Toxicity and tumors in female rats treated with different antitumor agents[a]

Agent	Dose (mg/kg/day)	No. of daily injections	No. tested	No. dead 0-30 days	At 150 days No. surviving	At 150 days No. with tumors
Myleran	30	1	10	10	0	
	20	1	25	10	15	0
	13.3	1	15	0	15	0
Mitomycin C	6	1	10	7	3	0
	4	1	15	10	2	0
	3	1	10	1	5	0
	2	1	16	0	16	0
Ethyl carbamate	1000	1	25	0	25	2
Hydroxyurea	2000	1	25	0	25	1
Methotrexate	5	5	11	5	6	0
	3.3	5	15	9	6	0
Actinomycin D	0.4	5	10	10	0	0
	0.27	5	15	15	0	0
	0.2	5	15	11	3	0
	0.13	5	15	7	7	0
Thioguanine	37.5	5	10	3	5	0
	25	5	10	1	9	0
	16.6	5	15	0	15	0
5-Fluoro-uracil	75	5	10	10	0	0
	50	5	10	3	7	0
	33.3	5	15	0	15	0

[a] CD rats, 5 weeks old, were given doses in isotonic saline by intraperitoneal injection.

The results of Table 2 show that most of the antitumor agents tested were without mammary tumor-inducing activity during the short 5-month period of observation. Even if the animals had been followed for a larger fraction of their expected life-span, it is unlikely that any of the agents would have proved more than weakly tumorigenic in mammary tissue.

We have conducted longer studies with Actinomycin D. Since Actinomycin D binds tightly to DNA, we were curious to learn whether such binding might provoke tumors if it persisted over long periods of time. We were also aware that significant numbers of mesotheliomas have been induced in the peritoneal cavity of rats treated repeatedly with intraperitoneal injections of Actinomycin D (14). No such tumors were present in mediastinum or thorax, nor did any appear in the peritoneum of rats receiving intravenous injections of the agent. This highly localized effect seemed reminiscent of our earlier finding that Actinomycin D is a local, contact poison causing necrosis and inflammation throughout the peritoneal lining after intraperitoneal injection, severe subdermal lesions if injected subcutaneously, and damage to veins and thrombophlebitis when injected intravenously (7). Possibly mesothelioma induction could be a nonspecific response to prolonged injury and regenerative hyperplasia in the peritoneal lining.

We chose to treat rats repeatedly over a 12- or 24-week period with the highest possible doses of Actinomycin D that could be given by intragastric intubation. Doses of 4 mg/kg/day, three times per week, were found to kill about 50% of treated rats within 14 days. However, doses of 1 and 2 mg/kg/day were tolerated, though the treated animals grew less rapidly than controls during the treatment period and throughout the period of observation after treatment. At the end of one year none of the animals given these doses had grossly observable tumors at any site (Table 3). The negative result leads us to question whether Actinomycin D can be considered a systemic carcinogen per se. Whether its local tumorigenic effects are due to a direct carcinogenic action or are secondary events remains a subject for further investigation.

Table 3. Toxicity and tumors in rats treated with repeated doses of Actinomycin D[a]

Sex	Dose (mg/kg/day)	Weeks of treatment	No. tested	At one year: No. surviving	At one year: No. with tumors
Female	2	12	12	11	0
Male	2	12	12	12	0
Male	1 2	12 12	10	10	0
Female	Control	12	12	12	0
Male	Control	12	12	11	0
Male	Control	24	11	11	0

[a]CD rats, 4-5 weeks old, given doses 3 times per week by intragastric intubation. Controls received isotonic NaCl.

During earlier investigations of cytotoxic effects of hydroxyurea we considered the possibility that it might have tumorigenic activity. The agent is known to be a highly selective inhibitor of DNA synthesis, a property it shares with certain other hydroxamic acid derivatives such as ethyl N-hydroxycarbamate. It is also, like the latter agent, acutely cytotoxic to cell renewal systems in vivo (9). Since ethyl N- hydroxycarbamate and its congener, ethyl carbamate, are highly active in inducing pulmonary adenomas in mice (1), we were curious to learn whether hydroxyurea might cause similar tumors. As shown in Table 4 we were disappointed to find that it does not.

Table 4. Pulmonary adenoma in mice treated with single doses of ethylcarbamate, ethyl N-hydroxycarbamate or hydroxyurea[a]

Agent	Dose (mg/kg)	No. tested	No. with tumors[b]	Tumors per mouse[b]
Ethyl carbamate	1000	15	15	13.2
	500	10	10	4.4
Ethyl N-hydroxy-carbamate	1000	10	10	4.4
	500	10	10	3.2
Hydroxyurea	1840	10	1	1
	920	10	2	1
Control		21	2	1

[a] Strain A, female mice weighing 17-25 g received single, intraperitoneal injections; controls received isotonic saline.

[b] At 11 weeks after injection.

Although the results of the above studies were essentially negative insofar as we did not detect any significant carcinogenic activity in antitumor agents, we have recently reported that Daunomycin can induce renal and genital tract tumors in female rats within one year after a single intravenous injection (13). BERTAZZOLI et al. have also described a significant increase in mammary tumors within one year in female rats receiving only one intravenous dose of the agent (2). Since the rats employed in both studies were Sprague-Dawley in origin, like those used in the negative tests reported above, the tumorigenic effects of Daunomycin may prove to be a unique property of this chemotherapeutic agent. Further study of its carcinogenicity is indicated.

COMMENT

About forty years ago HADDOW directed attention to the close association of tumorigenicity and cancer chemotherapeutic activity among many of the then known carcinogenic and antitumor agents (5). He surmised that the mechanisms of action involved were closely linked phenomena. In the intervening years there have been substantial additions to the list of chemical families that are recognizably carcinogenic, and numerous antitumor agents have been developed. The correlation between cancer chemotherapeutic activity and carcinogenicity no longer appears to be as close as it once seemed. Nevertheless, there are sufficient examples of the simultaneous presence of both properties to warrant continued interest in the question (4, 10, 11, 12).

Antitumor agents are in widespread use for the treatment of human disease. Were they restricted for use solely in the treatment of patients with inevitably fatal cancers, their potential for carcinogenic action would seemingly be a minor, academic concern. However, antitumor agents have other known or potential applications as immunosuppressives in organ transplantation and in the treatment of autoimmune diseases, as antiviral agents, and in the treatment of dermatoses such as psoriasis. Questions regarding the risk of cancer induction versus therapeutic benefit can become considerably more difficult to answer in these applications than in cancer therapy.

Continued study of the relationship between carcinogenicity and antitumor activity is of additional interest because it could contribute to further understanding of the mechanisms involved. In a recent publication we have briefly reviewed the evidence in support of the hypothesis that the proximate actions of carcinogens and of many antitumor agents are directed against DNA. We have also called attention to the remarkable fact that potent carcinogens such as DMBA and X-irradiation elicit selective cytotoxic effects in rapidly proliferating cell renewal systems of intact animals. The same systems are targets for the toxic effects of most clinically useful cancer chemotherapeutic agents. Presumably the common cytotoxic properties of both kinds of substances may be due to their capacity to cause derangements of nucleic acids which can be the cause of lesions in proliferating tissues (8). Nevertheless, clinically useful antitumor agents, taken as a group, are uncertain or weak carcinogens (4, 10, 11, 12). Almost certainly none can compare in potency with DMBA and other strongly carcinogenic substances. The main object of this report has been the provision of further evidence for this comparison.

REFERENCES

1. BERENBLUM, I., BEN-ISHAI, D., HARAN-GHERA, N., LAPIDOT, A., SIMON, E., TRAININ, N.: Skin initiating action and lung carcinogenesis by derivatives of urathane and related compounds. Biochem. Pharmacol. 2, 168 (1959).
2. BERTAZZOLI, C., CHIELI, T., SOLCIA, E.: Different incidence of breast carcinomas or fibroadenomas in Daunomycin or Adriamycin treated rats. Experientia 27, 1209 (1971).
3. BOND, V. P., CRONKITE, E. P., LIPPINCOTT, S. W., SHELLABARGER, C. J.: Studies on radiation-induced mammary gland neoplasia in the rat. Radiat. Res. 12, 276 (1960).
4. BROCK, N., SCHNEIDER, B.: Zur Frage der carcinogen Wirkung von Krebs-chemotherapeutica und chemischen Immunosuppressiva. Arzneimittel-Forsch. 21, 435 (1971).
5. HADDOW, A.: Cellular inhibition and the origin of cancer. Acta Un. int. Cancr. 3, 342 (1938).
6. HUGGINS, C.: Cancer and necrosis induced selectively by hydrocarbons. In: Horizons in Biochemistry, p. 497. New York: Academic Press 1961.
7. PHILIPS, F. S., SCHWARTZ, H. S., STERNBERG, S. S., TAN, C. T. C.: The Toxicity of Actinomycin D. Ann. N. Y. Acad. Sci. 89, 348 (1960).

8. PHILIPS, F. S., STERNBERG, S. S., MARQUARDT, H.: In vivo cytotoxicity of polycyclic hydrocarbons. Proc. 5th Int. Congr. Pharmacology, San Francisco Vol.2, p.75. Basel: Karger 1973.
9. PHILIPS, F. S., STERNBERG, S. S., SCHWARTZ, H. S., CRONIN, A. P., SODERGREN, J. E., VIDAL, P. M.: Hydroxyurea. I. Acute cell death in proliferating tissues in rats. Cancer Res. 27, 61 (1967).
10. PREJEAN, J. D., GRISWOLD, D. P., CASEY, A. E., PECKHAM, J. C., WEISBURGER, J. H., WEISBURGER, E. K., WOOD, H. B., JR.: Carcinogenicity studies of clinically used anticancer agents. Proc. Amer. Ass. Cancer Res. 13, 112 (1972).
11. PREJEAN, J. D., GRISWOLD, D. P., PECKHAM, J. C., CASEY, A. E., WEISBURGER, E. K., WEISBURGER, J. H.: Carcinogenicity of clinically used anticancer agents. Proc. Amer. Ass. Cancer Res. 14, 79 (1973).
12. SCHMÄHL, D., OSSWALD, H.: Experimentelle Untersuchungen über carcinogene Wirkungen von Krebs-Chemotherapeutica und Immunosuppressiva. Arzneimittel-Forsch. 20, 1461 (1970).
13. STERNBERG, S. S., PHILIPS, F. S., CRONIN, A. P.: Renal tumors and other lesions in rats following a single intravenous injection of Daunomycin. Cancer Res. 32, 1029 (1972).
14. SVOBODA, D., REDDY, J., HARRIS, C.: Invasive tumors induced in rats with Actinomycin D. Cancer Res. 30, 2271 (1970).

Adverse Reactions to Cytostatic Agents

N. S. Irey

The object of this paper is to present a broad spectrum of the morphologic changes that have been associated with cytostatic agents. This discussion is based on a retrospective study of biopsy and autopsy material from 155 human cases as seen by the practicing pathologist. These adverse changes are a measure of the failure of these drugs to preferentially inhibit or destroy neoplastic tissues while leaving the normal host tissues unaffected.

Such reactive changes in the tissues are not new, nor are they unique to cytostatic agents; in fact they are generally interchangeable with those related to the various forms of radiation injury, and are "radiomimetic."

For overall orientation, the basic diseases for which cytostatics were administered in this group of 155 cases fell into the categories and frequencies listed in Table 1. Note that 60% were reticuloendothelial malignancies, 25% were carcinomas, and slightly over 10% were nonmalignant conditions. The nonmalignant conditions are listed in Table 2 and were predominantly dermatologic problems.

Table 1. Basic diseases

52 - Leukemia	4 - Sarcomas
29 - Carcinoma	2 - Multiple myeloma
17 - Hodgkin's disease	2 - Gliomas
14 - Lymphomas	1 - di Guglielmo's disease
14 - Psoriasis	1 - Mycosis fungoides
5 - Renal transplant	1 - Letterer- Siwe disease

Table 2. Cytostatic drugs

Rx for Nonmalignant Disease:	
Psoriasis	- 14
Renal transplant	- 5
One case each of:	
Arthritis	
Exfoliative Dermatitis	
Lupus Erythematosus	

The cytostatic agents used, the antimetabolites being the most frequent, are listed in Table 3. Multiple cytostatic agents were utilized in the treatment of two-thirds of the patients in this series (Table 4), with sixty-one patients (40%) receiving in addition some form of concurrent steroid therapy. The four most frequent immediate causes of death in these 155 cases were, in order of frequency: pneumonia, septicemia, gastrointestinal hemorrhage, and pulmonary insufficiency.

Table 3. Antineoplastic agents

Antimetabolites	- 84
Alkylating agents	- 60
Alkaloids	- 39
Antibiotics	- 11
Miscellaneous	- 34
(155 cases)	

Table 4. Cytostatic drugs

Agents per patient	Number of patients
One	52
Two	55
Three	33
Four	12
Five	5
(In combination with steroids - 61)	

Table 5. Adverse reactions to cytostatic drugs

1. Toxicity: with degeneration and necrosis
2. a. Dysplasia
   b. Hyperplasia:
      parenchymal
      stromal
   c. "Pseudoneoplasia"
3. Chromosomal aberrations:
   a. Tumorogenic
   b. Teratogenic
   c. Mutagenic

Moving now to the adverse reactions found in these cases, Table 5 lists three major categories of pathologic alterations that were found in the host tissues. Of these three categories of changes, the second (dysplasias and hyperplasias), may be of particular difficulty to the pathologist in the interpretation of biopsy material. These alterations induced by cytostatic agents are frequently subtle and present a difficult differential diagnostic area in which overdiagnosis by the pathologist may give the patient an additional (malignant) diagnosis which may be incorrect.

The third major category of adverse reactions in Table 5 relates to chromosomal aberrations that can be induced by cytostatics, with serious consequences in either the somatic or the germ cells of the patient and resultant tumorogenesis in the host or in malformations in the host's conceptus.

For the first major category of adverse reactions (toxicity with degeneration and necrosis) in the normal tissues and organs of the patient, the five most frequent target organs were (in order of frequency): bone marrow, liver, lung, gastrointestinal tract (GI), and skin. It is not surprising that the three organs with the highest mitotic indices are included in this list, i.e., bone marrow, GI tract, and skin.

The degenerative changes in the bone marrow resulted, as would be anticipated, in the following conditions in the peripheral blood: pancytopenia, leukopenia, agranulocytosis, thrombocytopenia, and anemia. Serious secondary blood dyscrasias were seen in one-fifth of the cases in this series. This group was exclusive of those instances of peripheral blood abnormalities that could be accounted for on the basis of either primary or secondary malignancies involving the bone marrow.

The second most frequent site for adverse reactions of the degenerative and necrosis type was the liver. Microscopically, these were reflected in the findings of focal necrosis, cholestasis, portal fibrosis, and cirrhosis. Hepatic changes in one or more of these forms were almost as frequent as the abnormalities in bone marrow and peripheral blood. In several instances, extensive interconnecting periportal fibrosis was found, and in one instance the cirrhotic process was associated with esophageal varices, massive hemorrhage from which was the terminal event.

A case of colonic carcinoma is cited as an example of severe toxic changes in the gastrointestinal tract. This patient was treated with fluorouracil and developed severe hemorrhagic diarrhea terminally. Microscopically, the small bowel showed extensive mucosal atrophy, loss of villi, sparse glands, and very severe and striking submucosal edema. The associated inflammatory infiltrate was quite sparse and probably related to the severe and terminal pancytopenia, the latter being probably secondary to the cytostatic agent used.

Skin toxicity was found in eight of the cases, including instances of exfoliative dermatitis and severe bullous dermatitis. The exfoliative dermatitis was associated with multiple therapy (vincristine and chlorambucil). The bullous dermatitis was also associated with multiple agents (6-MP, methotrexate, vincristine, and prednisone).

A less frequent site of toxicity reactions to cytostatics was the kidney; there was one instance of uremia in a patient treated with a combination of fluorouracil and mitomycin for colonic carcinoma. The kidneys were the site of extensive interstitial fibrosis, reduction in tubules, and decrease in glomerular cellularity. These changes were radiomimetic, but no therapeutic radiation had been received.

Another rare site for adverse reactions to cytostatics was the central nervous system. One patient who received intrathecal methotrexate while in a leukemic remission subsequently developed quadraplegia, with terminal respiratory failure. Spinal cord sections revealed a necrotizing process which included loss of anterior horn cells. No demyelination was found. A second case was that of a leukemic who inadvertently received intrathecal vincristine, with cardiorespiratory failure on the fourth day following this therapy. Cord sections revealed acidophilic intracytoplasmic inclusion bodies of crystalline or crystalloid character. Special studies indicate that these inclusions result from either overproduction or reaggregation of the normal microtubules, and changes similar to these have been produced experimentally in rabbits receiving vincristine (7, 8).

Another type of adverse reaction to cytostatics which falls into the first category referred to in Table 5 is an important and relatively frequent one: an indirect effect secondary to the reduced immunologic capabilities of the host-opportunistic infections, including a variety of fungal infections. An illustrative case is that of a patient with lupus erythematosus who was treated with azathioprine and prednisone and who subsequently developed terminal candidiasis with widespread visceral dissemination. In this series of 155 cases, of the 35 in which the immediate cause of death was sepsis, there were related mycotic infections in three.

Another danger to patients in whom the immune response is suppressed is the possibility of complicating viral infections. An example in this series is that of a child with leukemia being treated with methotrexate and prednisone, who was exposed to a case of varicella. She subsequently developed disseminated varicella, with a terminal hemorrhagic diathesis and pulmonary candidiasis.

The next major group of adverse reactions to cytostatics is that relating to dysplasias and hyperplasias and the "pseudoneoplasias" (item 2 in Table 5). Examples of dysplastic changes were found in the following sites in this series of 155 cases: lung, gastrointestinal tract, skin, liver, lymph nodes, and pancreas. The most frequent site for dysplastic changes was the lung, and was seen in association with busulfan, bleomycin, melphalan, and cyclophosphamide. Morphologically, these alterations included pulmonary fibrosis and alveolar lining cell proliferation and atypicality.

These hyperplastic and dysplastic alterations in the parenchymal cells may have wide visceral distribution in association with these various cytostatic agents, the cervix uteri sometimes being affected. Their presence may complicate the interpretation of biopsy material, making it difficult to decide whether or not a premalignant or malignant process may be present.

Similar hyperplasia is also found in the stromal elements of the various viscera in some cases, including the liver and the heart. Myocardial interstitial fibrosis was noted in a leukemic patient who had received Daunomycin. Autopsy on this case revealed no coronary artery or valvular disease. Cardiac reactions of this type have an incidence of 4-10% in patients receiving Daunomycin and appear to be dose-related; similar myocardial fibrosis has been reproduced experimentally in rabbits (1, 4, 6).

Related to the cytostatically induced hyperplasias and dysplasias are the "pseudoneoplasms" that these agents occasionally produce. One patient with lung carcinoma treated with chlorambucil subsequently developed first anemia, and later leukopenia. During evaluation of the leukopenia a diagnosis of leukemia was made on the basis of the bone marrow studies. This was followed by aggressive therapy for leukemia with multiple cytostatic agents. Pancytopenia and sepsis terminated the case. Autopsy failed to reveal any evidence of leukemia, and re-evaluation of the bone-marrow material failed to substantiate the original diagnosis of leukemia.

The development of hyperplastic lymph nodes in patients receiving cytostatic agents can also present differential diagnostic problems. One patient in this series was receiving methotrexate for exfoliative dermatitis. This was followed by generalized lymphadenopathy. One node was biopsied, revealing blurred architecture and a hyperplasia and dominance of histiocytes and reticular lymphoblasts. Some observers thought this might represent a lymphoma, possibly an early monocytic leukemia.However, when the drug was stopped, the lymphadenopathy regressed and follow-up indicated that the patient returned to complete clinical and hematologic normality. Similar diagnostic difficulties have occasionally arisen in interpreting leiomyomata in the female genital tract during treatment with cytostatic compounds, because of the cellular atypism noted.

The third major category of cytostatically related adverse tissue reactions listed in Table 5 consists of changes secondary to chromosomal aberrations; an example of a tumorogenic complication is afforded by a renal transplant case who was treated for one year after the transplant operation with combined azathioprine and prednisone. After this year, neurologic symptoms and signs developed, with subsequent deterioration, coma, and death. Autopsy revealed multiple tumors in the brain and lung, diagnosed as reticulum-cell sarcoma. There has been a statistically significant increase in the frequency of a variety of neoplasms developing in patients treated with cytostatic and immunosuppressive agents, and this case appears to be an example of this. The increase may be related to the decreased immunologic surveillance capabilities of those receiving immunosuppressive agents (2, 3).

This series of 155 cases includes two which may reflect the capability of cytostatic drugs to produce teratogenic effects in the offspring of patients being treated with such agents, particularly if this therapy is given to the mother in the first trimester of her pregnancy. The first such instance is that of a child whose mother had received methotrexate in the first trimester for a carcinoma of the pyriform sinus. The child presented the picture of the Treacher-Collins syndrome (5). Autopsy at 2 1/2 years of age revealed poroncephaly and partial agenesis of the corpus callosum and fusion of the frontal lobes. While there are familial cases in the literature of the Treacher-Collins syndrome exhibiting a dominant mode of inheritance, a point favoring a drug relationship in this case is the coexistance of the multiple anomalies of the central nervous system, since these are not a part of the usual Treacher-Collins picture.

A second possible case of teratogenesis related to maternal cytostatic therapy is that of a woman who received a five-week course of chlorambucil during the first trimester for a fibrosarcoma. Her infant was stillborn in the eighth month, and had agenesis of the mandible and spade-like hands and feet.

Acknowledgement

The Registry of Tissue Reactions to Drugs is sponsored by the Food and Drug Administration (under Contract FDA 67-53) of the Department of Health, Education, and Welfare, and by the Armed Forces Institute of Pathology, and is under the auspices of Universities Associated for Research and Education in Pathology, Inc.

The opinions or assertions contained in this paper are the private views of the author and are not to be construed as official or as reflecting the views of the Department of the Army, Air Force, or Defense, or of the sponsors of the Registry of Tissue Reactions to Drugs.

REFERENCES

1. BONADONNA, G., MONFARDINI, S.: Lancet 1969 1, 837.
2. BURNET, P.: Lancet 1967 1, 1171.
3. Editorial: Ann. int. Med. 75, 310 (1971).
4. Leading Article: Brit. med. J. 1967 2, 587.
5. MCKENZIE, J., CRAIG, J.: Arch. Dis. Childh. 30, 391 (1955).
6. MARMONT, A. M., DAMASIO, E., ROSSI, F.: Lancet 1969 1, 837.
7. SCHOCHET, S. S., JR., LAMPERT, P. W., EARLE, K. M.: J. Neuropath. exp. Neurol. 27, 645 (1968).
8. SCHOCHET, S. S. JR., LAMPERT, P. W., EARLE, K. M.: Exp. Neurol. 23, 113 (1969).

The Changing Pattern of Hodgkin's Disease Seen at Autopsy

E. Grundmann and R. Fritzsche

We are now looking back on thirty years of cytostatic therapy. Hematoblastoses have been the principal field of application. A diagram outlining the present status of results obtained with combination therapy in Hodgkin's disease has been published elsewhere (4); six years after the start of a N. I. H. study in 1967, the surviving fraction for the group of risk was still over 0.5 in the entire group, and almost 0.6 in the complete remission group.

Such investigations concentrate on the surviving patients, duration of remissions, etc. Our study, however, is concerned with what happened in the case of patients who did not survive; whether their death was the oldfashioned "Hodgkin death" or whether the therapy was involved. The pathologist always has his place at the other side of the table.

Our study tries to compare and analyze material from two sample groups, the data collected under comparable conditions during two given periods, with the objective of defining any change in the terminal pattern of Hodgkin's disease. In particular we were anxious to test whether the more effective therapy of recent years has produced a change in the terminal pattern of this disease. Thus, our real interest was to find what a Hodgkin patient dies of, i.e. whether autopsy still reveals the typical massive involvement of the lymphoreticular organs, or have other phenomena come to the foreground, which could be caused by therapy. The last and most important question was whether there were any evidence of new malignant tumors being induced by cytostatic therapy of Hodgkin's disease, or of increased malignancy in the disease itself.

Hodgkin's disease is anything but homogeneous. Histologic classification of this disease is now performed according to the "RYE system" that was established chiefly by LUKES and BUTLER (10). Each histologic type seems to have its own "mean survival time." It must be kept in mind that modern therapy is adapted to the clinical stage in question, as defined by the Committee on Hodgkin's Disease Stage Classification in 1971. Despite these drawbacks, Hodgkin's disease seems to be better suited to a study of this kind than any other malignant tumor. The advantages are: (1) The comparatively high incidence: Hodgkin's disease accounts for about 50% of all lymphomas; (2) the exact histologic diagnosis; (3) the established and internationally adopted nomenclature.

The material of our investigation consists of all autopsies performed in the Institute of Pathology of Münster University from January 1, 1955, to August 31, 1973. These 16,037 autopsy cases happened to include exactly one hundred cases with a definite diagnosis of Hodgkin's disease. The hundred cases have been divided in two groups:

Group A includes autopsies performed from 1955 - 1964 (43 cases) and
Group B autopsies performed from 1965 - 1973 (57 cases).

They have been analyzed from various statistical, macroscopical, and histological aspects.

1. The mean survival time, defined as the span between diagnosis of the disease and death, is 35 months for the cases we studied. This period corresponds rather well with clinical data, which rather shocked us.

It must be realized that our material presents decidedly a negative selection, being collected from autopsies only. During studies at the Memorial Hospital in New York, CRAVER found an expected mean survival time of 36.8 months (5). An analysis of mortality statistics in Berlin yielded a mean survival time of 32 months (8). EDER and ZAGEL, in their study on autopsies in 1962, found 31 months (6). The statistically expected mean survival time is now considerably longer. High-voltage irradiation and different combined chemotherapies like the MOPP program with follow-up treatment have certainly increased the expected mean survival time for Hodgkin cases to over 48 months (3). FREI reports that 75% of all patients of the Southwest Cancer Chemotherapy Group have now been in remission for more than three years (7). Our autopsy material, negatively selected though it may be, shows an expected mean survival time of 22 months for group A (1955-1964), for group B (1965-1973) one of 42 months. Thus, the expected survival period has nearly doubled from one test period to the next.

2. Comparison of histologic types as found at biopsy or autopsy of the cases is hardly possible without serious reservations. We established, however, the following facts (Table 1):

Table 1. Histological classification according to LUKES and BUTLER (1966)
In 18 autopsies with scarred lymph nodes no classification was possible

	Group A		Group B		A + B	LUKES & BUTLER
Lymphocytic and histiocytic						
nodular	(Ia) 1= 4%		3= 5%		4= 5%	23= 6%
diffuse	(Ib) 5=19%	35%	4= 7%	16%	9=11%	40=11%
Nodular sclerosis	(II) 3=12%		2= 4%		5= 6%	149=39%
Mixed type	(III)3=12%		9=16%		12=15%	97=26%
Diffuse fibrosis	(IV) 4=15%		6=11%		10=12%	47=12%
Reticular type	(V) 10=38%		24=42%		34=41%	21= 6%
No Hodgkin tissue	-= 0%		8=15%		8=10%	- = 0%
Total cases	26		56		82	377

The type that has the highest clinical incidence, i.e. nodular sclerosis (type II), is less common among our autopsies. The incidence of types Ia, Ib, and II, which have by far the best survival expectancy, is 35% in our group A, but only 16% in group B. Thus in the earlier survey period of group A twice as many patients died of this type of Hodgkin's disease, whose prognosis is relatively favorable, than in the subsequent period of group B. Table 1 also shows that in group B 15% of the cases (8 of 57) histologically showed no longer any lymphogranulomatic tissue at all.

Another striking feature of our material is that there are 41 cases of the reticular type, whereas LUKES and BUTLER (10) found only 6% of this type among their biopsies. We know already that this type, the so-called Hodgkin sarcoma, is much more frequent among autopsies than among clinical patients (9). Other authors have established by means of sequential biopsy material that Hodgkin's disease with lymphocytic predominance has a tendency to develop into the lymphocytic depletion type, whereas nodular sclerosis seems to be more stable (12). In our autopsy material, nodular sclerosis is quite rare; it may have changed to other types between the first biopsy and the autopsy.

For 22 of our cases, we were able to compare the histologic slides made at the first diagnostic biopsy directly with the histologic findings at the autopsy. The result is shown in Fig. 1. In six cases the histologic type had not changed - one case of type Ia, two cases of type III, and all three cases of types IV and V. Twelve cases of types Ia to III had turned into the sarcoma type V. On the other hand, four cases of types Ia, II and III had been patients who, with all necessary reservations, can be considered "cured." The three cases of types IV and V had never reached this stage of so-called healing. It is striking that we have no proof of a type with a poor prognosis developing into a type with a favorable one. This supports the findings of STRUM and RAPPAPORT in their sequential biopsies (12). Other authors emphasize that increased malignancy occurs whenever Hodgkin tissue spreads and settles outside the lymph nodes. This can be confirmed by inference : in all cases of increased malignancy we found extensive foci of lymphogranuloma outside the lymph nodes.

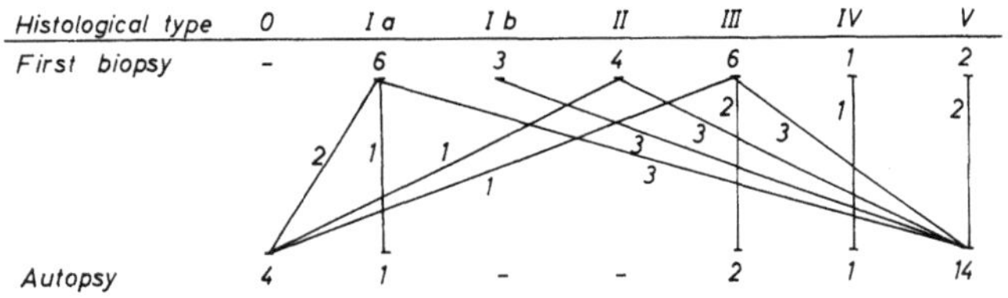

Fig. 1. Changes in histological types in Hodgkin's disease (LUKES and BUTLER) from first biopsy to autopsy (22 cases)

3. In order to formulate a statement on the dispersion of lymphogranulomatic foci and on the severity of the disease such as would offer a simple mode of tabulation, we adopted the system proposed by the Committee on Hodgkin's Disease Stage Classification. The results are shown in Table 2. There is a small difference between groups A and B; in group A, 39 of 43 cases died in the advanced stage IV, in group B, 47 of 56 cases died in stage IV. Table 2 compares the frequency of the four clinical stages as reported by PETERS (11) with our data collected from autopsies. While in the clinical study stage IV was found in only 13% of cases, we found stage IV in 87% of our autopsies. This may be due to the low survival expectancy for stage IV patients (less than two years according to PETERS). Moreover, the stage classification reflects the actual progression of the disease, so most patients will meet their end in stage IV.

4. The age-related incidence of Hodgkin's disease is demonstrated by several authors as a curve with two peaks, one around the 35th year of life and the other around the 55th. We checked our results against these findings and the outcome is shown in Fig. 2: Group A has one maximum between years 30 and 40 and

Table 2. Macroscopic classification of 99 Hodgkin's disease autopsies
In one further case no Hodgkin tissue was demonstrable

		Group A	Group B	A + B	after PETERS (1971)
Stage	I	1= 2%	1= 2%	2= 2%	246=39%
	II	1= 2%	3= 5%	4= 4%	122=20%
	III	2= 5%	5= 9%	7= 7%	175=28%
	IV	39=91%	47=84%	86=87%	81=13%
		43 cases	56 cases	99 cases	624 cases

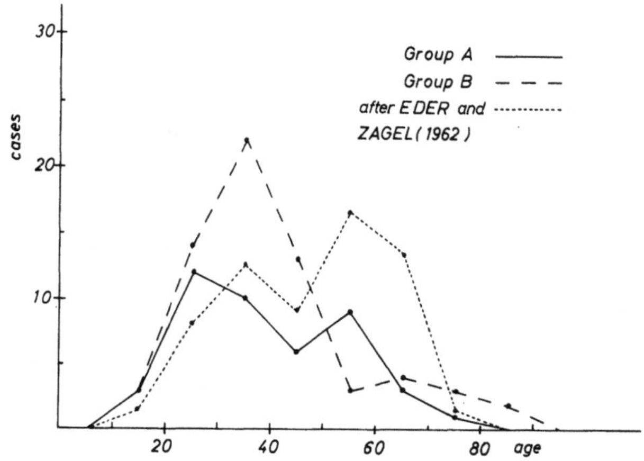

Fig. 2. Age-related distribution of lymphogranulomatosis in autopsies

another between 60 and 70. Group B has a steep maximum between 35 and 40, while between 65 and 70 there is only a barely perceptible elevation. We have drawn a dotted line in Fig. 2 to show the respective age distribution (6) for autopsy findings. Their results do not offer exact parallels since they only record the date of onset of symptoms and not the date of death. Nevertheless, the following conclusions appear obvious: (1) All three curves are two-peaked; (2) the percentage of younger patients dying of Hodgkin's disease increases from 1962 (6) to 1965 (group A) and again from 1965 to 1973 (group B), while the percentage of older patients decreases accordingly.

The possibility of changes in our recruiting area, or in the general pattern of the disease, or in the methods of diagnosis, can be disregarded. The duration of the disease, i.e. the mean distance between diagnosis and death, has become twice as long in our group B as it was in group A. This may be due to the success in therapy. The rising survival expectancy for the elderly will also explain a modified age distribution. The mean expected survival time for elderly patients in group A was 10 months, but it was 39 months in group B. This means that the elderly patients in the second group could expect to survive four times longer than those in the first.

5. The cause of death for Hodgkin patients can be, of course, an immediate consequence of the disease itself. In such cases the most prominent findings at the autopsy will be lymphomas, more or less definite and in various localizations. We have tabulated the implication of different organs in Table 3.

Table 3. Incidence of involvement of extralymphatic organs and tissues in Hodgkin's disease. In two cases no extralymphatic organ involvement

	Group A	Group B
Spleen	29=67%	39=71%
Liver	29=67%	30=56%
Lungs	19=44%	28=51%
Bone marrow	13=30%	24=44%
Bone	5=12%	3= 6%
Pleura	4= 9%	1= 2%
Skin	----	1= 2%
	43 cases	55 cases

In both groups, A and B, the organs most frequently involved are spleen and liver, where either large sarcoma nodes or diffused micronodular infiltration are found. The incidence of pulmonary involvement is strikingly high, most often taking the form of a perivascular or peribronchial lymphovascular invasion. Concomitant involvement of the pleura is rare, considering the number of pulmonary foci. On the other hand, bones and bone marrow are involved in more than one third of all cases. We usually refer to foci in bones if the compacta is destroyed.

Table 4. Specific death rates in Hodgkin's disease

	Group A	Group B
Typical Hodgkin death	24=56%	27=47%
secondary death	17=39%	20=35%
Death independent of Hodgkin's disease	2= 5%	10=18%
	43 cases	57 cases

All the cases cited above are listed as "Hodgkin death" in Table 4, regardless of the terminal concurrence of bronchopneumonia or of any other secondary disease. The second line in Table 4 reflects cases where therapeutic measures have provoked the final and fatal complications. Since it was not always possible to distinguish the roles played by the primary disease and by the therapy, we have placed all such cases under the heading "secondary death."

6. "Secondary death" includes three principal groups of symptoms (see Table 5):

a) Most striking is the damage to the bone marrow provoked by a treatment combining ionizing irradiation and cytostatics. In histological examination we see either cell-depleted marrow, often with severe reduction of trabeculae reflecting reactive osteoporosis, or extensive osteofibrosis. Small nests of lymphogranuloma, or at least some single cells, can be detected between the fibrils of connective tissue in such cases. This therapy-induced fibrosis is characterized by the accumulation of Hodgkin cells in small clumps that no longer possess their normal nuclear structure (with a vesicular pattern) but have pyknomorphous giant nuclei (Fig. 3). Another characteristic sequel of irradiation is the reactive densification of trabeculae with irregular lamellation.

Table 5. Secondary death in Hodgkin's disease

	Group A	Group B
Bone marrow damage	11	14
Intestinal hemorrhage	3	-
X-ray pulmonary fibrosis	-	6
Exacerbation of tuberculosis	1	-
No of cases:	15	20

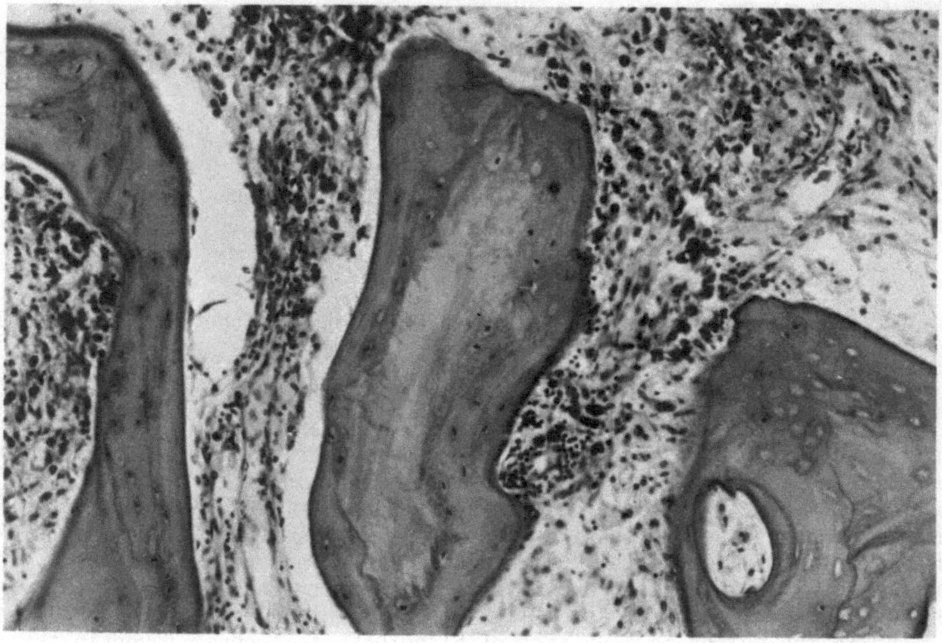

Fig. 3. Vertebral body with fibrous obliteration of bone marrow and pyknomorphic Hodgkin cells found after chemotherapy and irradiation in Hodgkin's disease. Irregular periostosis. Hematoxylin-Eosin x 80

More than 20% of all Hodgkin patients in our material died as a consequence of damage to the bone marrow. Two cases showed signs of sepsis with dense accumulation of bacteria in the blood vessels of lungs and spleen, while three other cases had developed the pneumonia typical with candida albicans.

b) X-ray-induced pulmonary fibrosis is another new complication encountered in group B. Histologically, the first sign is a fibrin coating of the alveolae. Eventually they are completely filled with masses of fibrin. Subsequent organization of this fibrin results in formation of granulation tissue, we get the picture of carnification. In the same alveolae, we often see Hodgkin cells lining the inner walls like a seam, while the lumen is scarred. The elastic lamellae appear densified due to shrinking. Since these cases are always histologic type V, we call this condition "carnifying Hodgkin's pneumonia" (Fig. 4).

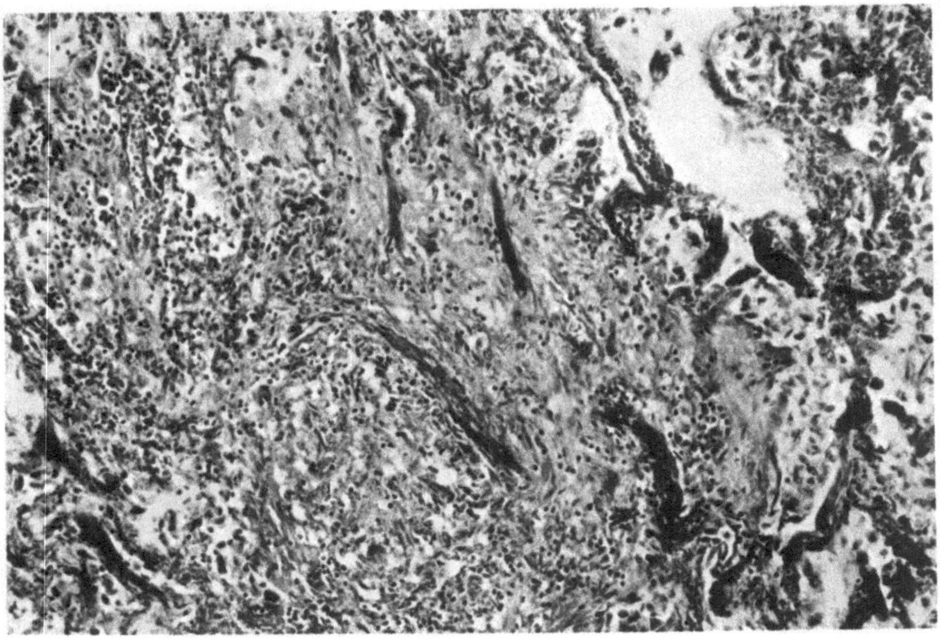

Fig. 4. Pulmonary fibrosis with residues of Hodgkin tissue (carnifying Hodgkin's pneumonia) after super-high-voltage irradiation.

7. Sequelae of therapy in lymph nodes and spleen are the well-known necroses and, above all, progressing fibrosis. In some cases, it may be difficult to identify the original histologic type by examination of the fibrotic lymph nodes. Nodular sclerosis can heal in a micronodular or in a more diffuse pattern, whereas the lymphocytic predominant diffuse type and primary diffuse fibrosis will end in diffuse hyalinization. This rule holds for lymph nodes as well as for spleen and liver. The splenic sinus remains intact and generally appears enlarged and well filled with blood. We may find endogenous pigment in the spleen as a vestige of bleeding; it is never found in the lymph nodes and rarely in the liver.

8. "Cured cases." In seven of the eight cases that could be described as "cured"from a pathologoanatomic aspect, we found large scars in the hilar lymph nodes and even in the lungs, in three cases in the spleen as well. The eighth case showed neither scars nor any other residues of Hodgkin tissue.

9. With regard to the actual question of a possible carcinogenic effect of cytostatics, our observations have led us to the following conclusions:

1. Despite reports that 3 - 3.5% of all Hodgkin patients develop another malignant tumor (1, 2), we have not found a single secondary carcinoma among our hundred autopsy cases.
2. We are not able to determine exactly whether the increasing incidence of prognostically unfavorable histologic types in our material is due to the sequelae of therapy or to autonomous features of Hodgkin's disease. We can only state that the sarcoma stage was found 40 times more frequently in our collection than in clinical reports (10). Other workers observed 2 sarcomas in 198 Hodgkin autopsies performed in the period from 1930 - 1948, and 14 sarcomas in 148 Hodgkin autopsies between 1949 and 1956 (13).

It is now accepted that 40% of all Hodgkin patients will die in the sarcoma stage, in spite of - or because of - the increased statistical chance of survival.

REFERENCES

1. ARSENEAU, J. C., SPONZO, R. W., LEVIN, D. L., SCHNIPPER, L. E., BONNER, H., YOUNG, R. C. CANELLOS, G. P., JOHNSON, R. E., DE VITA, V. T.: New Engl. J. Med. 287, 1119 (1972).
2. BERG, J. W.: J. nat. Cancer Inst. 38, 741 (1967).
3. BRUNNER, K. W.: Verh. dtsch. Ges. inn. Med. 79, 168 (1973).
4. CANELLOS, G. P., YOUNG, R. C., BERARD, C. W., DE VITA, V. T.: Arch. int. Med. 131, 388 (1973).
5. CRAVER, L. F.: Treatment of Hodgkin's Disease. In: Treatment of Cancer and Allied Diseases IX. Harper & Row (Hoeber Med. Div.): New York 1964.
6. EDER, M., ZAGEL, M.: Dtsch. med. Wschr. 87, 1960 (1962).
7. FREI, E.: Arch. int. Med. 131, 439 (1973).
8. GERHARTZ, H.: Verlängert d. zytostatische Therapie d. Lebenserwartung d. Hämoblastosen? In: Chemo- und Immunotherapie der Leukosen und malignen Lymphome. Vienna: Bohman 1969.
9. LENNERT, K.: Z. Krebsforsch. 78, 137 (1972).
10. LUKES, R. J., BUTLER, J. J.: Cancer Res. 26, 1063 (1966).
11. PETERS, M. V.: Cancer Res. 31, 1713 (1971).
12. STRUM, S. B., RAPPAPORT, H.: Arch. Path. 91, 127 (1971).
13. WÜST, G., JANSSEN, W.: Münch. med. Wschr. 98, 1395 (1956).

Tumor Inductions by Cytostatics in Man

W. Hunstein

By analogy with studies on ionizing radiation (48, 69), the title of this paper leads one to expect a number of individual case histories and statistical studies concerned with the induction of tumors by cytostatic drugs. The carcinogenic and leukemogenic effect of cytostatic drugs seems to be so surely proven in human beings that a discussion of this question seems hardly worth the effort. We know that cytostatic drugs have biologic effects that in 25 points are the same as these of ionizing radiation, and this knowledge has led to their classification as "radiomimetic" agents (13).

This makes it all the more surprising that in view of the large number of patients treated, tumor production by cytostatics is still the exception and not the rule. This paper does not deal with the accelerated and intensive tumor induction in recipients of kidney transplants because this is reviewed elsewhere (29, 50, 51, 15, 38, 3, etc.). This oncogenesis is multifactorial. There is a combined effect of cytostatic drugs, other immunosuppresssive drugs, irradiation, perhaps a graft-versus-host reaction and, as we have recently learned, apparently an infection with the tumor-producing Papova viruses (19, 39). Moreover, cases of tumor transfer during transplantation have been reported (23), as has the formation of a localized sarcoma at the site of injection of antilymphocyte serum (12).

The discussion of the subject in this paper is divided into three parts:

1. Presentation of cases published up to now (18, 27) with no claim to completeness;
2. Presentation of statistically proved increased tumor incidence and reviews;
3. Interpretation of observations and conclusions.

1. Most secondary, supposedly therapy-induced tumors have been described in connection with the administration of cyclophosphamide (Endoxan R). The cumulative doses vary from 7 to 140 g., the time of tumor induction between 14 months and 7 years. The following tumors have been described after treatment of multiple myeloma: 1 rectal carcinoma (53), 2 carcinomas of the stomach (17), 1 angiosarcoma (46); there are reports of the treatment of mammary carcinoma being followed by 1 ovarian carcinoma (54), 1 gallbladder carcinoma (55), and 2 acute leukemias (11); in some of these cases combined drug treatment was used. Acute leukemia has also been described during treatment of ovarian carcinoma (65). Recently a case of fibrosarcoma of the urinary bladder was seen concomitantly with Hodgkin's disease (58). The treatment of WALDENSTRÖM's macroglobulinemia has been followed by rectal carcinoma in one case (62), and lymphoreticular sarcomas in three cases (33).

The mustard derivative chlornaphazine has been implicated as a carcinogen of the urinary bladder with as short an induction time as 3 to 5 years after total doses of 80 - 100 g. (67, 37). The compound is a dichlorodiethylnaphthylamine. Its carcinogenic effect can be attributed to its naphthyl component. Therefore, it acts like a chemical and not as a cytostatic carcinogen. 2-Naphthylamine and related substances are potential carcinogens of the urinary bladder in human beings and animals.

Busulfan (Myleran R) is thought to have induced the following tumors in one case each: carcinoma of the breast (49), bronchiolar cell carcinoma (36), carcinoma of the bronchus (61). The combination of Myleran (busulfan) and Colcemid (demecolcine) is said to have produced a uterine carcinoma (66); the combination of busulfan and mercaptopurine has been followed by pancreatic carcinoma (2). Animal experiments have shown Myleran to be a fairly potent leukemogen (30).

The administration of the benzochinon-derivative Trenimon R over a period of 3 years for a myosarcoma is said to have produced monocytic leukemia (72).

Both an epithelial tumor (26) and a case of reversible reticulum cell hyperplasia (32) have been described after administration of amethopterin (Methotrexate R).

ANDERSON and VIDEBAEK (1) have reported the origin of several cases of stem cell leukemia after the treatment of multiple myeloma with melphalan (Alkeran R). The interval varied from 18 months to 4 years. Since then, similar observations have been published by other authors, some of them in connection with cyclophosphamide (35, 28, 56); in one instance the condition was observed after treatment for Waldenström's disease (52). A statistical evaluation of these publications has not yet been possible. Therefore, it is still not clear whether acute leukemia is the result of treatment or is the endstate of multiple myeloma after therapeutically prolonged survival (28). Polycentric lung carcinoma has been reported following treatment with melphalan (60).

2. Only one recent investigation in this group has received special attention (4). ARSENEAU and his group investigated their 425 cases of Hodgkin's disease for the appearance of further tumors. Fig. 1 shows their results. Radiation therapy or chemotherapy alone leads to no significant increase in tumor incidence, but the combination of the two does. Intensive chemotherapy alone does not give rise to any significant change. The majority of secondary tumors are entered under the heading "combined intensive chemotherapy plus intensive radiation" (cf. 8, 7).

In this connection a prospective study concerning the occurrence of secondary carcinomas in patients with hemoblastoses is significant (6). In 1561 cases of leukemia, 1871 of lymphosarcoma, 1028 of lymphogranuloma and 207 of myeloma 95 carcinomas were observed, among which there were 60 cases of asynchronous skin carcinomas alone, in 43 patients. The author concludes that "no single common cause for this increase was found, though a number of patients reported specific exposures ot carcinogenic situations." In his series of 4600 patients with tumors the chance of getting a second carcinoma was no greater than in the general population.

These results contrast with those of another study (25), which indicated that in men with chronic lymphatic leukemia the incidence of skin carcinoma was 13 times higher and the incidence of other carcinomas 15 times higher than in the general population (cf. 53). The patient sample was smaller in this study, and the number of females was too low for reliable statistical processing.

Risk of second malignant tumor according to treatment group

Group	No. of cases	Man-yrs of observation	2nd tumor Observed	2nd tumor Expected	Ratio of observed to expected
Without regard to intensity of therapy:					
Radiotherapy alone	134	575	4	1.17	3.4
Chemotherapy alone	98	257	3	0.70	4.3
Radiotherapy & chemotherapy	193	752	5	1.52	3.3
According to intensive therapy:					
IR without IC	149	562	4	1.05	3.8
IC without IR	110	371	3	0.94	3.2
IR + IC	35	108	3	0.10	29.0
No intensive therapy	131	543	2	1.28	1.6
Total cases studied	425	1584	12	3.38	3.5

Fig. 1. Incidence of secondary tumors in 425 patients with Hodgkin's disease (from ARSENEAU et al., 1972)

In another study of 1057 cases of hemoblastoses treated with cytostatic agents 10 secondary malignancies were found. This corresponds to a statistical expectation without cytostatics (27).

There are few reviews of the syntropy of different hemoblastoses. The simultaneous appearance of chronic lymphatic leukemia (primary) with Hodgkin's disease (secondary) in 21 cases was described as coincidental (42). Other authors have collected 27 cases in which acute leukemia has followed the onset of Hodgkin's disease (74, cf. 59).

In a study concerning multiple carcinomas in Hodgkin's disease it was not possible to confirm the elevated frequency of secondary carcinomas as compared with the expectancy for the general population (71).

These results indicate that (1) only intensive, and particularly combined, chemotherapy, especially when combined with X-irradiation, increases the risk of a secondary tumor in Hodgkin's disease, and (2) intensive melphalan medication seems to increase the risk of occurrence of acute leukemia in multiple myeloma; (3) all other publications describe isolated cases and do not confirm tumor induction by cytostatics in man.

This conclusion could be based on false population selection: tumor patients treated with cytostatic drugs do not survive to neocarcinogenesis. This interpretation is contradicted, however, by recent experience with transplant recipients.

It is thus necessary to examine the situation in patients treated with cytostatic drugs for indications other than malignancy. Some controlled studies have been run by the Paul Ehrlich Society, with a view to the cytostatic therapy of immunologic diseases, e.g. systemic lupus erythematosus, Sjögren's syndrome, rheumatoid arthritis and other collagenous diseases (cf. 47, 64, 70, 10). CHLUD reviews 720 cases of collagenous diseases treated intermittently since 1965 with benzochinon and podophyllin preparations without any tumor arising (9).

Moreover, patients with chronic aggressive hepatitis are treated with azathioprine, as are patients with ulcerative colitis and regional enteritis and those with nephrotic syndrome (one author reports one cervical carcinoma after cyclophospahmide therapy (51). MCEWAN and PETTY noted: " the worldwide use of azathioprine in nontransplant situations has yielded 3 published cases of neoplasms in over 4000 cases and 3 in a smaller number of placebo controls" (44).

Thereby it seems that the syntropy of immunologic diseases and tumors familiar in type-NZB mice (14, 24) can probably not be extrapolated to human beings. This syntropy is, however, often cited and expected, and there are incidental observations of it both with and without the administration of cytostatic drugs (57, 9, 43, 63). LIPSMAYER published a case of malignant cerebral lymphoma after treatment of SLE for 6 weeks (41): the validity of this was contested (64).

In contrast, malignant tumors do arise in immunodeficiency diseases (20) such as A-gammaglobulinemia, Wiskott-Aldrich syndrome, ataxia teleangectasia etc. with a spontaneous incidence of up to 5 - 10%.

3. The question of whether cytostatic drugs are largely carcinogenic in the human being must be left open. But all data from animal experiments and all our knowledge concerning the induction period for tumors due to ionizing radiation, which can extend over several decades, indicate that oncogenesis is a late sequel of radiation and alkylating agents.

The data on all patients who are receiving or have received cytostatic drugs should be collected, and if possible the patients should be followed up for the rest of their lives. Only in this way can we obtain the necessary statistical conclusion. This would also allow us to examine the question of mutation and cancer origin (34) and that of transplacental cancerogenesis (68).

As was stated in a leading article in the Lancet (40), "If we are to make progress in cancer prevention there must be more cooperation between laboratory worker and epidemiologist ... What we need is far more epidemiology and better record linkage so that we can avoid at least the therapeutic disasters."

REFERENCES

1. ANDERSEN, E., VIDEBAEK, A.: A stem cell leukaemia in myelomatosis. Scand. J. Haemat. 7, 201 (1970).
2. ANGUS, H. B., GUNZ, F. W.: Chronic granulocytic leukaemia and cancer. Blood 22, 88 (1963).
3. ARBUS, G. S., HUNG, R. H.: Hepatocarcinoma and myocardial fibrosis in an 8 3/4 year old renal transplant recipient. Canad. med. Ass. J. 9, 431 (1972).

4. ARSENEAU, J. C., SPONZO, R. W., LEVIN, D., SCHNIPPER, L. E., BRONNER, H. YOUNG, R. C., CANELLOS, G. P., JOHNSON, R. E., DE VITA, V. T.: Nonlymphomatous malignant tumors complicating Hodgkin's disease. New Engl. J. Med. 287, 119 (1972).
5. BASHOUR, B. N., MANCER, K., RANCE, C. P.: Malignant mixed mullerian tumor of the cervix following cyclophosphamide therapy for nephrotic syndrome. J. Pediat. 82, 292 (1973).
6. BERG, J. W.: The incidence of multiple primary cancers. J. nat. Cancer Inst. 38, 741 (1967).
7. BONADONNA, G., DELENA, M., BANFI, A., LATTUADA, A.: Secondary neoplasms in malignant lymphomas after intensive therapy. New Engl. J. Med. 289, 1242 (1973).
8. CASTRO, G. A. M., CHURCH, A., PECHET, L., SNYDER, L. M.: Leukemia after chemotherapy of Hodgkin's disease. New Engl. J. Med. 289, 103 (1973).
9. CHLUD, K.: Das Therapiekonzept der chronischen Polyarthritis. Therapiewoche 21, 3527 (1971).
10. Cooperating Clinics Committee of the ARA: A controlled trial of cyclophosphamide in rheumatoid arthritis. New Engl. J. Med. 283, 883 (1970).
11. DAVIS, H. L., PROUT, M. N., MACKENNA, P. J., COLE, D. R., KOBITZ, B. C.: Acute leukemia complicating metastatic breast cancer. Cancer 31, 543 (1973).
12. DEODHAR, S. D., KUKLINCA, A. G., VIDT, D. G., ROBERTSON, A. L., HAZARD, J. B.: Development of reticulum-cell sarcoma at the site of antilymphocyte globulin injection in a patient with renal transplant. New Engl. J. Med. 280, 1104 (1969).
13. DUSTIN, P.: Nature (Lond.) 159, 794 (1947).
14. EAST, J.: Immunpathology and neoplasms in New Zealand Black (NZB) and SJL/S mice. Progr. exp. Tumor Res. 13, 84 (1970).
15. Editorial: Transpalntation, Immunosuppression and Oncogenesis. J. Amer. med. Ass. 224, 1183 (1973).
16. ELSON, L. A., Radiation and radiomimetic chemicals. London: Butterworths 1963.
17. FASS, H.: Über die zytostatische Behandlung des Plasmozytoms. Med. Wschr. 16, 389 (1962).
18. FRAUMENI, J. F., MILLER, R. W.: Drug-induced cancer. J. nat. Cancer Inst. 48, 1268 (1972).
19. GARDNER, S.D., FIELD, A., COLEMAN, D., HULME, B.: New human papovavirus (B. K.) isolated from urine after renal transplantation. Lancet 1971 1, 1253.
20. GATTI, R. A., GOOD, R. A.: Occurrence of malignancy in immunodeficiency diseases. Cancer 28, 89 (1971).
21. GOERTTLER, K.: Modell und Wirklichkeit der iatrogenen Cancerogenese. Verh. dtsch. Ges. Path. 56, 138 (1972).
22. GREUL, W., HULAND, J., SCHÄFER, H. J.: Zur Frage der Langzeittherapie des Plasmazytoms. Dtsch. med. Wschr. 98, 496 (1973).
23. GROSS, L.: Transmission of cancer in men. Cancer 28, 785 (1971).
24. GRUNDMANN, E., HOBIK, H. P.: Lymphoretikuläre Sarkome bei immunologisch geschädigten Mäusen. Z. Krebsforsch. 79, 298 (1973).
25. GUNZ, F. W., ANGUS, H. B.: Leukemia and cancer in the same patient. Cancer 18, 145 (1965).
26. HARRIS, C. C.: Malignancy during Methotrexate and steroid therapy for Psoriasis. Arch. Derm. 103, 501 (1971).
27. HARTWICH, G.: Nebenwirkungen cytostatischer und immunsuppressiver Therapie. Fortschr. Med. 91, 357 (1973).
28. HOLLAND, J. F.: Epidemic acute leukemia. New Engl. J. Med. 283, 1165 (1970).

29. HOOVER, R., FRAUMENI, J. F.: Risk of cancer in renal transplant recipients. Lancet 1973 3, 55.
30. HUNSTEIN, W.: Ist Myleran (Busulphan) ein leukaemogenes Agens? Schweiz. med. Wschr. 95, 1437 (1965).
31. JEREMY, D.: Transplantation of malignant melanoma with cadaver Kidney. Transplantation 13, 619 (1972).
32. KELLETER, R., KÜHN, D., SCHNYDER, U. W., SCHROETER, R.: Lymphoretikuläre Hyperplasie nach dreijähriger Methotrexatbehandlung einer Psoriasis. Dtsch. med. Wschr. 97, 614 (1972).
33. KLEMM, D., MERKER, H., WESTERHAUSEN, M.: Akute Neuproliferation bei paraproteinämische Hämoblastosen unter langdauernder Cytostatikabehandlung. Dtsch. med. Wschr. 93, 2063 (1968).
34. KNUDSON, A. G.: Mutation and human cancer. Advanc. Cancer Res. 17, 317 (1973).
35. KYLE, R. A., PIERRE, R. V., BAYRD, E. D.: Multiple myeloma and acute myelomonocytic leukemia. New Engl. J. Med. 283, 1121 (1970).
36. KYUNG-WHAN, M., GYÖRKEY, .: Interstitial pulmonary fibrosis, atypical epithelial changes and bronchiolar cell carcinoma following busulfan therapy. Cancer 22, 1027 (1968).
37. LAURSEN, B.: Cancer in the bladder in patients treated with chlornaphazine. Brit. med. J. 3, 684 (1970).
38. LEB, D. E., HOWELL, R. S.: Carcinoma of the testis in a renal transplant recipient. Amer. J. med. Sci. 262, 171 (1971).
39. LECATSAS, G., PROZESKY, O. W., WYK, J. van: Papovavirus in urine after renal transplantation. Nature 241, 343 (1973).
40. Leading article: Transplacental carcinogenesis. Lancet 1973 2, 1425.
41. LIPSMEYER, E. A.: Development of malignant cerebral lymphoma in a patient with SLE treated with immunosuppression. Arthr. and Rheum. 15, 183 (1972).
42. LOKICH, J. J., MOLONEY, W. C.: Hodgkin's disease and chronic lymphatic leukemia. Oncology 26, 466 (1972).
43. MANNY, N., ROSENMAN, E., BENBASSAT, J.: Hazard of immunosuppressive therapy. Brit. med. J. 2, 291 (1972).
44. MCEWAN, A., PETTY, L. G.: Oncogenicity of immunosuppressive drugs. Lancet 1972 1, 326.
45. MICHLMAYR, G., GÜNTHER, R., LEDERER, B., HUBER, H.: Malignes Lymphom nach zweijähriger immunosuppressiver Therapie einer Periarteriitis nodosa. Med. Klin. 68, 180 (1973).
46. MICHOT, F.: Beitrag zum Problem des Plasmozytoms ohne Paraprotein. Dtsch. med. Wschr. 93, 2072 (1968).
47. MICHOT, F.: Erfahrungen in der Langzeitbehandlung von Kollagenkrankheiten mit Azathioprin (Imman R). Med. Klin. 63, 1262 (1968).
48. MOLE, R. H.: Late effects of radiation: carcinogenesis. Brit. med. Bull. 29, 78 (1973).
49. NELSON, B. M., ANDREWS, G. A.: Breast cancer and cytologic dysplasia in many organs after busulfan (Myleran). Amer. J. clin. Path. 42, 37 (1964).
50. PENN, I., STARZL, T. E.: Immunosuppression and cancer. Proc. 4th Int. Congr. Transplant. Soc. (in press).
51. PENN, I., STARZL, T. E.: Malignant tumors arising de novo in immunosuppressed organ transplant recipients. Transplantation 14, 407 (1972).
52. PETERSEN, H. S.: Erythroleukaemia in a Melphalan-treated patient with primary macroglobulinaemia. Scand. J. Haemat. 10, 5 (1973).
53. RENNER, K.: Kasuistischer Beitrag zur Frage der Neuentstehung maligner Neoplasmen unter cytostatischer Therapie. Strahlentherapie 142, 308 (1971).
54. RENNER, W. A.: Erfahrungen mit Endoxan und Mitarson bei einem metastasierenden Mamma Carcinom. Med. Klin. 58, 254 (1963).

55. RIECHE, K.: Zur Frage der Cancerogenität von Cytostatika. Arch. Geschwulstforsch. 34, 240 (1969).
56. RIEDLER, G. F., VORBURGER, E., MAIER, C.: Unreifzellige Leukosen und Myelom. Schweiz. med. Wschr. 102, 1592 (1972).
57. ROUZAUD, M., LEROUX, M. E., LAMISSE, F.: Erythromyêlose aigue aleicêmique et lêsions diffuses de pêriartêrite noueuse. Sêm. Hôp. Paris 45, 2831 (1969).
58. RUPPPRECHT, L., BLESSING, M. M.: Fibrosarkon der Harnblase nach siebenjähriger Chemotherapie einer Lymphogranulomatose im Kindesalter. Dtsch. med. Wschr. 93, 1663 (1973).
59. SCHAEFER, U. W., KANZLER, G.: Leukämie bei Morbus Hodgkin. Med. Klin. 67, 1024 (1972).
60. SCHEIDEGGER, S.: Lungenfibrose, rezidivierende Vasculitis und multizentrisches Lungencarcinom nach cytostatischer Therapie mit Alkeran. Verh. dtsch. Ges. Path. 56, 364 (1972).
61. SCHILLING, R. F., MEYER, O. O.: Treatment of chronic granulocytic leukemia with 1,4-Dimethansulfonyloxybutase (Myleran). New Eng. J. Med. 254, 986 (1956).
62. SCHMITT-KÖPPLER, A.: Die Umkehrwirkung eines Zytostatikums als mögliche Ursache eines Analkarzinoms. Therapiewoche 22, 1592 u. 1595 (1972).
63. SCHOLZ, G., REHN, K., HUNSTEIN, W.: Hodgkinsarkom bei immunsuppressiv behandeltem Erythematodes visceralis. Verh. dtsch. Ges. inn. Med. 79, 1376 (1973).
64. SHARON, E., PAOLINO, J. S., KAPLAN, D.: Lymphoma and Azathioprine. Arthr. Rheum. (N. Y.) 15, 558 (1972).
65. SMIT, C. G. S., MEYLER, L.: Acute myeloid leukaemia after treatment with cytostatic agents. Lancet 1970 2, 671.
66. STICH, W., LANGHAMMER, H.: Multiple Karzinome und Leukämie. Münch. med. Wschr. 109, 1597 (1969).
67. THIEDE, T., CHIEVITZ, E., CHRISTENSEN, B. C.: Chlornaphazine as a bladder carcinogen. Acta med. scand. 175, 721 (1964).
68. TOMATIS, R., MOHR, L. U., DAVIS, W.: Transplacental Carcinogenesis. International Agency for Research on Cancer. Scientific publication No. 4 (1973).
69. UNSCEAR: Ionizing radiation: levels and effects, Vol. II: Effects (a report of the United Nations Scientific Committee on the effects of atomic radiation to the General Assembly, with appendices). New York: United Nations 1972.
70. UROWITZ, M. B., GORDON, D. A., SMYTHE, H. A., PRUZANSKI, W., OGRYZLO, M. A.: Azathioprine in rheumtoid arthritis. Arthr. and Rheum. 16, 411 (1973).
71. WHITELAW, D. M.: Multiple primary carcinomas associated with Hodgkin's disease. Canad. med. Ass. J. 99, 291 (1968).
72. WILDHACK, R.: Monozytenleukämie mit γG-Paraproteinämie nach Röntgenbestrahlung und zytostatischer Behandlung eines Myosarkoms. Dtsch. med. Wschr. 95, 40 (1970).
73. ZWAAN, F. E., SPECK, B.: Acute myelomonocytic leukemia in a patient with Hodgkin's disease. Acta haemat. 49, 291 (1973).

Methodological Problems in the Quantitative Assessment of Carcinogenesis in Long-Term Studies

B. Schneider and N. Brock

1. INTRODUCTION

The question of carcinogenicity of cytostatics and of drugs in general, is a problem of vital importance to doctors, patients and drug research. The steadily increasing toxic risks of the human environment require a serious approach to this problem. This applies particularly to such poisons and drugs as exert their effect over a lengthy period of time, and which are thus very likely to produce mutagenic, cancerogenic and teratogenic effects. This problem can only be solved with the aid of suitable biometric and statistical methods which allow a clear-cut quantitative assessment of the toxic actions in long-term studies. The classic biometrical methods of evaluation, such as comparison of mean values or frequency comparison, which have so far been used, are not applicable, since the basic requirements (especially homogeneity) are not met in long-term studies. It is therefore necessary to develop new processes and models which are especially suited to the intricacies of long-term studies.

In recent years various research groups have tackled this problem; one team in particular, in the Biometric Branch of the National Cancer Institute, Bethesda (4), has contributed important preliminary studies, and other significant contributions have been made (2, 3). Our research group has also tackled this problem and developed new methods of evaluation (1, 5). In this text we report on the problems involved and on the new statistical methods.

2. THE PROBLEM OF THE COMPETITIVE RISKS DURING LONG-TERM STUDIES

A special problem during long-term studies is the fact that carcinogenesis may be overlayered and interfered with by other effects. In addition, the experimental animal or patient may die before a tumor develops. Therefore the tumor rates are distorted by the mortality risk. They do not allow direct conclusions as to the drug's carcinogenic effect. This would only be possible if the tumor induction times were considerably shorter than the survival time.

Comparison of the carcinogenic effect of compounds which do not differ only in their tumor induction time, but also in total mortality is even more complicated. The tumor rates observed after the individual preparations depend on both the carcinogenic effect and the lethal effect. It is therefore impossible to draw direct conclusions as to possible differences in the drugs' carcinogenic efficacy from the tumor rates alone. This is obviously due to the fact that the relation between tumor induction time and survival time is of particular importance in long-term studies. Thus, for quantitative assessment of the carcinogenic effect both the survival rate and the induction time must be determined for each particular animal and the results obtained with various drugs or dosages should be compared. In such a comparison the interrelation between the two factors involved should be carefully observed and analyzed. In the Anglo-American literature this factor is called a "problem of competing risk." Mathematical methods for dealing with this competing risk problem will now be described briefly:

3. MATHEMATICAL METHODS

The evaluation is based on the tumor induction time and on the survival time. It is necessary to state whether the observed induction and survival times or the crude induction and survival times are used. The crude induction and survival times are based on a group in which the effect is exerted to the full without any impairment.

The observed induction time will be designated x_1 and the observed survival time x_2. The crude induction time is designated y_1 and the crude survival time y_2. The animals are observed until a tumor develops or the animal dies.

The induction time x_1 is only observed if the crude induction time y_1 is smaller than the survival time y_2. Under these conditions an equation can be formulated in which the probability distribution of the observed induction time x_1 is related to the probability distributions of the crude induction time y_1 and the crude survival time y_2. This equation reads as follows:-

$$f_1(x_1) = \frac{p_1(x_1)}{\Pi_1} \left(1 - P_2[x_1] \right), \text{ where}$$

$f_1(x_1)$ indicates the probability density for the observed induction time x_1, $p_1(x_1)$ indicates the probability density for the crude induction time, and $P_2(x_1)$ the probability of a patient's or animal's death before the time x_1 without development of a tumor (distribution function of the crude survival time y_2); Π_1 is the probability of appearance of a tumor.

Before this formula can be used for statistical evaluation, additional assumptions must be made for the two distributions p_1 and P_2. As is well known, survival time and induction time do not usually follow the normal distribution pattern. Their distribution is asymmetric (since negative survival or induction times are not possible). In a first approximation it can be approached by means of an exponential distribution. This distribution is characterized by its average induction and survival times, from this point designated Θ_1 and Θ_2.

This can also be used for the calculation of the exponential distribution of the induction time x_1, whose mean value Δ is composed of the two mean values Θ_1 and Θ_2 according to the following equation:-

$$\frac{1}{\Delta} = \frac{1}{\Theta_1} + \frac{1}{\Theta_2} \qquad \text{(cf. SCHNEIDER, 1972).}$$

This formula shows how the influence of the carcinogenic effect and the competing influence of the lethal effect are intermingled during the observed induction time. If, in comparison to the mean crude induction time Θ_1, the mean crude survival time Θ_2 is very long, the addend $\frac{1}{\Theta_2}$ can be ignored and the observed mean induction time Δ is about the same as the crude induction time Θ_1. If, however, Θ_1 and Θ_2 are about the same, the observed induction time is only half the crude induction time. Thus shorter induction times are observed than have been seen in reality. Since various agents do usually not only influence the induction times, comparison of the observed induction times (and observed tumor rates) often gives a completely distorted picture of the drug's carcinogenic properties. Therefore it is important not to compare the carcinogenic effect of the individual agents on the basis of the observed induction times, but only on the corrected crude times.

Such a comparison can be effected by means of the usual procedures of mathematical statistics, especially the so-called maximum likelihood method. With its aid the medium crude induction times can be estimated on the basis of the observed induction and survival times, according to the following formula:-

$$\hat{\Theta}_1 = \bar{x}_1 + \frac{n_1}{n_2} \cdot x_2 \quad ,$$

where $\bar{x}_1$ is the observed medium induction time,

$\bar{x}_2$ is the observed medium survival time,

n_1 is the number of animals that have developed a tumor,

n_2 is the number of animals that have died without a tumor.

It should be noted that n_1 and n_2 are random figures and therefore the known statistical formula does not apply to the variance of the mean values $\bar{x}_1$ and $\bar{x}_2$. The appropriate formulas are given in the afore-mentioned paper by SCHNEIDER.

For long-term comparison of the carcinogenic activity of various agents and various doses, the mathematical model described above can be extended. In such a case the crude induction and crude survival times Θ_1 and Θ_2 must be assumed to be functions of agent and dose, and for this the following additive formula can be used to give an approximation:-

$$\Theta_{1jk} = \mu_1 + \alpha_{1j} + \beta_{1k} + \gamma_{1jk} \quad ,$$

where Θ_{1jk} is the mean crude induction time for the agent j and dose k,

μ_1 is the total average of the induction time,

α_{1j} is the influence of agent j on Θ_1,

β_{1k} is the influence of dose k on Θ_1,

γ_{1jk} is the influence of interaction between dose and agent on Θ_1.

Corresponding formulas apply to the mean survival time Θ_2.

The new parameters μ, α, β and γ can be assessed according to the maximum likelihood method. In addition, hypotheses can be tested, e.g. the assumption that there is no agent effect, no dose effect or no interaction. Testing methods for these hypotheses have recently been published (4).

4. CENSORED SAMPLES

In the foregoing mathematical considerations every experimental animal was assumed to be observed until a tumor occurred or until the animal died. Such long-term observations are often impossible in clinical cases, however, and each patient can only be observed for a restricted period of time. Such random observations are called censored samples. For the assessment of results this means that in addition to the occurrence of a tumor or death a third possibility must be taken into account, i.e. that during the period of observation neither tumor nor death occurs. The probability of this event can easily be calculated if the probability distribution for the crude tumor induction time and the crude survival time is known. If this probability function is designated P_1 and P_2, the probability that neither tumor nor death will occur during the observation period β_1 is expressed by the following formula:-

$$(1 - P_1[\beta_1]) \cdot (1 - P_2[\beta_t]).$$

If this formula is included in the maximum likelihood equation, the estimated value of the crude tumor induction time Θ_1 is slightly modified, because the influence of the restricted observation period must be included by adding the mean observation period $\bar{\beta}$, taking this average from all patients who have not responded:-

$$\hat{\Theta}_1^* = \hat{\Theta}_1 + \bar{\beta}.$$

5. USE IN LONG-TERM STUDIES

The biometric methods and models described above have been used in our comprehensive long-term studies for the detection of possible carcinogenic effects of antitumor agents. These studies are supported by the Federal Ministry for Research and Technology. In these studies the animal strains and the assay arrangements such as dosage, intervals between doses and duration of administration are systematically modified under controlled conditions. The studies are performed on rats of the BD II and Sprague-Dawley strains.

In the assay arrangement the duration of administration and dosage are modified. In long-term studies 2 different doses are given once weekly for 1 year, in short-term studies 3 different doses are given for a limited period of time. Each sample consists of 40 animals, 20 males and 20 females. The control group consists of 200 animals, 100 males and 100 females.

The test agents we used were modern cytostatics of the alkylating and antimetabolite types.

It is expected that these studies will not only allow the assessment of the pure carcinogenic potency in dependence on dose and agent, but in addition will give information on further toxic and and therapeutic effects with long-term use.

The results will also be of interest from a pharmacotherapeutic point of view, particularly the central question of whether agents with a wider margin of safety will allow a reduction of what has been referred to as long-term toxicity.

REFERENCES

1. BROCK, N., SCHNEIDER, B.: Arzneimittel-Forsch. (Drug Res.) 21, 435 (1971).
2. CHIANG, C. L.: Introduction to Stochastic Processes in Biostatistics. New York: Wiley 1968.
3. MOESCHBERGER, M. L., DAVID, H. A.: Biometrics 27, 909 (1971).
4. MYERS, M. H., HANKEY, B. F., MANTEL, N.: Biometrics 29, 257 (1973).
5. SCHNEIDER, B.: Arzneimittel-Forsch. (Drug Res.) 23, 1680 (1973).

Summary

E. Grundmann

The question as to whether cytostatic drugs might be carcinogenic has been presented and discussed in three experimental studies. The most extensive investigations were by J. H. WEISBURGER and coll. (New York, Alabama, Bethesda). They started with an exact determination of rate and localization for spontaneous tumors in their animal strains. Thirteen cytostatic compounds currently in clinical use were then given in the maximally tolerated dose (MTD) to groups of 25 male and 25 female animals (rats and mice) three times weekly, in most assays over a period of 6 months. Other identical groups of animals received 0.5 of the MTD. Each test involved 50 male and 50 female mice and the same number of rats. As positive controls, identical groups were given diethylnitrosamine, which induced tumors of liver, lungs and kidneys in the expected rates. The direct alkylating agents (Actinomycin D, Melphalan, Mitomycin D, Uracil mustard, Dibromomannitol and Dibromodulcitol) induced cancer in the peritoneal cavity, the site of the injections. Rats appeared to be more susceptible than mice. Other drugs (e.g. the cyclohexamide salt of phosphorodiamidic acid derivative, Natulan, DIC and streptozotocin) had a broad spectrum of carcinogenicity affecting a variety of organs. Several agents led to tumors in the hematopoietic and lymphatic systems in mice or rats or both. The correlation to the general immunosuppressive action is not quite clear. 6-Mercaptopurine induces lymphosarcomas in mice. Methotrexate, in contrast, has no carcinogenic effect, even though it exerts an immunosuppressive one. The same phenomenon has been observed in the case of prednisone.

The studies of D. SCHMÄHL (Heidelberg), carried out on a smaller scale with 46 BR rats, were also focused on the question whether the immunosuppressive effect might play some role, as well as the direct carcinogenicity of cytostatic compounds. One test group of animals received 7% of the LD_{50} once weekly over a period of 52 weeks. The other group received five applications, each of 17% of the LD_{50} at two-week intervals. The first mode of application approximated to the regime used in clinical therapy, the other to that used in postoperative chemoprophylaxis. The alkylating agents used (Myleran, Degranol, Dichloren, Mitomen, Endoxan, Thiotepa, Trenimon and Natulan) had a strong carcinogenic effect which was not observed with the antimetabolites 6-mercaptopurin, 5-fluorouracil, and Methotrexate. Whole-body irradiation had a carcinogenic effect comparable to that of the alkylating compounds. These substances were also tested for immunosuppressive effects (hemagglutination test and Jerne's plaque test). No correlation was found between the carcinogenic and the immunosuppressive effects. Further experiments failed to prove that carcinogenicity was increased by the simultaneous administration of cytostatic and strictly immunosuppressive drugs (e.g. hydrocortisone).

The third experimental study, by F. S. PHILIPS and S. S. STERNBERG (New York), concentrated on a single question, whether the carcinoma rate in rats higly susceptible to mammary carcinogenesis by 7,12-dimethylbenz(a)anthracene and X-irradiation, is increased further in short-term experiments by toxic doses of cytostatic compounds. The agents administered were: Myleran, Thioguanin, Mitomycin C, Methotrexate, Actinomycin D and 5-fluorouracil. All six compounds failed to induce mammary carcinomas in these rats. Prolonged treatment of rats with oral doses of Actinomycin D also failed to induce tumors. In another assay, high doses of hydroxyurea were administered to mice of a strain that shows a high rate of pulmonary adenomas after ethylcarbamate. Hydroxyurea had no carcinogenic effect in these experiments. The only cytostatic compound that could be proved to be carcinogenic under these conditions was Daunomycin, a cytostatic antibiotic which was not included in the experimental studies cited previously.

These experiments allow the conclusion that long-term administration of the cytostatic compounds in clinical use will have carcinogenic effects, and that alkylating agents play a leading role in this context. The immunosuppressive action of these compounds seems to be negligible. Two papers in this section discuss pathohistological changes caused by the use of cytostatics in clinic patients. The study by N. IREY (Washington) dealt with 150 cases, biopsies and autopsies. The conditions treated with cytostatics included 60% reticuloendothelial malignancies, 25% carcinomas, and some 10% nonmalignant diseases, among them psoriasis, arthritis, exfoliative dermatitis, lupus erythematosus, and immunosuppressive treatment following renal transplantation. Antimetabolites and alkylating agents were the compounds most used in treatment. The four most frequent immediate causes of death were pneumonia, septicemia, gastrointestinal hemorrhage and pulmonary insufficiency. The adverse reactions to cytostatic agents were divided into three main groups: immediate toxic effects are recognized in degeneration and necrosis. Stimulative reactions, i.e. stromal and parenchymal hyperplasias and dysplasias, and so-called pseudoneoplasms are more relevant to our question: these manifestations were found in the bone marrow and in the lymphatic system. Methotrexate, given for exfoliative dermatitis, provoked generalized lymphadenopathy. Histological observation revealed hyperplasia with predominance of histiocytes and reticular lymphoblasts. When the drug was stopped, the lymphadenopathy regressed, and follow-up examination indicated complete clinical and hematological normality. Busulphan, Bleomycin, Melphalan and Cyclophosphamide promoted dysplastic changes in the lungs, especially pulmonary fibrosis and atypical alveolar cell proliferations. Daunomycin induced myocardial interstitial fibrosis; these cardiac reactions have an incidence of 4-10% in patients receiving this drug. The third major category of adverse reactions related to cytostatics includes the changes secondary to chromosomal aberrations: tumorogenic, teratogenic, and mutagenic effects. Tumors occurring after combined therapy with azathioprine and prednisone after renal transplantation were mentioned in this context. The immunosuppressive effect was implicated in these cases. In others, a teratogenic effect of cytostatic drugs has been observed in the offspring of patients treated with such compounds, particularly if the therapy had been applied during the first trimester of pregnancy. Methotrexate is one example, Chlorambucil another.

The paper by E. GRUNDMANN and R. FRITZSCHE (Münster) concerns the impact of changes in the statistical patterns noted in autopsies on Hodgkin patients. There were two test groups: group A from 1955-1964, group B from 1965-1973, covering 100 Hodgkin autopsies. It appears that the mean expected survival time (defined as the span between first diagnosis and death of the patients) has doubled from group A to group B. In the age group of 50 and over, the survival time has even become four times longer. In contrast to clinical observations, a prevalence of Lukes type V (the reticular lymphocytic depletion type) was found among the autopsies. Of 22 cases where the histologic slides of first biopsies could be checked against those made at the autopsies, 12 had turned from Lukes type Ia - II into the sarcoma type V. Eight cases in group B had no lymphogranulomatic foci. Referring to the appropriate first biopsies, the authors found that these cases had started as Lukes types Ia, II and III, none of them from IV or V. Not a single secondary malignant tumor was observed in this material, but 40% of all Hodgkin patients died in the sarcoma stage. In comparison with results of other previous investigations, the relative frequency of Hodgkin sarcoma in autopsies has increased conspicuously in spite of - or because of? - the prolonged statistical survival expectancy. Both these facts may be a consequence of modern therapeutic methods.

These reports on pathohistological aspects made it apparent that any type of carcinogenicity related to compounds used in clinical practice has hitherto become manifest only in isolated cases. Malignant bladder tumors are obviously frequent after treatment with Chlornaphazine, a 2-naphthylamine mustard. While most other cytostatics require long-term administration before they take effect - a time that would considerably exceed the duration of normal clinical treatment - Chlornaphazine induces bladder carcinomas after a lapse of 3-5 years after even a short course of treatment. A review presented by W. HUNSTEIN (Heidelberg) dealt with relevant publications of recent years supporting a carcinogenic effect of cytostatic compounds. In Hodgkin's disease, neither irradiation therapy alone nor chemotherapy alone has promoted a significant increase in tumor incidence, but a low rate of malignant tumors has been observed in groups receiving a combination of intensive chemotherapy and intensive irradiation. Other large comprehensive studies, on several thousand patients undergoing intensive chemotherapy for hemoblastoses, have led to the conclusion that their risk of a secondary carcinoma was no greater than that in a comparable normal population. This observation must be qualified insofar as most tumor patients will not live beyond the period where a secondary carcinogenicity of cytostatic treatment could become manifest.

The conclusion to be drawn from the above reports is that, contrary to experimental experience and results, there is as yet no unbiased answer to the question of whether cytostatic drugs have been carcinogenic in human beings - with the so far isolated exception of Chlornaphazine. Certainly, all patients who receive or have received cytostatic drugs should be registered and subjected to further follow-up for as long as possible. Only by complying with this condition can we hope to find a reliable answer to this problem.

The study by B. SCHNEIDER and N. BROCK (Hannover/Brackwede) is particularly welcome in this context. They discuss mathematical, biometrical and methodological problems of projected long-term studies on the potential carcinogenic effects of cytostatics. These investigations are designed to yield information on further toxic effects, but also on therapeutic effects of cytotoxic compounds used in clinical treatment. Thus a fairly optimistic attitude is justified at the end of this first section.

Immune Suppression and Chemical Carcinogenesis *

R. Kroes, J. W. Weiss, and J. H. Weisburger

INTRODUCTION AND REVIEW

It is well known that a number of tumors arising in man are induced by chemical carcinogens. Some authors even state that the majority of tumors arising in man are due to chemical agents (17, 12, 13). Since publication of the first case reports concerning the possibility of development of tumors due to prolonged immunosuppression in transplantation patients (55), many studies on the subject have been initiated. It is not surprising that a number of these studies are designed to find out whether immunosuppression affects the action of chemical carcinogens.

The aim of this paper is to review the results of such animal studies and to elucidate the different results with reference to the various immunosuppressive agents used. In addition, some new results will be given, which indicate that it might be worthwhile to investigate the effect of immunosuppression on carcinogens that have not yet been studied.

EFFECT OF IMMUNOSUPPRESSION WITH ANTILYMPHOCYTE SERUM (ALS) OR ANTILYMPHOCYTEGLOBULIN (ALG) ON THE INCIDENCE AND LATENCY OF CHEMICALLY INDUCED TUMORS

Table 1. Effect of immunosuppression with ALS or ALG on the incidence of chemically induced tumors

Increased tumor incidence:	
Mice: 11 studies involving 28 different ALS-treated groups:	11/28
Rat: 4 studies involving 4 ALS-reated groups:	4/4
Hamster: 2 studies involving 2 ALS-treated groups:	2/2

* The experimental part of this work was performed while R. K. and J. H. W. were at the National Cancer Institute, N.I H. Bethesda, Md. R. K. was a recipient of a fellowship of the International Agency for Research on Cancer, Lyon. His present adress: National Institute for Public Health, PO Box 1 Bilthoven, The Netherlands.

Table 1 gives the effects of immunosuppression with ALS or ALG on tumor incidence found in studies in mice, rats and hamsters. From the mouse studies it is evident that in most groups (17/28) tumor incidence was not increased due to immunosuppression. In an attempt to find an explanation for this phenomenon we checked the influence of the dosage regime of ALS on the incidence of the induced tumors as well as the possible influence of the type of carcinogen or type of ALS.

Table 2. Influence of ALS or ALG dosage regime on the incidence of chemically induced tumors

		No. of groups with or without an increased incidence	
Dosage regime		+	-
Daily or several times per week starting at or around day 0, for a restricted period	:	9	2
Several times per week or once weekly throughout experiment	:	4	0
Weekly, starting at or around day 0, for a restricted period	:	2	2
Several times per week or weekly, starting later in the experiment	:	2	11
Only before day 0	:		2

Carcinogen administration was started at day 0

Table 2 shows the different dosage regimes for ALS and the results obtained. Because it involves only a few experiments, it is difficult to draw firm conclusions from this Table. There is an indication, however, that the timing and the number of doses has an influence on the effect of the carcinogen. It seems that the administration of ALS in the initiation period is particularly effective, as is continuous administration of ALS. The administration of ALS later in the experiment (2 weeks after the first carcinogen administration or later) seems to be rather ineffective, as is ALS treatment only before a carcinogen is given. In addition the number of doses administered per week seems to influence the results.

As can be seen from Table 3, the type of ALS does not seem to have any influence on the incidence of induced tumors. In addition, it is obvious that at least in these studies there is no evidence indicating that any one carcinogen is more influenced by ALS than another (Table 4). Two of the studies discussed above, both carried out with rats, gave evidence for the induction of a different type of tumor than expected in view of the carcinogen being used. In one (11), 7,12-dimethylbenzanthracene given orally induced nephroblastoma only in ALS-treated rats, while in the other (22) intravenous administration of NMU gave rise to bladder tumors in the ALS-treated rats, whereas neurogenic tumors were present in both ALS- and normal horse serum-treated rats.

The tumor systems studied were mostly induced subcutaneous sarcomas or skin tumors.

Table 3. Influence of ALS type on the incidence of induced tumors

	No. of groups with or without an increased incidence	
ALS type:	+	-
ALS (G) Rabbit	14	15
ALS Horse	2	1
ALS ?	1	1

Table 4. Influence of carcinogen on the incidence of induced tumors in ALS studies

	No. of groups with or without an increased incidence	
Carcinogen:	+	-
MCA (3-Methylcholanthrene)	5	9
DMBA (7,12-Dimethylbenz(a)anthracene)	9	8
Urethane	1	
NMU (Nitrosomethylurea)	1	
DENA (Diethylnitrosamine)	1	

Table 5. Effect of immunosuppression with ALS on the latent period of chemically induced tumors

	Shorter latent period
Mice: 8 studies involving 21 ALS-treated groups:	6/21
Hamster: 2 studies involving 2 ALS-treated groups:	2/2

In a number of studies mentioned above the latent period of the tumors was calculated. Table 5 gives a survey of the effect of immunosuppression with ALS on the latent period of chemically induced tumors. There is a strong indication that the ALS dosage regime does have an influence on the latent period of the induced tumors. It appears that continuous application of ALS, especially, shortens the latent period (Table 6). Like the tumor incidence, the latent period was unaffected by the type of ALS or the carcinogen used.

Table 6. Influence of ALS dosage regime on the latent period of chemically induced tumors

		No. of groups with or without a shorter latent period	
Dosage regime		+	-
Daily or several times per week starting at or around day 0[a], for a restricted period	:	1	3
Several times per week or weekly throughout experiment	:	4	0
Weekly, starting at or around day 0, for a restricted period	:	2	2
Several times per week or weekly, starting later in the experiment	:	1	8
Only before day 0	:	0	2

[a]Carcinogen administration was started at day 0

EFFECT OF IMMUNOSUPPRESSANTS OTHER THAN ALS ON THE INCIDENCE OR LATENT PERIOD OF CHEMICALLY INDUCED TUMORS

Table 7. Effects of immunosuppressive treatment with agents other than ALS on the incidence of chemically induced tumors

Immunosuppressive treatment	No. of exp. groups with incidence increased	unaffected	decreased
Azathioprine	2	1	3
Cortisone	2	2	1
Stress		5	
Thymectomy (neonatal)	9	3	1
Thymectomy (later)	2	2	2
Hormones	1[a]		4[b]
Carcino-chemotherapeutic agents	1[c]	7	2[d]
Total of 32 studies (mice: 20; rat: 8; hamster: 4) involving 50 experimental groups			

[a] progesterone.
[b] estradiol 1x, testosterone 3x.
[c] actinomycin D.
[d] vinblastine and cyclophosphamide.

Table 7 summarizes the studies carried out in recent years and the observed effect of the immunosuppressant used. It is obvious that interpretation of the results of these studies is even more difficult than interpretation of those obtained in the ALS studies. As far as can be seen from the table only neonatal thymectomy seems to induce an increased tumor incidence in most cases. It must be mentioned, however, that in most studies the supposed immunosuppression was not investigated or controlled, so that the existence of a genuine immunosuppression might be doubtful in at least some studies.

Table 8. Effects of immunosuppressive treatment with agents other than ALS on the latent period of chemically induced tumors

Immunosuppressive treatment	No. of groups with .... latent period		
	shorter	unaffected	longer
Azathioprine		2	2
Cortisone	1	1	
Stress	1[a]	4	
Thymectomy (neonatal)	9		
Thymectomy (later)	1		
Carcino-chemotherapeutic agents	4[b]	5	
Total of 16 studies (mice 10; rat 6) involving 30 experimental groups			

[a] Isolation of rats versus grouping.

[b] Biomycin 2 studies; fluorouracil 1 study; actinomycin-D 1 study.

Table 9. Effects of immunosuppressive treatment with agents other than ALS on chemically induced tumors. Influence of carcinogen on incidence or latent period

Carcinogen	No. of group with: Incidence			Latent period		
	>	0	<	<	0	>
DMBA (dimethylbenzanthracene)	4	10	12	5	2	2
MCA (methylcholanthrene)	5	5		5	4	
Urethane	6	2	1			
BP (benzo(a)pyrine)	2	2		3	2	
8-Aminoazotoluene		3		2	1	
DENA (diethylnitrosamine)		2			2	
NOHFAA	1	1			1	
DBA (dibenz(a,h)anthracene)		1		1		
Plastic s. c. implant	1					

Table 8 lists the effects of immunosuppression with agents other than ALS on the latent period. In this case it is even more evident that neonatal thymectomy is very effective in shortening the latent period of chemically induced tumors. There is no indication that any one carcinogen is more influenced by any immunosuppressant than another (Table 9).

MATERIALS AND METHODS

An experiment starting with 300 male Fisher rats was carried out to investigate the effect of ALG-induced immunosuppression on the carcinogenic effect of relatively low dosages of the liver carcinogen N-hydroxyfluorinylacetamide (NOHFAA), and of azoxymethane, which induces intestinal tumors. The experimental design is described in Table 10. The ALG and NRG used were obtained from the Microbiological Association, Bethesda, Maryland, U. S. A. and prepared according to the method of LEVEY and MEDAWAR (43). Separate allogenic skin graft experiments following the same dosage schedule as was used in the carcinogenicity study, but ceasing the treatment at day 7, and using 10 rats per group, indicated an average skin survival time for ALG-treated rats of 33.2 days, whereas saline controls and NRG-treated rats showed survival times of 10.4 and 9.5 days respectively. The same method with double the dose of NRG led to an average survival time of 11.1 days. In the carcinogenicity study complete histological examination was performed and liver, kidneys, spleen and, in the azomethane-treated groups, also the whole of the intestinal tract were studied histologically.

Table 10. Experimental design. In brackets: number of animals that died or were sacrificed in moribund state between weeks 16 and 28

Carcinogen	Treatment	No. of rats studied	No. of rats sacrificed at 20	26-28	32 weeks
NOHFAA in diet	Saline	30	15	15	
120 ppm	ALG	50	25	21	
for 16 weeks	NRG	40	20	20	
Azoxymethane 7.5 mg/kg b. w.	Saline	35	(8)^{x}	12	13
s. c. 1 x week	ALG	50	(27)	12	6
for 16 weeks	NRG	40	(8)	11	21
———	ALG	30	(26)		4
———	NRG	30	10	5	15

Dosage level and schedule of ALG/NRG i. p.

Day	-7	-3	0	3	7 etc.	2x/week until time of sacrifice
Dose (ml)	2.0	2.0	0.5	0.5	0.5 etc.	

PRELIMINARY RESULTS

In this study too, ALG-induced immunosuppression led to an increased tumor incidence and a shorter latent period or both, as is shown in Tables 11, 12 and 13.

Table 11. Effect of ALG on the tumor incidence in rats (receiving 120 ppm NOHFAA in the diet for 16 weeks) after 20 weeks. In brackets: Average number of lesions/animal/group

Number of rats	+ Saline 15	+ ALG 25	+ NRG 20
HNA[a]	15(2.3)	24(3.2)	20(2.8)
%	100	96	100
HEP[b]	6(1.5)	15(1.6)	4(1.0)
%	40	60	20
Mixed[c]	5(1)	15(1.2)	4(1)
%	33	60	20

[a] Hyperplastic nodule with atypicality.
[b] Hepatocellular carcinoma.
[c] Mixed lesions.

Table 12. Effect of ALG on the tumor incidence in rats (receiving 120 ppm NOHFAA in the diet for 16 weeks) after 26 weeks. In brackets: average number of lesions/animal/group

Number of rats	+ Saline 15	+ ALG 21	+ NRG 20
HNA[a]	15(3.2)	19(3.4)	18(3.4)
%	100	95	90
HEP[b]	10(2.0)	15(1.6)	14(1.9)
%	66	71	70
Mixed[c]	5(1.2)	11(1.1)	10(1.2)
%	33	52	50

[a] Hyperplastic nodule with atypicality.
[b] Hepatocellular carcinoma.
[c] Mixed lesion

NOHFAA-induced tumors were more frequent in ALG-treated rats after 20 weeks of experiments. However, the incidence of these tumors was the same in all groups after 26 weeks, thus indicating that ALG-treated rats only had a shorter latent period. Surprising results were obtained in the azoxymethane experiments. The incidence of intestinal tumors was relatively low, as was expected with the dosage used. In the ALG-treated rats, however, the incidence seemed

Table 13. Effect of ALG on the tumor incidence in rats (receiving azoxymethane 7.5 mg/kg b. w./week for 16 weeks). In brackets: percentages of tumor-bearing rats

	+ Saline	+ ALG	+ NRG
From 16-28 weeks			
Number of rats	8	27	8
Intestinal Ca	2(25)	2(7)	-(0)
Liver: angiosarcoma	-(0)	13[a](48)	1(12.5)
After 28 weeks			
Number of rats	12	12	11
Intestinal Ca	6(50)	1(7,5)	5(45)
Liver: angiosarcoma	-(0)	5[b](42)	3(27)
After 32 weeks			
Number of rats	13	6	22
Intestinal Ca	6(46)	3(50)	10[a](45)
Liver: angiosarcoma	-(0)	1(16)	1(4)

NRG controls (20): no tumors
ALG controls (30): no tumors

[a] One rat with two tumors of the same type
[b] Two rats with two tumors of the same type

to be even lower, but these rats, which usually died earlier, had a high incidence of angiosarcomas in the liver. These tumors were not found in the Saline-AOM control group. However, combined treatment with NRG and azoxymethane also gave rise to the development of a few angiosarcomas. These angiosarcomas were sometimes very anaplastic. One author (23) reported the development of hemangiosarcomas when rats were given low dosages of 1,2-dimethylhydrazine.

COMMENT

From a review of the literature it is apparent that immunosuppression can affect chemical carcinogenesis. Our own results seem to reinforce this idea. From the studies carried out in the past it is clear that ALS and ALG are particularly effective in enhancing tumor incidence and/or shortening the latent period. The action, however, depends very much on the time of administration. As has been shown, administration of ALS at or around day 0 (i.e. the day carcinogen treatment was started) was most effective in increasing tumor incidence. It has also been shown that administration of ALS more often than once weekly improved the results, whereas continuous application seemed particularly effective with respect to the latent period. In the majority of positive studies, the ALS treatment was started one week or 3 days before day 0, indicating that suppression of the immune system just before the initiation period is most effective. The same phenomena were noted in transplantation patients: immunosuppressive treatment just before the vascular anastomosis seemed to improve the "take" of the organ (45).

In some cases, as well as an increased tumor incidence or a shorter latent period, administration of ALS led to the formation of a tumor type not common with the carcinogen used. One possible explanation is that these tumors are more antigenic than the other types normally found to be induced. Under normal circumstances such a tumor will not develop because of the efficient elimination by the immune system. This immunosurveillance (61) is suppressed by efficient immunosuppression, with subsequent tumor development.

Immunosuppression by other means than ALS seems to be less effective, though neonatal thymectomy usually leads to an increased incidence and/or shorter latent period. Azathioprine was effective in only a minority of the studies, as was cortisone. It is surprising that, at least to our knowledge, no studies have been carried out with the combination of azathioprine and cortisone, a combination widely used for immunosuppressive treatment in man. It is evident that such studies are necessary, especially for the evaluation of the hazard of immunosuppressive therapy in man.

Chemical carcinogens are known to be immunosuppressive themselves. Dimethylbenzanthracene may inhibit the B-cell as well as the T-cell system, whereas methylcholanthrene usually affects primarily the B-cell system, as do most carcinogens. Suppression of the B-cell system may lead to a reduced number of "blocking antibodies" (34, 35, 18) and could thus theoretically lead to a lower tumor incidence. This is usually not the case, and it seems likely that in the balance of the immune system, the suppression of the T-cell system, most effectively achieved by means of ALS or ALG or neonatal thymectomy, has a particularly pronounced influence on the tumor incidence and/or the latent period of chemically induced tumors.

REFERENCES

1. References concerning the effect of immunosuppression by ALS or ALG on the incidence and/or latent period of chemically induced tumors: 6, 9, 11, 14, 15, 22, 24, 26, 28, 30, 33, 36, 64, 81, 84, 86.
2. References concerning the effect of immunosuppression by other means than ALS on the incidence or latent period of chemically induced tumors: 1, 2, 5, 20, 21, 25, 32, 37, 38, 42, 44, 47, 49, 50, 58, 59, 62, 63, 66, 69, 70, 71, 72, 73, 74, 75, 81, 82, 83, 85, 88.
3. References concerning immunosuppression by carcinogens: 3, 4, 7, 8, 10, 16, 19, 27, 29, 31, 39, 40, 41, 46, 48, 51, 52, 53, 54, 56, 57, 60, 65, 67, 68, 76, 77, 78, 79, 80, 87, 89.

1. ABEATICI, S., TERRACINI, B.: Tumori 57, 353 (1971).
2. ANDRIANOVA, M. M.: Vop. Onkol. 17, 63 (1971).
3. BALL, J. K.: J. nat. Cancer Inst. 44, 1 (1970).
4. BALL, J. K., DAWSON, D. A.: J. nat. Cancer Inst. 42, 579 (1969).
5. BALNER, H., DERSJANT, H.: J. nat. Cancer Inst. 36, 513 (1966).
6. BALNER, H., DERSJANT, H.: Nature 224, 376 (1969).
7. BARONI, C. D., BERTOLI, G., PESANDO, P., SCELSI, R.: Experientia 26, 899 (1970).

8. BARONI, C. D., SCELSI, R., PESANDO, P. C., MINGAZZINI, P.: Tumori 56, 269 (1970).
9. BARONI, C. D., SCELSI, R., PERONACE, M. L., UCCINI, S.: Brit. J. Cancer 28, 221 (1973).
10. BLUESTEIN, H. G., GREEN, I.: Nature 228, 871 (1970).
11. BOURGOIN, J. J., CUEFF, J., BAILLY, C., DARGENT, M.: Bull. Cancer 4, 429 (1972).
12. BOYLAND, E.: Progr. exp. Tumor Res. (Basel) 11, 222 (1969).
13. BRYAN, G. T., LOWER, G. M.: J. Milk Food Technol. 33, 506 (1970).
14. CARBONE, G., PARMIANI, G.: Tumori 57, 225 (1971).
15. CERELLI, G. J., TREAT, R. C.: Transplantation 8, 774 (1969).
16. CHANDRA, P., GERICKE, D., WACKER, A.: Z. Krebsforsch. 76, 40 (1971).
17. CLAYSON, D. B.: Europ. J. Cancer 3, 405 (1967).
18. CURRIE, G.: Brit. J. Cancer 28, Suppl. 1: 153 (1973).
19. DALE, M. M., HEDGES, J. R.: Brit. J. exp. Path. 54, 437 (1973).
20. DARGENT, M., BOURGOIN, J. J., NOEL, P., WEISSBROD, R.: Europ. J. Cancer 8, 605 (1972).
21. DELLA PORTA, G., COLNAGHI, M. I., PARMI, L.: Tumori 56, 121 (1970).
22. DENLINGER, R. H., SWENBERG, J. A., KOESTNER, A., WECHSLER, W.: J. nat. Cancer Inst. 50, 87 (1973).
23. DRUCKREY, H.: In: Carcinomas of the Colon and Antecedent Epithelium, Ed. BURDETTE, W. J., p. 267. Springfield, Ill.: Thomas 1970.
24. FISHER, J. C., DAVIS, R. C., MANNICK, J. A.: Surgery 68, 150 (1970).
25. FRANKEL, H. H., YAMAMOTO, R. S., WEISBURGER, E. K., WEISBURGER, J. H.: Toxicol. appl. Pharmacol. 17, 642 (1970).
26. FRIEDRICH - FRESKA, H., HOFFMANN, M.: Nature 223, 1162 (1969).
27. GERICKE, D., CHANDRA, P., WACKER, A.: Z. Krebsforsch. 75, 85 (1971).
28. GIUNTA, J. L., SHKLAR, G.: Oral Surg. 68, 150 (1970).
29. GORELIK, L. S., KAGAN, L. F.: Probl. Eksp. Genet. 259, 61 (1972).
30. GRANT, G. A., ROE, F. J. C.: Nature 223, 1060 (1969).
31. GRYSCHEK, G., PASTERNAK, G.: Acta biol. med. gen. 27 195 (1971).
32. GUILLON, C., GENTIL, A., LASNE, C., CHOUROULINKOV, M. I.: Cancérologie 270, 1066 (1970).
33. HARAN-GHERA, N., LUZIE, M.: J. nat. Cancer Inst. 46, 103 (1971).
34. HELLSTRÖM, I., HELLSTRÖM, K. E., SJÖGREN, H. O.: Cellular Imm. 1, 18 (1970).
35. HELLSTRÖM, I., HELLSTRÖM, K. E., WARNER, G. A.: Int. J. Cancer 12, 348 (1973).
36. HUNT, P. S., HOLYOKE, E. D.: Ajebak 51, 417 (1973).
37. JOHNSON, S.: Brit. J. Cancer 22, 755 (1968).
38. KALIS, N., FULLER, J. L.: J. nat. Cancer Inst. 41,967 (1968).
39. KEARNEY, R., HUGHES, L. E.: Brit. J. Cancer 24, 319 (1970).
40. KRASKOVSKII, G. V., GORELIK, L. S., KAGAN, L. F.: Probl. Eksp. Genet. 117, 23 (1971).
41. LAPPE, M. A., STEINMULLER, D. S.: Cancer Res. 30, 674 (1970).
42. LAW, L. W.: Nature (Lond.) 205, 672 (1965).
43. LEVEY, R. H., MEDAWAR, P. B.: Proc. nat. Acad. Sci. (Wash.) 56, 1130 (1966).
44. LEVY, I. S., RWOMUSHANA, J. W., POLLIACK, A.: Europ. J. Cancer 6, 187 (1970).
45. MCGEOWN, M. G.: Lancet 1973 2, 310.
46. MATSUOKA, Y., SENOH, H., KAWAMOTO, T., KOHMO, T., HAMAOKA, T., KITAGAWA, M.: Nature New Biol. 238, 273 (1972).
47. MILLER, J. F. A. P., GRANT, G. A., ROE, F. J. C.: Nature (Lond.) 199, 920 (1963).
48. NAKASHIMA, S., ONO, S.: Gann 63, 111 (1972).
49. NEMOTO, N., KATO, N., MIZUNO, D., TAKAYAMA, S.: Gann 62, 293 (1971).

50. NISHIZUKA, Y., NAKAKUKI, K., USUI, M.: Nature (Lond.) 205, 1236 (1965).
51. OTTONEN, P. O., BALL, J. K.: J. nat. Cancer Inst. 50, 491 (1973).
52. OUTZEN, H. C., PREHN, R. T.: Cancer Res. 33, 408 (1973).
53. PARMIANI, G.: J. nat. Cancer Inst. 47, 569 (1971).
54. PARMIANI, G., COLNAGHI, M. I., DELLA PORTA, G.: Brit. J. Cancer 25, 354 (1971).
55. PENN, I., HAMMLND, W., BRETTSCHNEIDER, L., STARZL, T. E.: Transplant. Proc. 1, 106 (1969).
56. PEROCCO, P., FRANCESCII, C., DI MARCO, A. T., PRODI, G.: Proc. Soc. exp. Biol. 136, 1024 (1971).
57. PHILLIPS, J. M.: Int. J. Cancer 9, 39 (1972).
58. POLLIACK, A., CHARUZY, I., LEVY, I. S.: Path. Microbiol. 35, 348 (1970).
59. POLLIACK, A., LEVY, I. S., PFEFFERMANN, R.: Brit. J. Cancer 26, 368 (1972).
60. POTEL, J.: Arzneimittel-Forsch. (Drug Res.) 15, 527 (1965).
61. PREHN, R. T.: Progr. exp. Tumor Res. 14, 1 (1971).
62. PYLEVA, Z. A.: Pat. fiziol. exp. ter. 14, 54 (1970).
63. PYLEVA, Z. A., VYSHESLAVOVA, M. Ya.: Byull. eksp. Biol. Med. 69, 75 (1970).
64. RABBAT, A. G., JEEJEEBHOY, H. F.: Transplantation 9, 164 (1970).
65. SALOMON, J. C., GUEGUEN, S., LAZAR, P.: Path. Biol. 18, 65 (1970).
66. SANFORD, B. H., SOO, S. F.: J. Immunol. 110, 595 (1973).
67. SCHERF, H. R.: Akt. Probl. Geb. Cancerol. X, 34 (1970).
68. SCHERF, H. R.: Z. Krebsforsch. klin. Onkol. 77, 189 (1972).
69. SCHMÄHL, D., WAGNER, R., SCHERF, H. R.: Arzneimittel-Forsch. (Drug Res.) 3, 403 (1971).
70. SHEEHAN, R., SHKLAR, G., TENNENBAUM, R.: Arch. Path. 21, 264 (1971).
71. SHEEHAN, R., SHKLAR, G.: J. dent. Res. 50, 981 (1971).
72. SHELLABARGER, C. J., SOO, K. A.: Cancer Res. 33, 1567 (1973).
73. SHISA, H.: Mie med. J. 9, 101 (1969).
74. SHISA, H.: Mie med. J. 9, 111 (1969).
75. SHKLAR, G., TURBINER, S.: J. dent. Res. 50, 985 (1970).
76. SKAZAL, A. K., HANNA, M. G.: Nat. Cancer Inst. Monogr. 35, 173 (1972).
77. STJERNSWARD, J.: Antibiot. et Chemother. (Basel) 15, 214 (1969).
78. STUTMAN, O.: Science 166, 620 (1969).
79. STUTMAN, O.: Israel J. med. Sci. 9, 217 (1973).
80. TANO DI MARCO, A., FRANCESCHI, C., XERRI, L., PRODI, G.: Cancer Res. 31, 1446 (1971).
81. TRAININ, N., LINKER-ISRAELI, M.: J. nat. Cancer Inst. 44, 893 (1970).
82. TURBIN, N. V., KRASKOVSKI, G. U., PORUBOVA, G. M., KOGAN, L. F.: Doklady Akademii Nauk 193, 1400 (1970).
83. TURBINER, S., SHKLAR, G., CATALDO, E.: Oral Surg. 29, 130 (1970).
84. WAGNER, J. L., HAUGHTON, G.: J. nat. Cancer Inst. 46, 1 (1971).
85. WHITMIRE, C. E., SALERNO, R. A., RALSTEIN, L. S.: Proc. Soc. exp. Biol. (N. Y.) 141, 890 (1972).
86. WOODS, D. A.: Nature 224, 276 (1969).
87. YAMASHITA, U., MATSUOKA, Y., KITAGAWA, M.: Gann 64, 317 (1973).
88. YASUHIRA, K.: Gann 60, 57 (1969).
89. ZSCHIESCHE, W., SCHULZ, W. D.: Z. Krebsforsch. 75, 277 (1971).

Experimental Investigations on Immunodepressive Properties of Carcinogenic Substances in Male Sprague-Dawley Rats

H. R. SCHERF and D. SCHMÄHL

The finding during the nineteen-fifties that carcinogens depress the immune response led to the hypothesis that the rise of malignomas might be correlated with the impairment of the immunocompetent system (1-3). This hypothesis was confirmed by systematic investigations of these relationships by STJERNSWÄRD, and especially by the comparison of the activities of carcinogenic and noncarcinogenic hydrocarbons, which revealed that in contrast to noncarcinogenic substances, carcinogens caused immunosuppression (4-6).

Subsequent years saw the appearance of many publications comparing the immunodepressive and carcinogenic activities of carcinogenic compounds. In particular, 3-methylcholanthrene (7-15), 7,12-dimethylbenz(a)anthracene (16-20), ethylurethane (21-28), 4-nitrochinoline-1-oxide (29-31), and ethylnitrosourea were tested for immunosuppressive effects. The influence of carcinogenic substances and their noncarcinogenic derivatives on the immune mechanism was investigated by means of several immunological methods, such as determination of antibody titer during the primary and secondary immune response, the so-called plaque test or agar-plaque technique according to Jerne, and also skin and tumor transplantations. Most investigators reported positive correlations between carcinogenic and immunosuppressive activities (e.g. 14, 25, 26), in contrast to others who obtained negative results or confirmed these findings only in part (9, 23, 27, 29, 36).

Recently this problem has become topical again following clinical investigations by PENN and his co-workers (37-38), who found that in patients treated with immunosuppressive compounds after organ transplantation, malignomas, and particularly lymphomas, developed more frequently than in the controls. Experiments by SCHMÄHL and OSSWALD demonstrated in rats the carcinogenic effect of some substances that are used in antineoplastic or immunosuppressive therapy in man (39, 40). These clinical and experimental data caused us to investigate whether antimetabolites, alkylating agents, alkaloids and antibiotics tested for their carcinogenicity in rats are immunosuppressive to the same extent as they are carcinogenic (Table 1). In addition, the influence of N-nitroso compounds and polycyclic hydrocarbons on the immunocompetent system was tested, and there are also plans to test the aromatic amines. We used dosages of subacute toxicity and also dosages just high enough to induce cancer.

EXPERIMENTS

In the first experiment with cytostatic substances the animals received single injections of 40% of the LD50 of these compounds. The doses given were thus

Table 1. Survey of the cytostatic substances used, their toxicologic data and the dosages applied in the experiment

Substance	LD_{50} (mg/kg)	40% LD_{50} (mg/kg)	7% LD_{50} (mg/kg)
Methotrexate	14.00	5.60	0.98
5-Flourouracil	500.00	200.00	35.00
6-Mercaptopurin	250.00	100.00	17.50
Cyclophosphamide	190.00	76.00	13.50
Trenimon	0. 50	0.20	0.035
Dichloren	1.70	0.68	0.11
Thio-Tepa	15.00	6.00	1.05
Natulan	350.00	140.00	24.50
Myleran	1.80	0.72	0.07
Degranol	56.00	22.40	3.92
Vinblastin	2.00	0.80	0.14
Proreside	140.00	56.00	9.80
Colcemid	1.70	0.68	0.07
Mitomycin	3.00	1.20	0.21
Sanamycin	100.00	40.00	7.00
X - rays	700 r	280 r	49 r

equitoxic. Immediately after administration of the cytostatics all rats were immunized by inoculation of sheep red blood cells and examined for their immune reaction by means of the plaque test described by Jerne for 12 days and the hemagglutination test for 6 weeks (41).

In a second experiment, 7% of the LD_{50} was given once weekly for 14 weeks. After the last injection the rats were immunized and examined for their immune reaction as described above.

A single injection of 40% of the LD_{50} of mercaptopurine, methotrexate or cyclophosphamide led to significant suppression of hemagglutinin production. The two antimetabolites caused a decreased antibody titer persisting through an observation period of 6 weeks (Fig. 1). In contrast to this, cyclophosphamide showed such potent activity that for one week after injection no measurable antibody titer could be obtained in the treated animals. This effect, however, was reversible and two weeks after the beginning of the experiment a rapid increase in the hemagglutinin titer was observed (Fig. 2).

A single injection of 0.2 mg/kg triazichone and subsequent immunization resulted in a clear increase of the immune response. The mass of antibodies produced in the treated animals two and three weeks after immunization was 8 times higher than that produced in the controls.

In the agar-plaque test, too, after a single injection of 40% of the LD_{50} only some of the substances tested showed immunosuppressive activity. This was the case with the antimetabolites, the alkylating agents, cyclophosphamide and dichlorene as well as the antibiotics. The antimetabolites and the alkylating agents in this test method were clearly different in their mode of action.

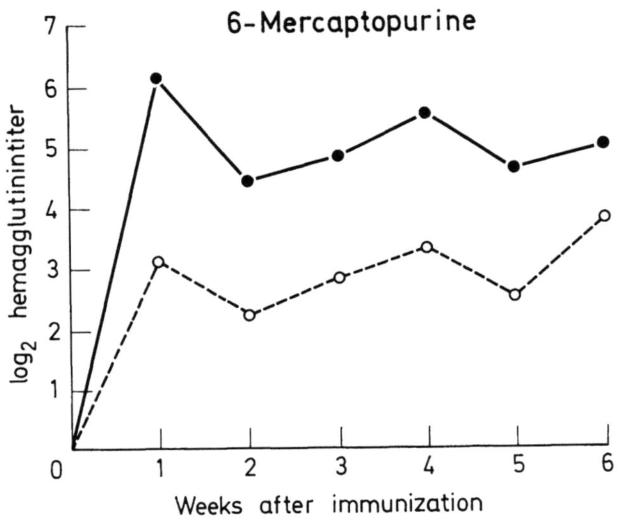

Fig. 1. Result of the hemagglutination test after a single injection of 40% of LD_{50} of 6-mercaptopurine. _________ Controls; ------ titer in treated animals

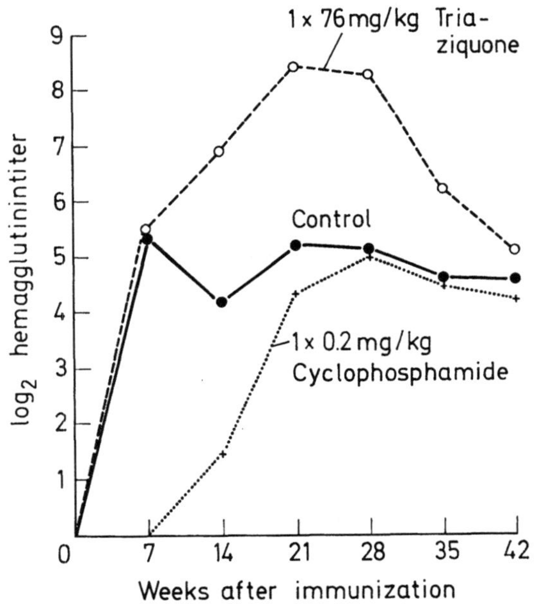

Fig. 2. Hemagglutinin titer after a single injection of 40% of LD_{50} of the specified substances

The antimetabolites inhibit the proliferation of plaque-forming spleen cells during the first four days of experiment, resulting in a reduction of plaque rate and a shift in the maximum of the proliferation course (Fig. 3). Administration of the alkylating agents had no perceptible effect for the first

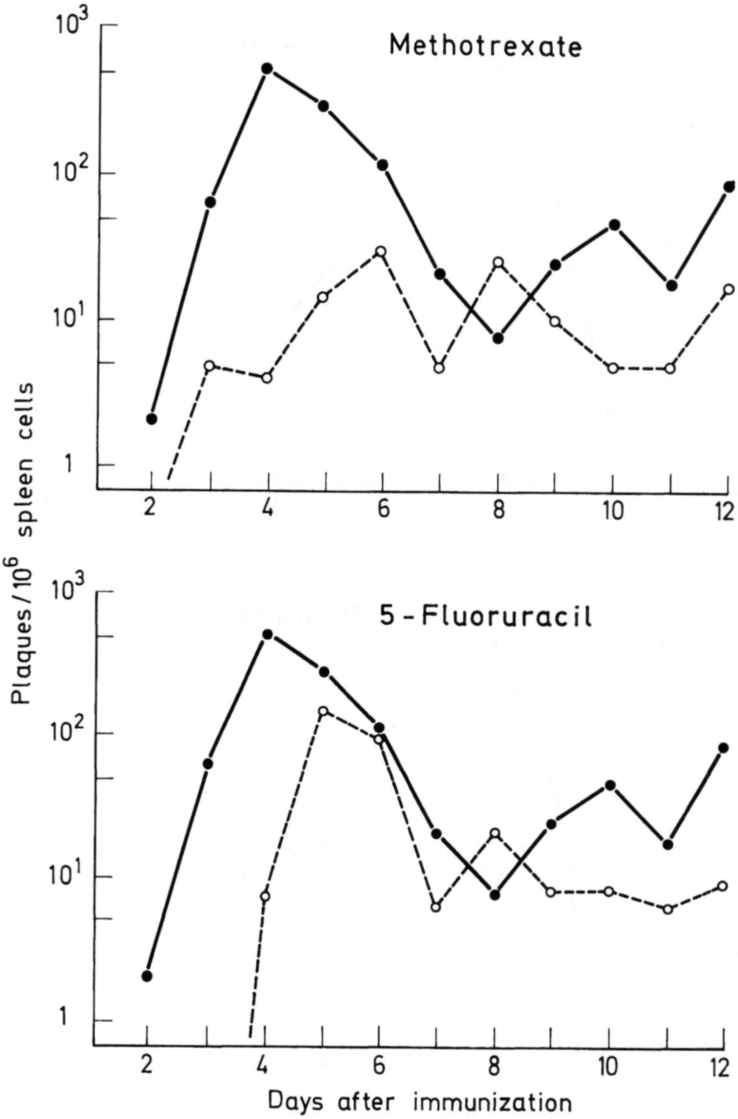

Fig. 3. Influence of a single injection of 40% of LD_{50} of the specified compounds on the kinetics of the plaque-forming spleen cells. ______ Controls; ------ results after treatment

three days after immunization. Differences between treated animals and controls could not be distinguished before the fourth day (Fig. 4). At this time a reduction in the number of IgM plaques was caused which, however, did not persist for long and in the animals treated with cyclophosphamide or dichloren gave way to a new increase of the IgM antibody-producing cells on the fifth and sixth days respectively. In this experiment triaziquone also had a significantly stimulating effect. In the rats treated with antibiotics the course of proliferation of the IgM-producing spleen cells was the same as in the controls; there was merely a depression of the plaque rate, which lasted throughout the test.

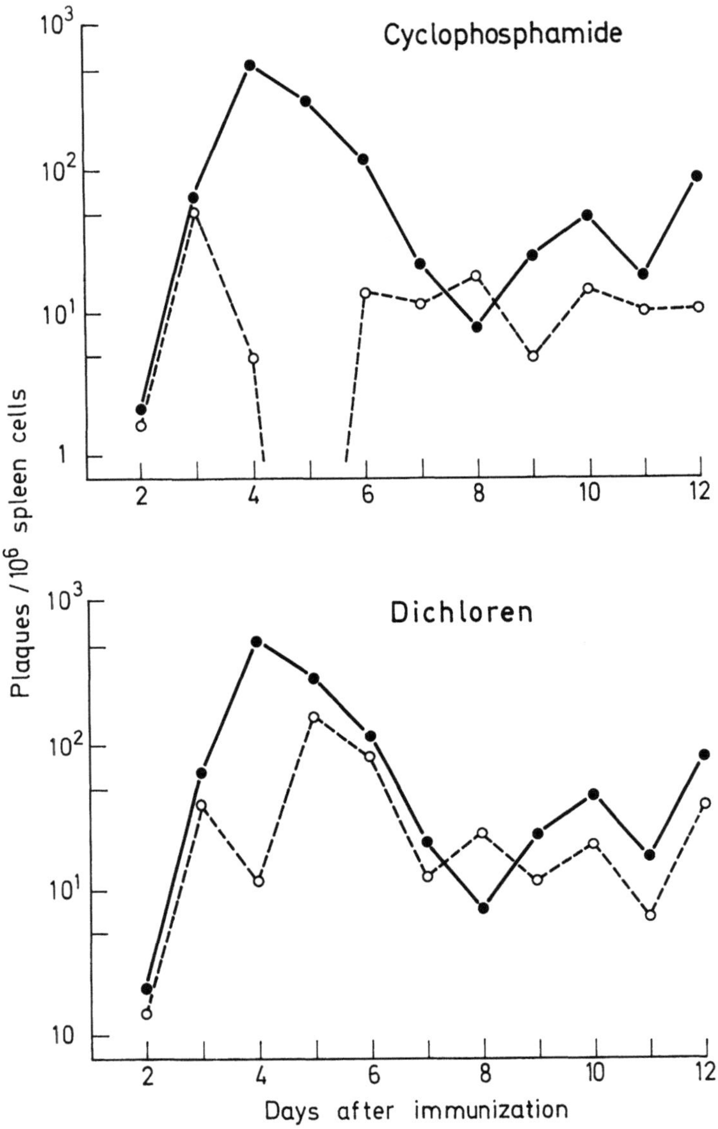

Fig. 4. Influence of a single injection of 40% of LD_{50} of the specified compounds on the kinetics of the plaque-forming spleen cells. ——— Controls; ------ results after treatment

In a second experiment, 7% of the LD_{50} of the same substances was administered to rats once weekly for 14 weeks. This is the dosage usually given in clinical therapy. Investigation of the immune response yielded the following findings: a suppression of the hemagglutinating antibody production was caused by the antimetabolite fluorouracil, the alkylating agents (except Myleran) and the alkaloids and x-rays, which resulted in reduced antibody production throughout the observation period (Fig. 5). The agar-plaque technique yielded different findings with this dosage. Compared to the controls a strong reduction of the plaque-forming spleen cells was produced only by triaziquone and cyclo-

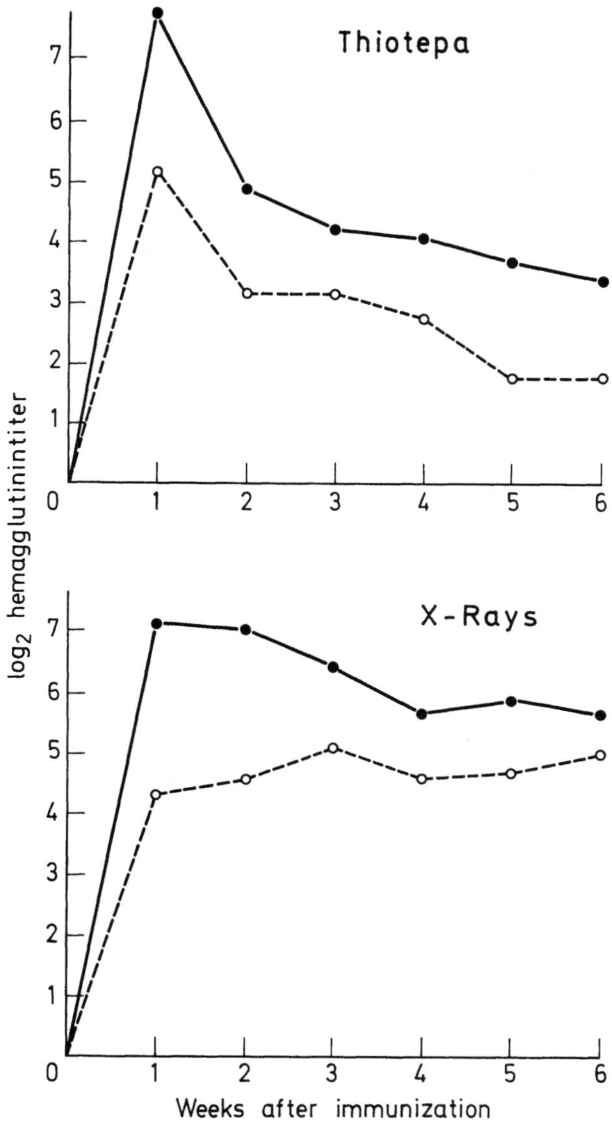

Fig. 5. Hemagglutinin-titer after injection of 7% of LD_{50} once weekly for 14 weeks. ______ Controls; ------ titer in the treated group

phosphamide. At the maximum of the proliferation course, on day 4 and 5 after immunization, only 50% and 12% respectively of the plaque-forming cells were detected in the spleen of triaziquone- and cyclophosphamide-treated animals (Fig. 6). The other alkylating agents, i.e. dichlorene and Myleran, the antimetabolites methotrexate and 6-mercaptopurine and the antibiotics had only a slight activity, because injection of these compounds depresses the hemolysin-producing spleen cells in the area of the maximum proliferation to 60-70% of the control level.

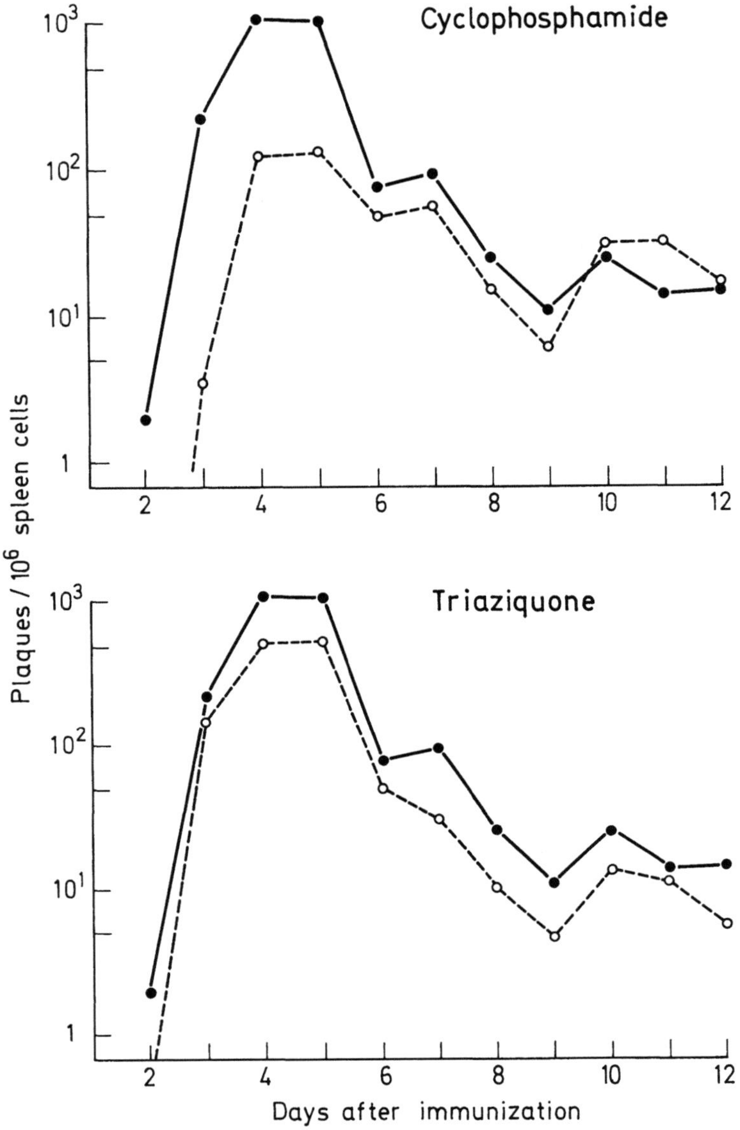

Fig. 6. Effect of the application of 7% of LD_{50} once weekly for 14 weeks on number of plaque-forming spleen cells. Controls; ------ titer in the treated animals

We attempted to summarize the results of these experiments in such a way as to allow comparison of them with the findings of SCHMÄHL and OSSWALD (Table 2) for the purpose of finding out whether those of the 16 tested compounds that induce cancer in rats can also reduce the activity of the immune system, especially after chronic application, more than the substances that have no carcinogenic effects. However, no clear answer to this question could be obtained in this study.

Table 2. Immunosuppressive and carcinogenic activity of cytostatics and x-rays. HA = Hemagglutination test; APT = Agar-plaque technique; + = weak activity; ++ = marked activity; - = no activity

Substances	Immunosuppression				Carcino-genicity
	1 x 40% LD_{50}		14 x (7% LD_{50}/week)		
	H A	APT	H A	APT	
Methotrexate	+ +	+ +	-	+	-
5-Fluorouracil	-	+ +	+	-	-
6-Mercaptopurine	+ +	+ +	-	+	-
Cyclophosphamide	+ +	+ +	+ +	+ +	+ +
Trenimon	-	-	+	+ +	+ +
Dichloren	-	+ +	+ +	+	+ +
Thiotepa	-	-	+ +	-	+ +
Natulan	-	-	+ +	-	+ +
Myleran	-	-	-	+	+
Degranol	-	-	+ +	+	+
Vinblastin	-	-	+	-	-
Proresid	-	-	+	-	-
Colcemid	-	-	+	-	-
Mitomycin C	-	+	-	+	+ +
Sanamycin	-	+	-	+	-
X - rays	-	-	+ +	-	+ +

Cyclophosphamide, which is a strong immunosuppressive agent, is also a potent carcinogen. Natulan and Thiotepa, which are also carcinogens, caused immunosuppression only in the hemagglutination test in rats treated with 7% of the LD_{50} for 14 weeks. The antibiotics mitomycin C and sanamycin had the same immunosuppressive effects, but only mitomycin C had any carcinogenic activity. A strong correlation between carcinogenic and immunosuppressive activity of the antineoplastic chemotherapeutics was thus not detected.

In a further experiment, four N-nitroso compounds that are carcinogenic in rats were tested for immunosuppressive properties. We used dimethylnitrosamine and N-nitroso-morpholine, which are both liver carcinogens, ethyl-n-butyl-nitrosamine, which induces carcinomas of the esophagus after oral, rectal and intravenous application, and methylnitroso-urea, which produces malignomas of the forestomach and the nervous system.

Four groups of rats were formed, each of which received 5%, 2.5%, 1.25% or 0.625% of the LD_{50} of one of the N-nitroso compounds once weekly. The treatment extended over 12, 18 or 24 weeks (Table 3). After they had received the last injection the animals were immunized. Five days later, at the time of maximum proliferation, the number of IgM-producing spleen cells was determined (42), since previous experiments had demonstrated that the course of proliferation is the same in treated and control animals and that only the number of plaque-forming spleen cells depends on the treatment and can be changed. To allow comparison of results they were all calculated as percentages of the control values (Table 4).

Table 3. Acute toxicity of the N-nitroso compounds used (LD_{50}) and the single doses of the four dosage groups. The compounds were injected once weekly, each in four equitoxic doses (based on the LD_{50}) for 12, 16, and 24 weeks respectively in 4 different groups of rats. The data are determined as mg/kg body weight

N-nitroso compounds	LD_{50}	Single week doses 5%	2.5%	1.25%	0.625%
Dimethyl-nitrosamine	45	2.25	1.12	0.56	0.28
Ethyl-n-butyl-nitrosamine	380	19.0	9.5	4.75	2.37
N-nitroso-morpholine	320	16.0	o.0	4.0	2.0
Methylnitroso-urea	110	5.5	2.75	1.37	0.68

The various N-nitroso compounds had very different effects on the immune system, even though they were administered in comparable toxic doses and over the same period. This test revealed that after injection of the highest dose for 12 weeks, only methylnitroso-urea caused a clear reduction of the plaque-forming spleen cells. After 18 and 24 weeks of experiment the reactions of rats treated with high doses of dimethylnitrosamine and ethyl-n-butyl-nitrosamine also showed significant differences form the controls. N-nitroso-morpholine had the weakest immunosuppressive activity.

The doses that did not influence the immune response in our experiment are nevertheless carcinogenic. The lowest total dose of dimethylnitrosamine that is still carcinogenic when given in divided doses distributed over the whole lifespan of a rat is 70mg/kg, and the lowest total dose of N-nitroso-morpholine is 180 mg/kg (43). If the mean lifespan of a rat is about 140 weeks, it can be caluclated that a weekly dose of 0.5 mg/kg dimethyl-nitrosamine or 1.3 mg/kg N-nitroso-morpholine can induce tumors. A comparable dose of of 0.56 mg/kg/week of dimethyl-nitrosamine, which was used in our experiments, led to a decrease in the numbers of plaque-forming spleen cells. The minimum carcinogenic dose of N-nitroso-morpholine, 1.3 mg/kg, which was substantially exceeded in this experiment, had no effect on the immunocompetent system of the rats.

N-nitroso compounds can be both carcinogenic and immunosuppressive, but there is no correlation between the two activities.

Recently we have performed immunological tests in rats after inoculation of polycyclic hydrocarbons. We applied 3-methylcholanthrene, 3.4-benzo(a)pyrene and the noncarcinogenic benzo(e)pyrene in doses of 6.0, 0.6 and 0.06 mg/animal. The immune reaction was investigated by means of the agar-plaque technique and the hemagglutination test. Up to now, the preliminary results indicate that none of the substances has any suppressive effect on the immune response of the rats.

While in the past we have tested merely the influence of carcinogenic compounds on the humoral immunity, in future we will also examine their activities on the cellular immune response.

Table 4. Number of plaque-forming cells per 10^6 spleen cells as percentage of the control value (arithmetic mean of 5 animals ± standard error) after injections of 4 N-nitroso compounds in different dosages (see Table 3) for 12, 18, and 24 weeks. Control 1 is the control value corresponding to the dosage groups 5% and 2.5% of the LD_{50}. Control 2 is the control value of the rats treated with 1.25 and 0.625% of LD_{50} of the N-nitroso compounds. The data marked with [a] are significantly different from the controls (t - test)

Substance	Doses as % of LD_{50}	Time of treatment 12	18	24
Dimethyl-nitrosamine	5	100±41	33±5[a]	44±9[a]
	2.5	111±33	62±13	49±8[a]
	1.25	123±30	58±9	47±14[a]
	0.625	152±35	70±11	54±15
Ethyl-n-butyl-nitrosamine	5	78±25	30±9[a]	37±6[a]
	2.5	148±25	52±13	53±13
	1.25	73±21	94±14	66±13
	0.625	92±23	81±23	60±31
N-Nitroso-morpholine	5	58±16	46±9[a]	58±16
	2.5	82±27	74±28	68±13
	1.25	84±21	119±19	67±21
	0.625	105±48	78±38	71±42
Methyl-nitroso-urea	5	20±8[a]	23±8[a]	10±4[a]
	2.5	71±22	48±15[a]	31±8[a]
	1.25	106±18	55±7	54±16
	0.625	96±25	51±21	83±31
Control 1	-	100±41	100±18	100±14
Control 2	-	100±21	100±24	100±27

DISCUSSION

In recent years, some investigators have reported a clear correlation between carcinogenic and immunosuppressive effects of carcinogenic substances (1-11, 15-24, 27, 28, 30, 31, 33-35) and of immunosuppressants (37, 38), whereas other investigators have failed to confirm a direct relationship between the two activities (9, 14, 23, 25, 26, 29, 36, 41, 42).

The different results are due partly to the different test systems used, as the dosages of carcinogens given and timing of antigen inoculation are different. However, this does not explain the different immunological activities of carcinogenic substances in comparable studies, i.e. by BALL, or in the present case. Such findings might lead to the conclusion that the immune status, which may be influenced by the carcinogen, does not play an important role in the chemical induction of tumors, especially since a defective immune system does not explain all the phenomena of tumor formation and growth (i.e. enhancement) (44, 45).

The findings of quantitative carcinogenesis also seem to suggest that there is no close correlation between carcinogenic and immunodepressive activity, since it has been shown that chronic application of lower doses of carcinogens causes a wider distribution of tumor localization than high doses (46). If the immunocompetent system were involved in tumorigenesis, high doses, which lead more readily to immunosuppression, would result in a broader distribution of malignomas. However, this is not so. The contradictory findings obtained after thymectomy, lymphadenectomy and injection of antilymphocytic serum and corticosteroids with simultaneous or subsequent application of a carcinogen confirm the present findings (47-56).

The results of viral carcinogenesis are not affected by these reflections: in this case an injury to the immune system can be of decisive importance in the formation of tumors (57, 58).

REFERENCES

1. MALMGREN, R. A., BENNISON, B. E., MC KINLEY, T. W., Jr.: Proc. Soc. exp. biol. (N. Y.) 79, 484 (1952).
2. DAVIDSOHN, I., STERN, K., SABET, L.: Proc. Amer. Ass. Cancer Res. 2, 102 (1956).
3. PREHN, R. T., MAIN, J. M.: J. nat. Cancer Inst. 18, 769 (1957).
4. STJERNSWÄRD, J.: J. nat. Cancer Inst. 35, 885 (1965).
5. STJERNSWÄRD, J.: J. nat. Cancer Inst. 36, 1189 (1966).
6. STJERNSWÄRD, J.: J. nat. Cancer Inst. 38, 515 (1967).
7. STUTMAN, O.: Science 166, 620 (1969).
8. SALOMON, J. C., GUEGUEN, S., LAZAR, Ph.: Path. Biol. 18, 65 (1970).
9. CHANDRA, P., GERICKE, D., WACKER, A.: Z. Krebsforsch. 76, 40 (1971).
10. ZSCHIESCHE, W., SCHULZ, W. D.: Z. Krebsforsch. 75, 277 (1971).
11. GERICKE, D., CHANDRA, P., WACKER, A.: Z. Krebsforsch. 75, 85 (1971).
12. DURAN-REYNALS, M. L.: J. nat. Cancer Inst. 48, 9 (1972).
13. LILLY, F., DURAN-REYNALS, L. M.: J. nat. Cancer Inst. 48, 105 (1972).
14. BRAI, M., PATRUCCO, A., OSLER, A. G.: J. Immunol. 109, 317 (1972).
15. REES, J. A., SYMES, M. O.: Int. J. Cancer 11, 202 (1973).
16. BALL, J. K., DAWSON, D. A.: J. nat. Cancer Inst. 42, 579 (1969).
17. BARONI, C. D., SCELSI, R., PESANDO, P. C.: Tumori 56, 269 (1970).
18. KEARNEY, R., HUGHES, L. E.: Brit. J. Cancer 24, 319 (1970).
19. DI MARCO, A. T., FRANCESCHI, C., XERRI, L., PRODI, G.: Cancer Res. 31, 1446 (1971).
20. MATSUOKA, Y., SENOH, H., KAWAMOTO, T., KOHMO, T., HAMAOKA, T., KITAGAWA, M.: Nature New Biol. 238, 273 (1972).
21. PARMIANI, G., COLNAGHI, M. I., DELLA PORTA, G.: Proc. Soc. exp. biol. (N. Y.) 130, 828 (1969).
22. LAPPE, M. A., PREHN, R. T.: Cancer Res. 30, 1357 (1970).
23. PARMIANI, G.: Int. J. Cancer 5, 260 (1970).
24. LAPPE, M. A., STEINMULLER, D. S.: Cancer Res. 30, 674 (1970).
25. PARMIANI, G.: J. nat. Cancer Inst. 47, 569 (1971).
26. PARMIANI, G., COLNAGHI, M. I., DELLA PORTA, G.: Brit. J. Cancer 25, 354 (1971).
27. PEROCCO, P., FRANCESCHI, C., DI MARCO, A. T., PRODI, G.: Proc. Soc. exp. biol. (N. Y.) 136, 1024 (1971).
28. DI MARCO, A. T., FRANCESCHI, C., PRODO, G.: Cancer Res. 32, 1569 (1972).
29. PHILLIPS, J. M.: Int. J. Cancer 9, 39 (1972).
30. NAKASHIMA, S., ONO, S.: Gann 63, 111 (1972).
31. OUTZEN, H. C., PREHN, R. T.: Cancer Res. 33, 408 (1973).

32. KUPFER, M., KUPFER, G., BERGER, U.: Naturwissenschaften 56, 216 (1969).
33. YOKORO, K., IMAMURA, N., TAKIZAWA, S.: Gann 61, 287 (1970).
34. GRYSCHEK, G., PASTERNAK, G.: Acta biol. med. germ. 27, 195 (1971).
35. GRYSCHEK, G., PASTERNAK, G.: Acta biol. med. germ. 29, 907 (1972).
36. BALL, J. K.: J. nat. Cancer Inst. 44, 1 (1970).
37. PENN, I., HAMMOND, W., BRETTSCHNEIDER, L.: Transplant. Proc. 1, 106 (1969).
38. PENN, I.: Malignant tumors in organtransplant recipients. In: Recent Results in Cancer Research, Vol. 34, p. 51. Berlin, Heidelberg, New York: Springer 1970.
39. SCHMÄHL, D.: Dtsch. med. Wschr. 92, 1150 (1967).
40. SCHMÄHL, D., OSSWALD, H.: Arzneimittel-Forsch. 20, 1461 (1970).
41. SCHERF, H. R., KRÜGER, C., KARSTEN, C.: Arzneimittel-Forsch. 20, 1467 (1970).
42. SCHERF, H. R.: Z. Krebsforsch. 77, 189 (1972).
43. SCHMÄHL, D.: Z. Krebsforsch. 74, 457 (1970).
44. GLEICHMANN, H., GLEICHMANN, E.: Klin. Wschr. 51, 255 (1973).
45. GLEICHMANN, E., GLEICHMANN, H.: Klin. Wschr. 51, 260 (1973).
46. DRUCKREY, H., SCHILDBACH, A., SCHMÄHL, D., PREUSSMANN, R., IVANKOVIC, S.: Arzneimittel-Forsch. 13, 841 (1963).
47. FRIEDRICH-FRESKA, H., HOFFMANN, M.: Nature 223, 1162 (1969).
48. COLE, J. L., FOLEY, W. A.: Radiation Res. 39, 391 (1969).
49. CERILLI, G. J., TREAT, R. C.: Transplantation 8, 774 (1969).
50. WOODS, D. A.: Nature 224, 276 (1969).
51. FISHER, J. C., DAVIS, R. C., MANNICK, J. A.: Surgery 68, 150 (1970).
52. TRAININ, N., LINKER-ISRAELI, M.: J. nat. Cancer Inst. 44, 893 (1970).
53. SCHMÄHL, D., WAGNER, R., SCHERF, H. R.: Arzneimittel-Forsch. 21, 403 (1971).
54. FRANKEL, H. H., YAMAMOTO, R. S.: Toxicol. appl. Pharmacol. 17, 462 (1970).
55. BOLTON, P. M.: Oncology 27, 430 (1973).
56. DENLINGER, H. R., SWENBERG, J. A., KOESTER, A., WECHSLER, W.: J. nat. Cancer Inst. 50, 87 (1973).
57. VANDEPUTTE, M.: Transplant. Proc. 1, 100 (1969).
58. GRUNDMANN, E., HOBIK, H. P.: Z. Krebsforsch. 79, 298 (1973).

The Significance of Immunosuppression and Antigenic Stimulation in the Development of Malignant Lymphomas

G. Krueger

Every cancer therapist must expect immunosuppressive side effects when using the usual chemotherapeutic compounds. Before any discussion of the risk of malignant lymphoreticular disease secondary to such immunosuppression, I shall summarize the various ways in which carcino-chemotherapeutic agents can interfere with the immunologic reactivity of an individual; these are shown in Table 1.

Which of the possible responses are in fact acting in a patient depends upon the nature of the compound, the dose and route of administration, and probably also upon the state of metabolic and immunologic activity of the patient. In addition, the type of antigen, its availability and its immunogenicity may influence the response to chemotherapeutic drugs. Despite some current evidence for all these influences, detailed investigations are needed to clarify the underlying mechanisms.

The most prominent effect of carcino-chemotherapeutic compounds on the immune response is immunosuppression. Any attempt to relate tumor development to induced immunosuppression (as in this paper) involves consideration of other untoward cancerogenic effects of chemotherapeutic measures and of supportive treatment, and these are summarized in Table 2.

Most important of all, perhaps, is the immediate carcinogenic potential of chemotherapeutics. In this context, it may be recalled that Alexander Haddow demonstrated a biphasic activity of polycyclic hydrocarbons, which are able to induce tumors as well as to inhibit their growth, as early as 1935. The converse is also true with many carcino-chemotherapeutics.

An exact evaluation of the various mechanisms leading to cancer is especially difficult in man, since polychemotherapy is widely used and may include: immunosuppressants, carcinogens, and cocarcinogens. We are forced, therefore, to turn to animal experiments to gain some insight into the relationship that may exist between immunosuppression as achieved by cancer chemotherapy and tumor development.

It is of considerable interest with regard to tumor pathogenesis that in acquired or in inherited immune deficiency syndromes (including the status after allografting), the incidence of malignant lymphomas is increased significantly more than that of any other type of malignant tumors. This fact has been documented in several publications (21, 13) and it is not easily explained by the assumption that immunosuppressive treatment increases the incidence of malignant tumors solely by interfering with the host's immunologic surveillance. In order to test the mechanism of "immunologic tumor develop-

Table 1. Effect of carcino-chemotherapeutic agents on the immune response

Mechanisms of Action	Compounds (Examples)	References
I. Immunosuppression:		
a) Depression of the function of immunocompetent tissues	virtually all compounds	MIHICH, 1971; CAMIENER and WECHTER, 1972; KRUEGER, 1972.
b) Decrease in immunogenicity of tumor cells	probably mutagenic and carcinogenic agents; secondary to isoantigenic variation, selection, and mutation.	for general principles see KLEIN, 1971; SOUTHAM, 1971.
II. Immunostimulation:		
a) Increased tumor immunogenicity	Pyrazole-4-carcoxamide and derivatives	NICOLIN et al., 1973.
b) Action of the drug as hapten or as immunogen	L-Asparaginase, Ribonuclease, Daunorubicin, Azathioprine	LORKE and TETTENBORN, 1970; REIS and SCHMIDT, 1970; KRUEGER, 1972.
c) Induction of auto-antibody formation and of immune complexes	X-rays, some toxic drugs (needs further study)	for general principle see SARGENT et al., 1966; FLAD et al., 1969.

Table 2. Untoward carcinogenic effect of carcino-chemotherapy and supportive treatment

Type of Activity	Compounds (Examples)	References
I Carcinogenicity of chemotherapeutic compounds	alkylating agents, stilbestrol, methotrexate, procarbazine, X-ray	BOYLAND, 1967; SCHMÄHL, 1967, 1970; CASTRO et al., 1973.
II Carcinogenic impurities and additives of drugs	urethane (formerly used as solvent and sedative), metals (chromium, nickel), antibiotics	SCHRAMM et al., 1966; HUEPER, 1967; DICKENS, 1967; BOYLAND, 1967.
III Cocarcinogenic action of cancer chemotherapeutic compounds	hormones	DONTENWILL, 1966; POEL, 1967.

Table 3. Immunosuppressive chemotherapy and lymphoma development in the mouse

Mouse strain	Compound	Additive	Humoral immune response	Cellular immune response	Lymphoma incidence	Latent period (mo.)
BALB/c, DBA/2	azathioprine	antigens	increased	inhibited	32-66%	5-7
C57B1	azathioprine	---	decreased	inhibited	3-12%	ca.7
DBA/2	methotrexate	antigens	slightly increased	inhibited	12%	5-8
	methotrexate	---	decreased	inhibited	0%	-
DBA/2	triethylene melamine	antigens	inhibited	inhibited	0%	-
	triethylene melamine	---	inhibited	inhibited	0%	-
BALB/c, C57B1	cyclophosphamide	antigens	mildly decreased	inhibited	30%	4-6
	cyclophosphamide	---	decreased	inhibited	-10%	6-8
BALB/c, C57B1,	---	antigens	positive	positive	2-4%	above 18

Azathioprine: 5-15 mg/kg/day in drinking water; Methotrexate: 3 mg/kg/day in drinking water
Triethylene melamine: 0.3 mg/kg/day in drinking water Cyclophosphamide: 3/ mg/kg twice weekly i.p.
Antigens: 0.1 mg H37Ra tubercle bacteria in adjuvant every other week s.c. or
bovine serum albumin, daily i.p., 0.2 ml of a 10% solution.
Assessment of immune response: micro-hemagglutination tests and foot pad tests with histological evaluation.

ment" further, we devised and conducted a line of experiments imitating the model cases presented by human pathology. In these experiments, inbred mice were subjected simultaneously to immunosuppression and immunostimulation. The results, which are published in part elsewhere (17, 16, 14), are summarized in Table 3.
In additional preliminary studies, ribonuclease of bovine origin was administered to mice in a dose of 5 mg/mouse/day for more than 2 months. Decreases of varying intensity in the humoral and cellular immune response were documented, but no lymphoma development occurred. Our results indicating increased lymphoma induction with cyclophosphamide and simultaneous antigenic stimulation have been confirmed in part by another study (29).

The experimental data show that all five chemotherapeutic agents tested had a significant immunosuppressive effect. Nevertheless, only when the mice were stimulated simultaneously and persistently with antigens was lymphoma development regularly observed. In addition, when both the humoral and the cellular immune responses were suppressed to the same degree, as in the mice receiving triethylene melamine, no lymphomas were seen, but the animals usually died even during the latent period.

There are two exceptions from the above observations:

1. Of DBA mice receiving azathioprine, malignant lymphomas were observed in up to 12%;
2. Of BALB/c mice treated with cyclophosphamide lymphomas were observed in up to 10%.

In accordance with other results (25), it must be assumed that cyclophosphamide is probably a carcinogen besides having immunosuppressive effects. As far as we know, no carcinogenic activity has yet been unequivocally demonstrated for azathioprine. Since DBA mice treated with azathioprine alone were also carrying large quantities of C-type particles, it might be assumed that this virus provided the antigen necessary for concomitant persistent antigenic stimulation of the immune system.

We have offered a theory to interpret our experimental results, namely the induction of malignant lymphomas by concurrent persistent antigenic stimulation and immunosuppression (15); it is summarized in Fig. 1.

The effects of both stimulatory and inhibitory measures are separated into their interference with cell proliferation and interference with cell differentiation, i.e. cell function. Four main reaction patterns are possible:

1. Functional inhibitors have equally weak effects on both cell proliferation and cell differentiation, causing a decreased immunological reactivity (the clinical result is repeated and chronic infection);
2. functional inhibitors interfere equally effectively with cell proliferation and cell differentiation, thus causing the death of the subject (clinically usually a result of widespread infections, sepsis, and shock);
3. functional inhibitors interfere primarily with cell proliferation, ultimately causing the death of the subject;
4. functional inhibitors interfere primarily with cell differentiation, i.e. cell function, causing progressive cell proliferation to overcome the functional defect. Clinically the result is a lymphomatous growth of cells in immuno-(in)competent tissues.

Functional inhibitors may be carcino-chemotherapeutic drugs, as shown above. Various other measures that include a depression of immune responsiveness

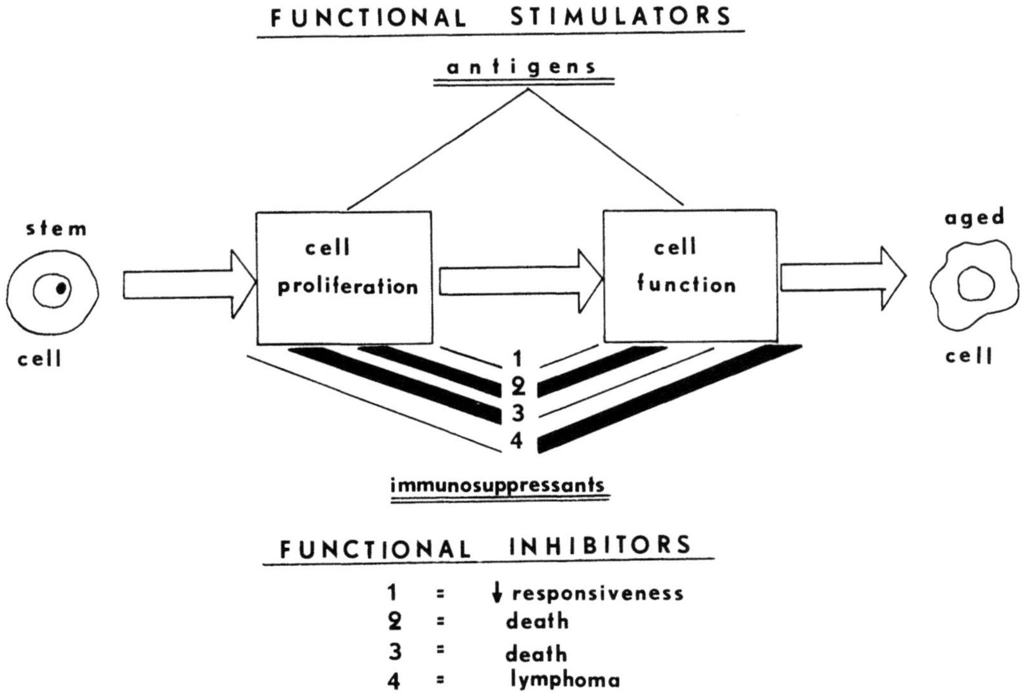

Fig. 1

can also have similar effects. Such measures include the induction of specific tolerance and stimulation with the tolerogen, which in experimental animals has actually caused malignant lymphomas (30). This "functional" scheme also includes "oncogenic" viruses, which decrease the host's immune responsiveness, probably secondary to lymphoid cell transformation (and act as stimulating antigens at the same time).

In our own experience, the intensity of persistent antigenic stimulation is also decisive in the degree of immunosuppression and the pathogenesis of malignant lymphomas.

I will now try to deduce from the animal experiments the situations in which the risk of lymphoma development in cancer patients is greatest.

It may be that only patients with a long survival time after initiation of cancer treatment are at risk. The shortest latent period for lymphoma induction in our mice receiving immunosuppressive treatment was 4 months, which corresponds to about 10-15 years of human life.

Patients must be kept on extended maintenance therapy with immunosuppressive drugs to be included in the risk group. It is not yet known for how long this therapy must be maintained to become dangerous for the patient, but it is likely to be more than one year, and more probably several years.

The cancer patient's state of reduced immunologic reactivity is accompanied by persistent immunologic stimulation. Repeated infection by environmental organisms is probably sufficient to guarantee such stimulation, especially since the depressed immunologic reactivity may favor the persistence of normally neutralized infectious agents. The frequent demonstration of cytomegalo viruses and herpes viruses in cancer patients is probably indicative of this.

Immunosuppression is not complete in the risk group, i.e. humoral and cellular reactivity cannot be present simultaneously, since death secondary to sepsis would be inevitable. In fact, as the experimental lymphoma induction in tolerant animals suggests (30) the immunologic nonreactivity might be limited to one or a few antigens in an otherwise normoreactive person. A similar specific defect is known in Wiskott-Aldrich syndrome in man, where the response to polysaccharide antigens is inadequate (4); up to 15% of patients with this syndrome suffer from malignant lymphomas that develop during the course of the disease (15). Furthermore, it is our impression that a defective cellular immune response may make an organism more liable to the induction of lymphomas than an impaired humoral immune response. This is in keeping with FUDENBERG's theory (9) that a defective cellular immune surveillance is a pacemaker for autoimmune disease and lymphoreticular malignancy.

To our knowledge, no statistical evaluation is yet available on any coincidence of immunosuppressive cancer chemotherapy in man with subsequent development of malignant lymphomas. We have to rely, therefore, on individual publications of such cases, which are quite scarce. TERBRÜGGEN published 3 cases of reticulum-call sarcoma following 18 months' to 4 years' maintenance therapy with Trenimon R (tris-ethyleneimino benzochinone) for carcinomas of the breast, bronchus, and colon (31). The second primary tumor was observed between 1 and 4 years after the cytostatic maintenance therapy was discontinued.

Similarly, atypical reticulum-cell proliferation and reticulum-cell sarcoma have been observed following chemotherapy for leukemia. These phenomena were interpreted at the time as the consequence of a therapeutically induced metamorphosis of the primary disease. The possibility that reticulum-cell sarcoma is a second primary following immunosuppressive chemotherapy cannot yet be excluded. Much easier to interpret is the observation of a second primary leukemia in a patient treated with chemotherapy and bone-marrow transplantation for his primary leukemia (7). The second leukemia involved the donor's bone-marrow cells, which were cytogenetically distinct from the host cells. It was thought that a persistent oncogenic virus had caused the primary leukemia and might also have transformed the donor cells. Another possibility in this case, however, is that induced immunosuppression had favored this process of leukemogenesis, as discussed in our theory.

Finally, we have observed two patients who were treated with the mildly immunosuppressive streptozotocin for malignant islet-cell tumors. Both patients showed atypical reticular stem cell hyperplasia in the bone marrow, with circulating atypical cells in the blood. They died of the primary tumor and sepsis, however, before a clear-cut diagnosis of malignant lymphoma or leukemia could be made.

In conclusion, it appears possible that malignant lymphoreticular disease occurs in cancer patients receiving long-term immunosuppressive chemotherapy. But the risk of suffering from malignant lymphomas is low for these patients compared to the risk of dying from their primary tumor or from sepsis secondary to extensive immunologic paralysis. If carcino-chemotherapy continues to advance at the same pace as it has in recent decades, resulting in much longer survival times, malignant lymphomas may become one of the more frequently expected side effects of treatment.

REFERENCES

1. BOYLAND, E.: Biochemical Aspects of Carcinogenesis with Special Reference to Alkylating Agents and Some Antibiotics. In: Potential Carcinogenic Hazards from Drugs (Ed. R. TRUHAUT), p. 204. UICC Monograph No. 7. Berlin, Heidelberg, New York: Springer 1967.
2. CAMIENER, G. W., WECHTER, W. J.: Immunosuppression Agents, Procedures, Speculations and Prognosis. Progr. Drug Res. 16, 67 (1972).
3. CASTRO, E. B., ROSEN, P. P., QUAN, S. H. Q.: Carcinoma of Large Intestine in Patients Irradiated for Carcinoma of Cervix and Uterus. Cancer 31, 45 (1973).
4. COOPER, M. D., CHASE, H. P., LOWMAN, J. T., KRIVIT, W., GOOD, R. A.: Immunologic Defects in Patients with Wiskott Aldrich Syndrome. In: Immunologic Deficiency Diseases in Man (Eds. D. BERGSMA, R. A. GOOD, J. FINSTAD, P. A. MIESCHER, R. T. SMITH, J. L. NUSSER). Birth Defects Original Article Series Vol. 4, No. 1, p. 378. New York: National Foundation-March of Dimes 1968.
5. DICKENS, F.: Drugs with Lactone Groups as Potential Carcinogens. In: Potential Carcinogenic Hazards from Drugs (Ed. R. TRUHAUT), p. 144. UICC Monograph No. 7. Berlin, Heidelberg, New York: Springer 1967.
6. DONTENWILL, W.: Erzeugung von Tumoren durch endogenhormonelle Faktoren. In: Hdb. exp. Pharmacol., Vol. 16 No. 13, p. 74. Tumors II (Eds. O. EICHLER, A. FARAH, H. HERKEN, A. D. WELCH), Berlin, Heidelberg, New York: Springer 1966.
7. FIALKOW, P. J., THOMAS, E. D., BRYANT, J. J.: Leukemic Transformation of Engrafted Human Marrow Cells in Vivo. Lancet 1971 1, 251.
8. FLAD, H.-D., PLAYFAIR, J. H. L., GHAFFAR, A., MIESCHER, P. A.: Strain Differences in Liver Autoantibody Response of Inbred Mice. Proc. Soc. exp. Biol. (N.Y.) 131, 121 (1969).
9. FUDENBERG, H.: Genetically Determined Immune Deficiency as the Predisposing Cause of "Autoimmunity" and Lymphoid Neoplasia. Amer. J. Med. 51, 295 (1971).
10. HADDOW, A.: Influence of Certain Polycyclic Hydrocarbons on the Growth of the Jensen Sarcoma. Nature (Lond.) 136, 868 (1935).
11. HUEPER, W. C.: Carcinogenic Hazards from Arsenic and Metal Containing Drugs. In: Potential Carcinogenic Hazards from Drugs (Ed. R. TURHAUT), p. 79. UICC Monograph No. 7. Berlin, Heidelberg, New York: Springer 1967.
12. KLEIN, E.: Parental Variants. Transplant. Proc. 3, 1167 (1971).
13. KRUEGER, G. R. F.: Morphology of Chemical Immunosuppression. In: Advances in Pharmacology and Chemotherapy (eds. S. GARATTINI, F. HAWKING, A. GOLDIN, I. J. KOPIN), p. 1. New York: Academic Press 1972.
14. KRUEGER, G. R. F.: Host Response During the Latent Period and the Growth of an Immunologic Induced Mouse Lymphoma. Beitr. Path. 142, 132 (1972).
15. KRUEGER, G. R. F.: Chronic Immunosuppression and Lymphomagenesis in Man and Mice. Nat. Cancer Inst. Monogr. 35, 183 (1972).
16. KRUEGER, G. R. F., HEINE, U. I.: Morphogenesis of Two Immunologically Induced Mouse Lymphomas. Cancer Res. 32, 573 (1972).
17. KRUEGER, G. R. F., MALMGREN, R. A., BERARD, C. W.: Malignant Lymphomas and Plasmacytosis in Mice under Prolonged Immunosuppression and Persistent Antigenic Stimulation. Transplantation 11, 138 (1971).
18. LORKE, D., TETTENBORN, D.: Experimental Studies on the Toxicity of Crasnitin in Animals. In: Experimental and Clinical Effects of L-Asparaginase (Eds. E. GRUNDMANN, H. F. OETTGEN), p. 174. Recent Results in Cancer Research Vol. 33. Berlin, Heidelberg, New York: Springer 1970.
19. MIHICH, E.: Preclinical Evaluation of the Interrelationships Between Cancer Chemotherapy and Immunity. Natl. Cancer Inst. Monogr. 34, 90 (1970).

20. NICOLIN, A., VADLAMUDI, S., GOLDIN, A.: Increased Immunogenicity of Murine Lymphatic Tumors by Pyrazole-4-Carboxamide, 3(or 5)-Amino (NSC 1402; PCA). Cancer Chemother. Rep. 57, 3 (1973).
21. PENN, I., STARZL, T. A.: A Summary of the Satus of De Novo Cancer in Transplant Recipients. Pransplant. Proc. 4, 719 (1972).
22. POEL, W. E.: Progesterone and Mammary Carcinogenesis. In: Potential Carcinogenic Hazards from Drugs (Ed. R. TRUHAUT), p. 162. UICC Monograph No. 7. Berlin, Heidelberg, New York: Springer 1967.
23. REIS, H. E., SCHMIDT, C. G.: The Antigenicity of E.coli-Asparaginase. In: Experimental and Clinical Affects of L-Asparaginase (Eds. E. GRUNDMANN, H. F. OETTGEN), p. 194. Recent Results of Cancer Research Vol. 33. Berlin, Heidelberg, New York: Springer 1970.
24. SARGENT, A. U., MYERS, J., RICHTER, M.: The Immune Response to Circulating Autologous Hepatocellular Antigens. J. Immunol. 96, 268 (1966).
25. SCHMÄHL, D.: Karzinogene Wirkung von Cyclophosphamid und Triazichon bei Ratten. Dtsch. med. Wschr. 92, 1150 (1967).
26. SCHMÄHL, D.: Entstehung, Wachstum und Chemotherapie maligner Tumoren. Aulendorf: Cantor 1970.
27. SCHRAMM, T., BIELKA, H., GRAFFI, A.: Geschwulsterzeugung durch chemische Substanzen. In: Hdb. exp. Pharmacol. Vol. 16, Nr. 12; Tumors I (Eds. EICHLER, A. FARAH, H. HERKEN, A. D. WELCH), p. 1. Berlin, Heidelberg, New York: Springer 1966.
28. SOUTHAM, C. M.: Immunological Research in Human Neoplasia: Present Status and Prospects. 1971.
29. STÜCK, B.: Auftreten von Leukosen nach kombinierter Gabe Cyclophosphamid und Freund Adjuvans im Tierversuch. Paper presented at 2nd Internat. Conference on Chemotherapy of Leukemia and Malignant Lymphomas, Vienna/ Austria, March 19-23, 1972.
30. SUCIU-FOCA, N., DUMITRESCU, V., LAZAR, C., NACHTIGAL, M.: Host and Tumor Modifications Associated with Serial Heterotransplantation of Tumors through Immunologically Tolerant Animals. Cancer Res. 30, 1681 (1970).
31. TERBRÜGGEN, A.: Neoplastische Retikulose nach zytostatischer Dauerbehandlung von radikal operierten Karzinomen. Verh. dtsch. Ges. Path. 49, 241 (1965).
32. VAUGHAN, J. H.: Autoallergic Diseases: Concepts and General Considerations. In: Immunological Diseases, Vol. 2 (Eds. M. SAMTER, D. W. TALMAGE, B. ROSE, W. B. SHERMAN, J. H. VAUGHAN), p.987. Boston: Little, Brown & Co. 1971.

Malignant Disease in Immunodeficient States in Man *

I. Penn

In recent years great interest has been aroused in the relationship between the immune status of the individual and the development of cancer. A wide variety of animal experiments have demonstrated that states of immunodeficiency are associated with an increased incidence of malignancies (37). Similar evidence is accumulating in man (36-42, 45, 48, 49). Before reviewing this data it is pertinent to summarize some current ideas regarding cancer and immunity.

CANCER AND IMMUNITY

Throughout our lives we are repeatedly exposed to potentially oncogenic agents in the environment. These include sunlight, ionizing radiation, agents in ingested food and liquids, medications, air pollutants, industrial chemicals, viruses, and other agents. Every day our bodies produce massive numbers of new cells to replace those lost through normal wear and tear. Under the influence of environmental agents a number of these cells undergo mutations, some of which are potentially malignant. When neoplasms develop at least some of them are believed to acquire new antigens, known as tumor-specific antigens, which are foreign to the host (16, 26, 27, 43). Many investigators now believe that a major activity of the lymphoreticular system is to exert an immunologic surveillance function (5, 6, 54) whose purpose is to recognize tumor-specific antigens and to eliminate, or at least restrict the growth of, malignant cells. Cell-mediated immunity appears to be a major factor in immunologic surveillance (5, 6, 48), but humoral factors may also play a role. Immunologic surveillance is weakest at the two major periods of cancer incidence, in infancy and early childhood, when the lymphoreticular system is immature, and in old age when it becomes effete (19). Immunologic surveillance may also be impaired in a number of naturally occurring states of immunodeficiency. These rare disorders are characterized by defects in cell-mediated or humoral immunity or both, and the incidence of malignancy is roughly 10, 000 times greater in a sample of patients with these conditions than in the general age-matched population (20). These disorders include infantile X-linked agammaglobulinemia (Bruton type); severe combined immunodeficiency

* This work was supported by research grants from the Veterans Administration, by grants RR-00051 and RR-00069 from the general clinical research centers program of the Division of Research Resources, National Institutes of Health, and by grants AI-10176-01, AI-AM-08898, AM-07772, and HE-09110 of the United States Public Health Service.

(lymphopenic agammaglobulinemia of the Swiss or X-linked types), Wiskott-Aldrich disease, "common variable" forms of immunodeficiency (late onset, acquired, sporadic, hypo-or dysgammaglobulinemia), ataxia-telangiectasia, and deficiency of IgA (20, 25). The host's resistance to malignancy may also be impaired by various forms of cancer therapy, including radical surgical procedures (12, 15, 59), radiotherapy (12, 30, 31, 52, 59) and cancer-chemotherapy (39, 40, 42). As this symposium is concerned with special problems of cancer-chemotherapy we shall concentrate on the development of malignancies in patients treated with this form of therapy or with immunosuppressive agents, many of which are derivatives of cancer chemotherapeutic drugs. In some of the groups to be described there is unequivocal evidence of an increased incidence of cancer, while in others there are data suggestive of such a relationship.

IMMUNE DEFICIENCIES AND CANCER IN ORGAN HOMOGRAFT RECIPIENTS

Immunosuppressive therapy is given to an organ homograft recipient to prevent rejection of the transplant by depressing the cell-mediated and humoral immune functions of the lymphoreticular system of the host. Among the measures used are a number of pharmacologic agents, including azathioprine, cyclophosphamide, corticosteroids, actinomycin C or D, antilymphocyte globulin, and other less commonly used agents (Table 1). Various combinations of these agents are used in different transplant centers. The largest doses are given during the first few months after transplantation, when problems with rejection are most frequently encountered. The resultant depression of the lymphoreticular system has undesirable side effects, including a greater risk of infectious complications and an increased incidence of malignancy.

Since 1968 we have maintained an informal Tumor Registry in Denver to record all cancers encountered in organ homograft recipients either before or after transplantation (36-42, 45, 48). Physicians from transplant centers throughout the world have generously contributed information concerning their patients. This report presents data collected up to November 1973.

Cancers have been encountered in three groups of organ homograft recipients: a) patients in whom a neoplasm arose de novo at some time after transplantation; b) recipients in whom a tumor was accidentally transmitted with the transplant; c) individuals with malignancies present before transplantation.

(a) De-Novo Cancers

Long-term studies of renal homograft recipients treated at the University of Colorado Medical Center and the Denver Veterans Administration Hospital have demonstrated a 5 to 6% incidence of de-novo malignancies following transplantation (36, 38-42, 45, 48). This frequency is about 100 times greater than that in the general population in the same age range (37). At present the Denver Tumor Registry has records of 184 patients with de-novo cancers. One hundred eighty one were recipients of kidney transplants and three were given cardiac homografts. One hundred thirty two types of epithelial cancer occurred in 125 patients (68%) and 61 mesenchymal tumors were found in 60 recipients (32%), with one patient having both an epithelial cancer and a mesenchymal tumor. The majority of the mesenchymal tumors were lymphomas. A most unusual feature of these tumors was their predilection for the central

Table 1. Immunosuppressive agents used in organ transplant recipients and in various disease states

Condition treated	Number of cases	Agent used[b]	Number of cases
Organ transplantation[a]	184	Azathioprine	183
		Prednisone	183
		A. L. G.	56[c]
		Actinomycin	48
		Cyclophosphamide	6
		Other agents	3
Psoriasis	22	Methotrexate	21
		Aminopterin	3
		Other agents	3
Chronic renal disease	9	Azathioprine	6
		Cyclophosphamide	4
		Other agents	6
Rheumatoid arthritis	7	Cyclophosphamide	5
		Methotrexate	2
		Chlorambucil	2
		Azathioprine	2
		Prednisone	5
		Other agents	1
Systemic lupus erythematosus	4	Azathioprine	4
		Prednisone	4
		Cyclophosphamide	1
Chronic cold agglutinin disease	2	Chlorambucil	2
		Melphalan	1
		Cyclophosphamide	1
		Azathioprine	1
		Corticosteroids	1
Dermatomyositis or polymyositis	2	Prednisone	2
		Azathioprine	1
		A. L. G.	1
Ulcerative colitis	1	Azathioprine	1
		Prednisone	1
Macroglobulinemia with renal insufficiency	1	Cyclophosphamide	1

[a]Other immunosuppressive measures included local irradiation of the transplant (57), splenectomy (49), thoracic dust fistula (8), thymectomy (8), thymic irradiation (2), endolymphatic irradiation (2), total-body irradiation (1) and extracorporeal irradiation of the blood (1). The patients in the table are those with de-novo cancers. Similar immunosuppressive therapy was used in patients with transplanted cancers and with cancers present before transplantation.

[b]In most cases more than one agent was used.

[c]Two patients received A. L. G. after the appearance of the neoplasms.

nervous system (45). Of 53 patients with lymphomas, 26 had brain or spinal cord involvement. In 21 instances the central nervous system was the only area affected by the tumor.

Most of the cancers occurred in young people (average age 38, range 8 to 70 years) with 60% of the patients under the age of 40 years. The average time of appearance of the tumors after transplantation was 28 months, with the epithelial neoplasms manifesting at 31 and the mesenchymal malignancies at 21 months.

The most common epithelial tumors involved the skin, the lip, and the cervix of the uterus. These had a relatively good prognosis as 73 of the 84 patients (87%) are still living, as opposed to 10 of 41 (24%) with other types of carcinoma and 11 of 59 (19%) with mesenchymal malignancies.

(b) Transplanted Cancers

Transplantation of a malignant tumor from one healthy human to another is unlikely to be successful (46) as the host's immune defenses recognize the neoplastic cells as "foreign" and destroy them. However, chronic immunosuppressive therapy hampers the defense mechanisms so that any malignant cells present in the transplanted organ may survive and grow and ultimately invade the surrounding tissues and spread widely. Forty-seven renal or cardiac recipients were given organs obtained from donors who had cancer at the time of donation or who developed evidence of neoplasia within a few months. In nearly every case the homograft appeared to be grossly free of cancer. However, in some cases full autopsy examinations of the cadaver donors after removal of the homografts revealed cancers in the contralateral kidneys and in several instances these findings prompted removal of the transplants (37, 41). No evidence of malignancy was found in 30 of the recipients, either at autopsy or during follow-up, which ranged from 3 to 38 months. Apparently, either the grafts were free of cancer or transplanted malignant cells were unable to become established in the recipients. In four other patients malignant cells were found in transplanted kidneys removed within the first three weeks after transplantation. In two more recipients the kidneys and adjacent structures were involved by malignancy, and 11 additional patients had widespread cancers. Seven of these eleven died of the transplanted tumors and in an eighth metastatic malignancy contributed to the patient's death. In the remaining three patients immunosuppressive therapy was stopped and the cancers disappeared. Apparently these recipients' immune defenses recovered and destroyed the foreign tumors (29, 58, 60). Experiences of this kind have convinced most transplant surgeons of the advisability of avoiding the use of organs from donors with cancer, except in the case of primary tumors of the central nervous system which rarely spread to other areas of the body (44, 57).

(c) Cancers Present Before Transplantation

Thus far we have provided unequivocal evidence that the immunosuppressive agents can cause de-novo tumors and permit the growth and dissemination of transplanted neoplasms. However, the effect of these agents on patients with pre-existing cancers is not clearly defined (40-42). We have collected data on 73 patients who had cancers for 5 years or less before transplantation. The neoplasm did not involve replacement of the organ in 21 of the 73 patients. In the remaining 52 recipients transplantation was performed specifically for treatment of carcinoma of one or both kidneys (31 cases), primary or metastatic cancer of the liver (19 cases), carcinoma of the larynx (1 case) or recurrent desmoid tumor of the small bowel (1 case). When transplantation was performed as definitive treatment of a malignancy the lesion was localized and there appeared to be a reasonable prospect of obtaining a "cure."

Recurrent or metastatic cancer occurred in 26 patients (36%). In several of the liver transplant recipients metastases appeared within a few months and grew very rapidly, massive deposits appearing in the homograft itself (48, 49). No evidence of tumor was found in 43 recipients (59%) followed for 2 to 90 months. Four patients (5%), one of whom had metastases of a preexisting carcinoma of the ureter, developed de-novo cancers of an entirely different kind from their original malignancies, and in one patient (1%) a non resected tumor remained unchanged. At present it is not possible to state whether the 36% incidence of recurrent and metastatic tumors represents the natural history of the original malignancies or is an actual increase caused by the immunosuppressive agents.

CANCERS IN NONTRANSPLANT PATIENTS TREATED WITH IMMUNOSUPPRESSIVE AGENTS

From a review of the literature and personal communication with many physicians (40-42) we have collected data suggesting that nontransplant patients with various diseases (psoriasis, chronic renal disease, rheumatoid arthritis, systemic lupus erythematosus, chronic cold agglutinin disease, dermatomyositis,polymyositis, ulcerative colitis, and macroglobulinemia) treated with immunosuppressive agents may have an increased incidence of cancer. Unfortunately the number of patients at risk is not known so no accurate figures regarding the incidence of this complication in this group of patients can be provided. Forty-nine cancers were reported in 48 patients on immunosuppressive therapy. Some of the cancers may have developed quite independently of this treatment, as they appeared in patients with auto-immune diseases, in which an increased incidence of malignancy has been reported by some workers (22), although it has not been confirmed by others (35). Similarly, the development of carcinoma of the colon in a patient with ulcerative colitis may be totally unrelated to the immunosuppressive therapy, as this cancer is a well-recognized complication of chronic ulcerative colitis. However, psoriasis is not a disorder commonly associated with cancer unless the patient has been treated with an oncogenic agent such as arsenic. The appearance of cancers in 22 psoriatic patients who received chronic treatment with methotrexate or aminopterin (Table 1) must therefore be looked upon with considerable suspicion.

DEVELOPMENT OF NEW MALIGNANCIES IN PATIENTS WITH CANCER TREATED WITH CHEMOTHERAPY

Patients with one cancer sometimes develop second or third neoplasms. In some instances these merely represent a naturally increased predisposition to malignancy (32). In other cases the natural history of the neoplasms is evolution into related types of cancers. Examples are the development of lymphatic leukemias in patients with solid lymphomas. In addition, some of the tumors may have been caused by radiotherapy, which has proven oncogenic effects (8, 9). Finally, many of the agents used in cancer-chemotherapy have immunosupressive properties and may, paradoxically, be oncogenic (40, 42). Circumstantial evidence has accumulated to suggest that cancer-chemotherapeutic agents, while controlling the original tumors, may contribute to the development of new malignancies. Previously we described a series of 124 patients who developed 128 new cancers while receiving chemotherapy (42). The series has now increased to 140 new malignancies in 135 patients (3, 7, 13, 14, 28, 34, 50, 55). Two examples of unusual alterations of the natural history of neoplasms during cancer-chemotherapy are shown in Tables 2 and 3. The first was the development of acute leukemias in patients treated for multiple myeloma. The second was the occurrence of solid lymphomas in patients receiving cytotoxic therapy for chronic granulocytic leukemias.

Table 2. Development of second cancers in patients receiving cancer chemotherapy

Initial cancer	Number of patients
Multiple myeloma	31
Major agent used	
Melphalan	29
Cyclophosphamide	4
Other agents	3
Second cancer	
Acute leukemia	29[a]
Miscellaneous carcinomas	3[a]

[a]One patient developed acute leukemia and a basal cell carcinoma.

Table 3. Development of second cancers in patients receiving cancer chemotherapy

Initial cancer	Number of patients
Chronic granulocytic leukemia	31
Major agent used	
Busulfan	23
Second cancer	
Reticulum cell sarcoma	22
Lymphosarcoma	3
Hodgkin's disease	2
Carcinoma of vulva	1
Carcinoma of breast	1
Carcinoma of pancreas	1
Carcinoma of lung	1

Little statistical information is so far available regarding the risk of development of new cancers in patients while on treatment with chemotherapy. Some idea may be gained from the series of 425 cases of Hodgkin's disease reported by ARSENEAU et al. (3), in which there was a statistically significant increase in the incidence of additional cancers. The expected number was 3.4 cases, whereas 12 cases were observed.

DISCUSSION

This study indicates that the immunosuppressive and cancer-chemotherapeutic agents are two-edged swords. While they provide beneficial effects in the disorders for which they are being used, they may also expose the patients to the risk of developing cancer. In most cases this probably occurs through a weakening of immunologic surveillance function of the lymphoreticular system, which allows malignant mutations to survive and become overt cancers. However, we must consider several other possible mechanisms for the development of the neoplasms. One is a direct oncogenic effect of the agents used. In animal experiments these agents may cause chromosome breaks, mutagenic, teratogenic and oncogenic changes (41). In man, chromosome breaks, nuclear abnormalities, cytologic dysplasia, and teratogenic effects have also been noted (41). The alkylating agent chlornaphazine appears to have direct oncogenic effects in man, causing the development of bladder cancers (Table 4). This is not surprising, as it is excreted in the urine as a metabolite β-naphthylamine, which has been incriminated as the cause of the bladder cancer in aniline dye workers (17, 53, 56).

Table 4. Development of second cancers in patients receiving cancer chemotherapy

Initial cancer	Number of patients
Polycythemia rubra vera	11
Hodgkin's disease	2
Major agent used	
Chlornaphazine	13
Second cancer	
Papilloma or carcinoma of bladder	12[a]
Carcinoma of kidney	1
Carcinoma of prostate	1[a]

[a]One patient developed carcinoma of the bladder and prostate

Another possible mechanism of oncogenesis is that the immunosuppressive and cancer-chemotherapeutic agents may enhance the effects of various environmental oncogens such as sunlight, radiation, and chemical carcinogens. This mechanism has been demonstrated in animal experiments (37).

The agents have also been shown to permit oncogenic viruses to become established and cause malignant tumors in studies in experimental animals (37). It is possible that they play a similar role in man, particularly as virus infections with potentially oncogenic viruses including EB virus, herpes hominis II virus and polyomavirus are common in immunosuppressed patients and those receiving cancer-chemotherapy (1, 2, 11, 37, 47, 51).

The findings in the present study indicate the need for caution in the use of immunosuppressive and carcino-chemotherapeutic agents. In organ transplant recipients the dosage of the former agents should be kept at the lowest level compatible with good organ function. In view of the danger of these agents in permitting the growth and dissemination of accidentally transplanted tumor cells, organs should not be obtained from donors with cancer, except possibly in the case of primary cancers confined to the central nervous system. Nontransplant patients with benign diseases such as psoriasis or rheumatoid arthritis should not be treated with immunosuppressive agents unless other forms of therapy have failed to provide relief. In patients with advanced malignancies there is no reason to restrict the use of the appropriate carcino-chemotherapeutic agents, as the risk of the development of new malignancies is far outweighed by the months or even years of control of the original neoplasms. In this respect, intermittent treatment appears to be less dangerous than continuous and prolonged chemotherapy (10, 18, 21, 23). However, the use of cancer-chemotherapy as an adjuvant to surgery or radiotherapy in patients who do not have advanced malignancies is open to question. In many instances, chemotherapy has failed to prevent recurrences or metastases (4, 24, 33), and it is possible that by hampering the host's immune responses, chemotherapy may have actually permitted the survival of residual cancer cells. More studies are needed to clarify this point. In addition, further research is needed to find means of increasing the patient's immune response to his cancer with various types of immunotherapy.

ACKNOWLEDGEMENT

Except where cited in the references, all data in this paper were obtained from our own clinical material, or from personal communication, or are cited in previous papers by the author (References 36-42, 45, 48). I wish to express my gratitude to numerous colleagues in many countries who generously sent me details regarding their patients.

REFERENCES

1. ALLEN, D. W., COLE, P.: Viruses and human cancer. New Engl. J. Med. 286, 70 (1972).
2. ARMSTRONG, D.: Infectious complications in cancer patients treated with chemical immunosuppressive agents. Transplant Proc. 5, 1245 (1973).
3. ARSENEAU, J. C., SPONZO, R. W., LEVINE, D. L., SCHNIPPER, L. E., BONNER, H., YOUNG, R. C., CANELLOS, G. P., JOHNSON, R. E., DE VITA, V. T.: Nonlymphomatous malignant tumors complicating Hodgkin's disease. Possible association with intensive therapy. New Engl. J. Med. 287, 1119 (1972).

4. BRUNNER, K. W., MARTHALER, T., MULLER, W.: Unfavourable effects of long term adjuvant chemotherapy with endoxan in radically operated bronchogenic carcinoma. Europ. J. Cancer 7, 285 (1971).
5. BURNET, F. M.: Cancer: A biological approach. Brit. med. J. 1957 1, 779, 841.
6. BURNET, F. M.: Immunological surveillance in neoplasia. Transplant. Rev. 7, 3 (1971).
7. BURNS, C. P., STJERNHOLM, R. L., KELLERMEYER, R. W.: Hodgkin's disease terminating in acute lymphosarcoma cell leukemia. A metabolic study. Cancer 27, 806 (1971).
8. Case records of the Massachusetts General Hospital. Case 47-1972. New Engl. J. Med. 287, 1085 (1972).
9. CASTRO, E. B., ROSEN, P. P., QUAN, S. H. Q.: Carcinoma of large intestine in patients irradiated for carcinoma of cervix and uterus. Cancer 31, 45 (1973).
10. CHEEMA, A. R., HERSH, E. M.: Patient survival after chemotherapy and its relationship to in vitro lymphocyte blastogenesis. Cancer 28, 851 (1971).
11. COLEMAN, D. V., GARDNER, S. D., FIELD, A. M.: Human polyomavirus infection in renal allograft recipients. Brit. med. J. 1973 3, 371.
12. CRILE, G., Jr.: Biological considerations in the treatment of cancer. Cleveland Clin. Quart. 39, 145 (1972).
13. DAVIS, H. L., Jr., PROUT, M. N., MCKENNA, P. J., COLE, D. R., KORBITZ, B. C.: Acute leukemia complicating metastatic breast cancer. Cancer, 31, 543 (1973).
14. DURANT, J. R., TASSONI, E. M.: Coexistent DiGuglielmo's leukemia and Hodgkin's disease. A case report with cytogenetic studies. Amer. J. med. Sci. 254, 824 (1967).
15. FISHER, B., FISHER, E. R., FEDUSKA, N.: Trauma with the localization of tumor cells. Cancer 20, 23 (1967).
16. FOLEY, E. J.: Antigenic properties of methyl cholanthrene-induced tumors in mice of strain of origin. Cancer Res. 13, 835 (1953).
17. FRAUMENI, J. F., Jr., MILLER, R. W.: Drug-induced cancer. Editorial. J. nat. Cancer Inst. 48, 1267 (1972).
18. FREI, E. III: Combination cancer therapy. Presidential Address, 63rd Annual Meeting of the American Association for Cancer Research. Cancer Res. 32, 2593 (1972).
19. GATTI, R. A., GOOD, R. A.: Aging, immunity and malignancy. Geriatrics 25, 158 (1970).
20. GATTI, R. A., GOOD, R. A.: Occurrence of malignancy in immunodeficiency diseases. A literature review. Cancer 28, 89 (1971).
21. GEORGE, R. P., POTH, J. L., GORDON, D., SCHRIER, S. L.: Multiple myeloma-intermittent, combination chemotherapy compared to continuous therapy. Cancer 29, 1665 (1972).
22. GOLDENBERG, G. J., PARASKEVAS, F., ISRAELS, L. G.: Lymphocyte and plasma cell neoplasms associated with auto immune diseases. Semin. Arthr. and Rheum. 1, 174 (1971).
23. HERSH, E. M., GUTTERMANN, J. U., MAVLIGIT, G., MCCREDIE, K. B., BODEY, G. P., FREIREICH, E. J., ROSSEN, R. D., BUTLER, W. T.: Host defense, chemical immunosuppression and the transplant recipient. Relative effects of intermittent versus continuous immunosuppressive therapy with reference to the objectives of treatment. Transplant. Proc. 5, 1191 (1973).
24. HIGGINS, G. A., Jr.: Use of chemotherapy as an adjuvant to surgery for bronchogenic carcinoma. Cancer 30, 1383 (1972).
25. HOERNI, B., LAPORTE, G.: Immunological disorders in the aetiology of lymphoreticular neoplasms. Rev. europ. ètud. clin. biol. 15, 841 (1970).
26. HUMPHREY, L. J.: Tumor immunity. J. surg. Res. 10, 493 (1970).

27. KLEIN, G.: Tumor antigens. Ann. Rev. Microbiol. 20, 223 (1966).
28. LACHER, M. J., SUSSMAN, L. N.: Leukemia and Hodgkin's disease. Ann. int. Med. 59, 369 (1963).
29. LANARI, A., RODO, J. E., BARCAT, J. A., MOLINS, M., MORANDO, G. G., AGUERO, M. T., BLANCO, O. L.: Cuatro casos de desarrollo de un cancer del dader en el rinon injertado. Medicina 32, 79 (1972).
30. MEYER, K. K.: Radiation induced lymphocyte immune deficiency: A factor in the increased visceral metastases and decreased hormonal responsiveness of breast cancer. Arch. Surg. 101, 114 (1970).
31. MEYER, K. K., MACKLER, G. L., BECK, W. C.: Increased IgA in women free of recurrence after mastectomy and radiation. Arch. Surg. 107, 159 (1973).
32. MOERTEL, C. G., DOCKERTY, M. B., BAGGENSTOSS, A. H.: Multiple primary malignant neoplasms. I. Introduction and presentation of data. Cancer 14, 221 (1961).
33. MOORE, F. D.: New problems for surgery. Science 144, 388 (1964).
34. NEWMAN, D. R., MALDONADO, J. E., HARRISON, E. G., Jr., KIELY, J. M., LINMAN, J. W.: Myelomonocytic leukemia in Hodgkin's disease. Cancer 25, 128 (1970).
35. OLEINICK, A.: Leukemia or lymphoma occurring subsequent to an auto-immune disease. Blood 29, 144 (1967).
36. PENN, I., HAMMOND, W., BRETTSCHNEIDER, L., STARZL, T. E.: Malignant lymphomas in transplantation patients. Transplant. Proc. 1, 106 (1969).
37. PENN, I.: Malignant Tumors in Organ Transplant Recipients. Berlin, Heidelberg, New York: Springer 1970.
38. PENN, I., HALGRIMSON, C. G., STARZL, T. E.: De novo malignant tumors in organ transplant recipients. Transplant. Proc. 3, 773 (1971).
39. PENN, I., STARZL, T. E.: Malignant tumors arising de novo in immunosuppressed organ transplant recipients. Transplantation 14, 407 (1972).
40. PENN, I., STARZL, T. E.: The effect of immunosuppression on cancer. In: Seventh National Cancer Conference Proceedings, p. 425-436. Philadelphia: Lippincott 1973.
41. PENN, I.: Malignancies in recipients of organ transplants. In: The Role of Immunological Factors in Viral and Oncogenic Processes. Seventh Miles International Symposium. (Eds. BEERS, R. F., jr., TILGHMAN, R. C., BASSETT, E. G.) Baltimore, Maryland, May 31 and June 1, 1973. Johns Hopkins Med. J. 3, 211-221 (1974).
42. PENN, I.: Occurrence of cancer including alimentary tract cancer in immune deficiencies. Cancer 34, 858-866 (1974).
43. PREHN, R. T., MAIN, M. M.: Immunity to methylcholanthrene induced sarcomas. J. nat. Cancer Inst. 18, 769 (1957).
44. RUBINSTEIN, L. J.: Extracranial metastases in cerebellar medulloblastoma. J. path. Bact. 78, 187 (1959).
45. SCHNECK, S. A., PENN, I.: De novo cerebral neoplasms in renal transplant recipients. Lancet 1971 1, 983.
46. SOUTHAM, C. M.: Host defense mechanisms and human cancer. Ann. Inst. Pasteur 107, 585 (1964).
47. SPENCER, E. S., ANDERSEN, H. K.: Clinically evident, non-terminal infections with herpes viruses and the wart virus in immunosuppressed renal allograft recipients. Brit. med. J. 1970 3, 251.
48. STARZL, T. E., PENN, I., PUTNAM, C. W., GROTH, C. G., HALGRIMSON, C. G.: Iatrogenic alterations of immunologic surveillance in man and their influence on malignancy, Transplant. Rev. 7, 112 (1971).
49. STARZL, T. E., GILES, G., LILLY, J. R., TAGAKI, H., MARTINEAU, G., SCHROTER, G., HALGRIMSON, C. G., PENN, I., PUTNAM, C. W.: Indications for orthotopic liver transplantation: With particular reference to hepatomas, biliary atresia, cirrhosis, Wilson's disease and serum hepatitis. Transplant. Proc. 3, 308 (1971).

50. STEINBERG, M. H., GEARY, C. G., CROSBY, W. H.: Acute granulocytic leukemia complicating Hodgkin's disease. Arch. int. Med. 125, 496 (1970).
51. STEVENS, D. A.: Immunosuppression and virus infections. Transplant. Proc. 5, 1259 (1973).
52. STJERNSWÄRD, J., JONDAL, M., VANKY, F., WIGZELL, H., SEALY, R.: Lymphopenia and change in distribution of human B and T lymphocytes in peripheral blood induced by irradiation for mammary carcinoma. Lancet 1972 1, 1352.
53. THIEDE, T., CHRISTENSEN, B. C.: Bladder tumors induced by chlornaphazine. Acta med. Scand. 185, 133 (1969).
54. THOMAS, L.: In: Discussion of MEDAWAR, P. B., Reactions to homologous tissue antigens in relation to hypersensitivity. In: Cellular and Humoral Aspects of the Hypersensitive States (Ed. LAWRENCE, H. S.), p. 530. New York: Paul Hoeber 1959.
55. VAN HOVE, W., HAMERS, J., DEMEULENAERE, L.: Acute leukemia in myeloma. Lancet 1973 2, 570.
56. VIDEBAEK, A.: Chlornaphazine (Erysan(R)) may induce cancer of the urinary bladder. Acta med. scand. 176, 45 (1964).
57. WILLIS, R. A.: The spread of tumours in the human body, p. 100. St. Louis: C. S. Mosby 1952.
58. WILSON, R. E., HAGER, E. B., HAMPERS, C. L., CARSON, J. M., MERRILL, J. P., MURRAY, J. E.: Immunologic rejection of human cancer transplanted with a renal allograft. New Engl. J. Med. 278, 479 (1968).
59. WOODRUFF, M. F. A.: Immunological aspects of cancer. Lancet 1964 2, 265.
60. ZUKOSKI, C. F., KILLEN, D. A., GINN, E., MATTER, B., LUCAS, D. O., SEIGLER, H. F.: Transplanted carcinoma in an immunosuppressed patient. Transplantation 9, 71 (1970).

The Effect of Cytostatic Therapy on Cellular Immunity *in vitro* *

M. Winnewisser, H. Theml, and H. Begemann

INTRODUCTION

At a time when chemotherapy of tumors with combined cytostatic agents is becoming a routine treatment and the range of effectiveness of such therapy is becoming evident as an increasingly large number of patients is treated, we can turn our attention to the body's own immunological surveillance and possible ways of influencing it. With this in mind, it is evident that the problems resulting from drug-induced suppression of cellular and humoral immunity must be taken into consideration as well as the positive therapeutic effect (i.e. tumor regression or stoppage of tumor growth). However, there are as yet no standardized methods for determining the degree of immunosuppression in man and thus facilitating the determination of dosage of the cytostatic agents.

In animal experiments the transformation rate of the small recirculating lymphocytes in vitro is considered to be a good indicator of the level of cellular immunity (1). The responsiveness depends on an intact thymus-dependent mechanism of reaction (2, 3) and can be stimulated nonspecifically with phytohemagglutinin (PHA).

The purpose of this study was to try to determine the effects of cytostatic therapy on the human cellular reaction (4). The degree of stimulation obtained with PHA in vitro was used as the criterion of effectivity.

MATERIALS AND METHODS

Thirteen patients with various malignant solid tumors were selected, who had undergone neither chemical nor radiological treatment and in whom surgical measures were impossible. Sex and age and also kind and size of tumor were disregarded. All patients received a massive dose of a combination therapy consisting of vincablastine sulfate, cyclophosphamide and amethopterine. The dosages were: Velbe[R] 5 - 10 mg; Endoxan[R] 500 mg; Methotrexate[R] 25 - 50 mg. This single massive dose was repeated at intervals of 10 to 21 days.

---

* Supported by grants from the Deutsche Forschungsgemeinschaft.

At regular intervals blood samples were taken, the lymphocytes isolated on Leukopak columns after heparin sedimentation, cultured by Rabinowitz's method (modified by Flad (5)) and then examined for their responsiveness to phytohemagglutinin stimulation (PHA: Wellcome; 0.0025 ml/10^6 lymphocytes). The incorporation rate of tritiated thymidine after 72 hours of culture (1 μCi/ml culture medium and 2 hours of incubation) was used as a measure of the degree of transformation of one million lymphocytes in one sample; this rate was determined by liquid scintillation counting.

The cultures were prepared with Eagle's Minimal Essential Medium (MEM) and unactivated fetal calf serum from Difco; no autologous plasma was used.

RESULTS

The PHA response of lymphocytes from tumor patients (Fig. 1) prior to therapy was lower than that of lymphocytes from healthy controls (shaded area) in 10 of 13 patients; the lymphocytes of the three remaining patients showed "normal" values.

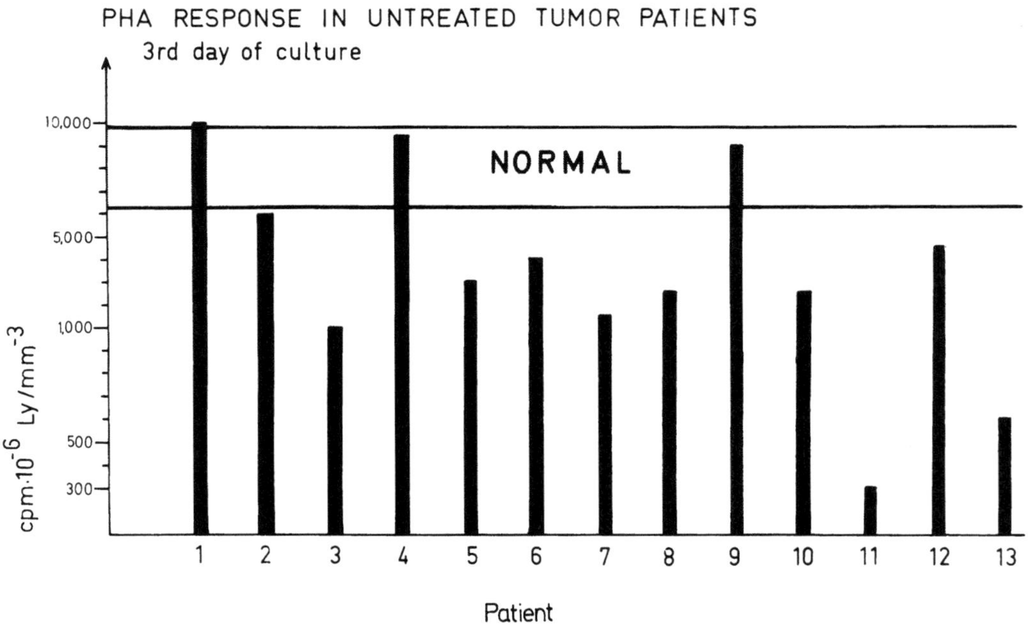

Fig. 1. 1. Bronchial carcinoma with metastasis; 2. Prostate carcinoma with metastasis of bone marrow; 3. Seminoma with metastasis; 4. Mammary carcinoma with metastasis of bone marrow; 5. Bile-duct carcinoma with hepatic metastasis; 6. Mammary carcinoma with metastasis of bone marrow; 7. Hepatic metastasis with unknown primary tumor; 8. Colon carcinoma with metastasis; 9. Sarcoma of the bone marrow with lung metastasis; 10. Primary hepatic carcinoma; 11. Hypernephroma with brain metastasis. 12. Hepatic metastasis with unknown primary tumor; 13. Carcinoma of colon with metastasis

A diminished response to lymphocyte stimulation in tumor patients has been reported by a number of authors (6, 7, 8, 9); there seems to be a direct correlation with the stage of the disease but not with size or kind of tumor.

During cytostatic treatment there was a characteristic change in the rate of response, as shown in Fig. 2 for two of the patients: shortly after administration of the cytostatic agents the capacity for stimulation was depressed for a short time. After some time (between 9 to 35 days after chemotherapy), the depressed responsiveness gave way to an overshoot reaction to PHA as compared with the pretreatment values.

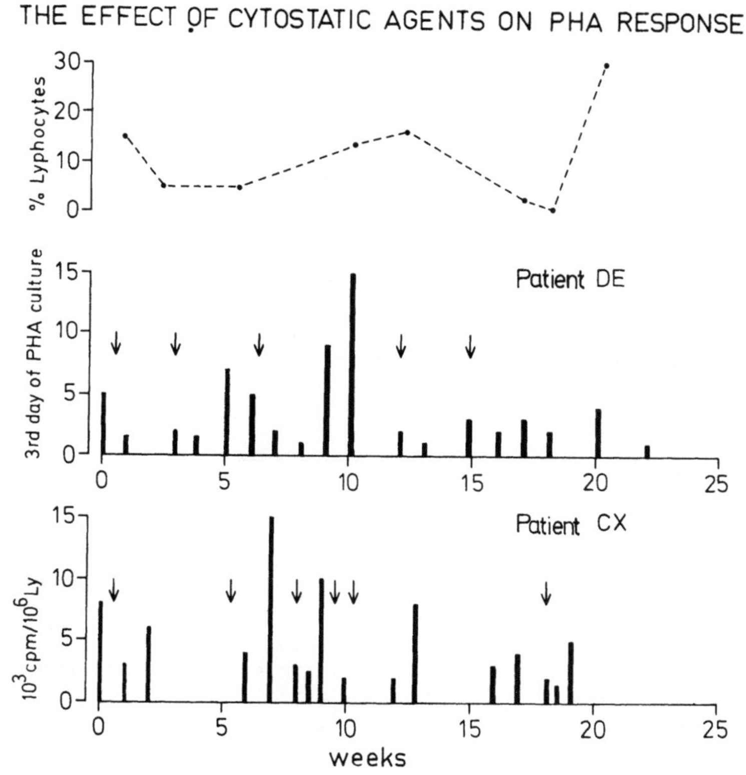

Fig. 2. PHA-induced stimulation of the lymphocytes of two patients during chemotherapy. Drug administration is indicated by an arrow on each occasion. The peripheral lymphocyte count belongs to DE

If the drug combination was repeated at very short intervals this overshoot reaction failed to occur.

This high responsiveness of lymphocytes to antigenic stimulation in vitro not long after chemotherapy was observed by a good number of authors (8, 10, 11, 12, 13). This overshoot can occur after the first dose but can just as well occur first after the second or third dose. The degree of this PHA-induced responsiveness varies, but appears to decrease in the advanced stages of disease, and the associated defect in ability to respond increases. This observation led CHEEMA et al. (4) to employ the degree of this "rebound effect" as a prognostic indicator for patient survival time. No direct correlation with tumor size could be established, at least during the early stages of the disease. A correlation between peripheral lymphocyte count and nucleosid incorporation was determined only after a peripheral lymphopenia of 500 lymphocytes/mm^3 blood was observed.

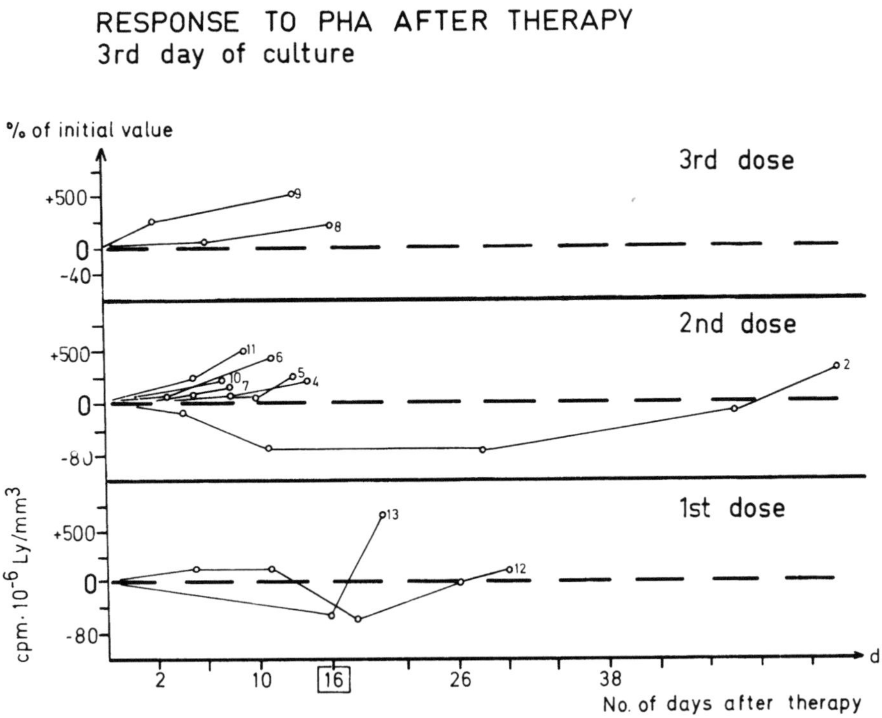

Fig. 3. "Overshoot reaction" after administration of massive dose. The pretreatment value was taken as zero for each patient, and the degree of overshoot is expressed as a percentage of this value. The numbers (2 - 13) indicate patients with different kinds of tumor, as shown in legend to Fig. 1

The relationship between drug administration and rebound effect over time is shown in Fig. 3: for each patient the pretreatment value was taken as zero and the degree of overshoot expressed as a percentage of this value. The appearance of this rebound phenomenon was observed between days 4 and 21 after drug administration, the mean being day 16.

The three patients whose initial levels of lymphocyte responsiveness were "normal" showed no overshoot reaction to PHA stimulation during therapy; they "only" reached subnormal to normal values (Fig. 4).

DISCUSSION

We have attempted to find an explanation for the impaired responsiveness *per se* in most of the tumor patients and the "rebound effect" in nearly all of the patients some time after administration of cytostatic drugs.

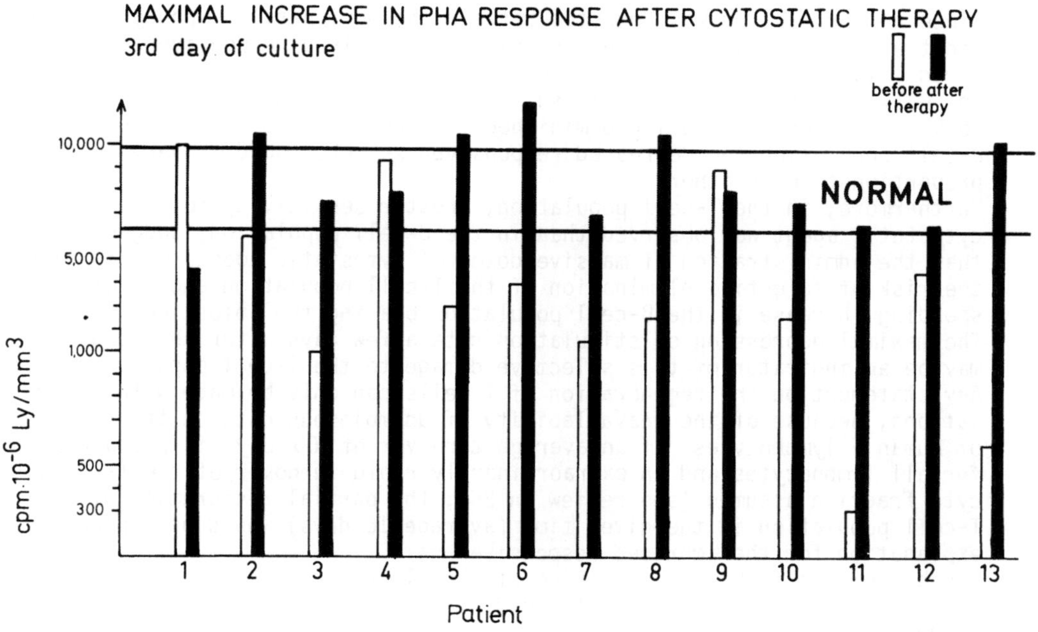

Fig. 4. Each of the numbers 1 - 13 represents a patient with a different kind of tumor, as shown in legend to Fig. 1

It is known that the PHA-induced transformation in vitro reflects the non-specific cellular immunity. Three possible explanations for the impaired response to PHA are under discussion:

1. Many authors (6, 15, 16, 17, 18) assume that patiens with tumors have some factor in their plasma which has a depressive effect on responsiveness to PHA, PPD or tuberculine. We tried to eliminate this factor by washing the cells several times and using only fetal calf serum and no autologous plasma in preparing the cultures.

2. Also to be considered are the so-called "blocking factors" of a tumor, which may be capable of blocking all the antigenic sensitive receptors on the surface of the lymphocytes (19). This "coating effect" (20) may also be directed against tumor-specific antigenic receptors. The literature includes a number of reports indicating that after surgical removal of a tumor the level of antigen-induced stimulation of lymphocytes in vitro is higher (9, 21, 22, 23).
   It is also conceivable that the tumor causes an abnormal change in the "intrinsic factor" and that this affects the ability of PHA to induce the formation of messenger RNA (18, 24).

3. Another possibility under discussion is whether a change in the cell population caused by the tumor might be responsible for the impaired responsiveness to PHA.
   The ability to respond to PHA stimulation is very characteristic of the thymus-dependent T-lymphocyte population but has not as yet been observed in bone marrow-dependent B lymphocytes (2, 3).

Since no correlation was detected between the peripheral lymphocyte count and the degree of stimulation, the cause of impaired responsiveness may be a reduction in the proportion of PHA-sensitive lymphocytes as compared to the B lymphocytes. This view is supported by STJERNSWÄRD's study (25) on leukemic children, in which diminished T-lymphocyte population, increased B-cell population and decreased responsiveness were found to vary in direct proportion to each other.
Furthermore, in the T-cell population, greater sensitivity to x-rays and cytostatic agent was observed than in the B-cell population, suggesting that the administration of massive doses of cytostatic agents may involve the risk of selective elimination of the T-cell population and a corresponding increase in the B-cell population bearing the "blocking factors." The maximal depression of stimulation rate a few days after chemotherapy may be an indicator of this selective damage to the T-cell population.
Any statement on the regeneration of T cells can only be made with reservations, because of the unavailability of unambiguous data on the turnover of human T lymphocytes. If an average turnover of 60 days is postulated for all lymphocytes and an extraordinarily rapid turnover of the T-lymphocyte fraction assumed (see review in 26), the partial restoration of the T-cell population in the given time (average 16 days) would be a plausible explanation for the improved responsiveness.
Furthermore, a temporary unmasking of the blocked antigen-sensitive receptors by the cytostatic agent could be responsible for increased responsiveness.

The absence of the rebound phenomenon when the dosage of the cytostatic drug is too massive has great significance for practicing physicians. Therefore we suggest that the administration of cytostatic drugs be governed by the appearance of the "overshoot response" to PHA, in order to reduce the damage to the cellular immunity mechanism to a minimum and thus to encourage the body's own immunological surveillance. The same data also indicate the optimal timing for the use of active immunotherapy (specific or nonspecific) during a phase of increased susceptibility to immunization.

REFERENCES

1. MILLS, J. A.: Immunol. 97, 239 (1966).
2. JANOSSY, G., GREAVES, M. F.: Clin. exp. Immun. 9, 483 (1971).
3. ROITT, J. M., GREAVES, M. F., TORRIGIANI, G., BROSTOFF, J., PLAYFAIR, J. H. L.: Lancet 1973 2, 1254.
4. BEGEMANN, H., THEML. H., WINNEWISSER, M.: Verh. dtsch. Ges. inn. Med. 78, 112 (1972).
5. FLAD, H. D., HOCHAPFEL, G., FLIEDNER, T. M., HEIMPEL, H.: Acta haemat. 44, 21 (1970).
6. GARRIOCH, D. B., GOOD, R. A., GATTI, R. A.: Lancet 1971 1, 892.
7. NAGEL, G. A.: Schweiz. med. Wschr. 101, 13: 470 (1971).
8. HERSH, E. M., OPPENHEIM, J. J.: Cancer Res. 27, 98 (1967).
9. WATKINS, S. M.: Lancet 1973 2, 1254.
10. MAKINODAN, T., SANTOS, G. W., QUINN, R. P.: Pharmacol. Res. 22, 189 (1970).
11. TALIAFERRO, W. H., TALIAFERRO, L. G.: J. infect. Dis. 95, 134 (1954).
12. MERRIT, K., JOHNSON, A. G.: Proc. Soc. exp. Biol. (N. Y.) 115, 1132 (1964).
13. BORELLA, L., GREEN, A. A., WELSTER, R. G.: Blood 40, 47 (1972).
14. CHEEMA, A. R., HERSH, E. M.: Cancer 28, 851 (1971).

15. WHITTAKER, M. G., REES, K., CLARK, C. G.: Lancet 1971 1, 892.
16. SILK, M.: Cancer 20, 2088 (1967).
17. SAMPLE, F. W., GERTNER, H. R., CHRETIEN, P. B.: J. nat. Cancer Inst. 46, 1291 (1971).
18. AL-SARRAF, M., VAITKEVIEINS, V. K.: Lancet 1971 2, 314.
19. KOHOUT, J., SCHNETZ, E.: Med. Klin. 2, 43 (1973).
20. STJERNSWÄRD, J.: J. nat. Cancer Inst. 40, 13 (1968).
21. KLEIN, G., SJÖGREN, H. O., KLEIN, E., HELLSTRÖM, K. E.: Cancer Res. 20, 1561 (1960).
22. STJERNSWÄRD, J., CLIFFORD, P., SING, S., SVEDMYR, E.: E. Afr. Med. J. 45, 7, 484 (1968).
23. MARROW, R. H., PIKE, M. C., KISIUDE, A.: Brit. med. J. 1967 4, 323.
24. COOPER, H. L., RUBIN, A. D.: Science 152, 516 (1966).
25. STJERNSWÄRD, A. J., ROWFOUD, G. F., LEE, M. R.: Lancet 1972 1, 687.
26. TREPEL, F.: In Der Lymphozyt, p. 127. Vienna: Pietschmann 1972.

The Balance of Host Immunocompetence in Chemical Carcinogenesis and "Nonspecific" Immunotherapy *

M. G. Hanna, jr., A. K. Szakal, and L. C. Peters

INTRODUCTION

The recognition that host immunocompetence can limit the development of malignant clones has arisen both from teliologic arguments and from data derived from investigations in experimental systems. Several familiar correlations have been cited as evidence for the role of immunosurveillance in cancer, such as the variability in tumor incidence that accompanies age-associated changes in immunocompetence, the increased tumor incidence associated with chronic or induced immune deficiencies, and the general suppression of immunity to alloantigens during treatment with certain chemical carcinogens.

In addition, there is some clinical evidence of tumor-reactive host immunologic factors. This includes histologic evidence of immunologic reactivity to tumors, in the form of perivascular infiltration and regional lymph node response (1-3); reports of spontaneous regressions (4, 5); correlations of skin reactivity with metastases (6); and the demonstration that in some leukemic patients with good tumor response delayed hypersensitivity responses convert from negative to positive during chemotherapy, whereas in a number of unresponsive patients they are converted from positive to negative (7). These reports, plus the reproducible detection in vitro, and occasionally in vivo, of a range of host immunity to autochthonous tumors (8-11), currently strengthen the conclusion that malignancies are not autonomous in their growth, and that immune components are among the primary tumor-limiting host factors. Most of the evidence, however, suggests that the immune system affects the latency but not the total incidence of tumors.

At present, the major questions concern the ability of antigenic tumors to develop and the nature of the immune status of the host against its own primary tumor. Reasonable estimates are that not more than 5% of human cancer can be associated with viruses and less than 5% with radiation. On the other hand, an increasing percentage of spontaneous cancers in man, especially lung cancers, can be associated with environmental factors, presumably in the form of chemical carcinogens (12). Thus, information about the success of antigenic tumors should continue to be developed from models based on chemical carcinogenesis. In the past, only a few histologic types of tumors and carcinogenic agents have been utilized in such studies; however, variability of antigenic

* Research jointly sponsored by the National Cancer Institute and the U. S. Atomic Energy Commission under contract with the Union Carbide Corporation.

expression on chemically induced tumors has been demonstrated. Results have suggested that some chemically induced tumors are deficient in tumor-associated rejection antigens, and it has been shown that tumors can vary at their inception from weakly to highly antigenic, and that there is an inverse relationship between latency and antigenicity (13, 14). This variability in antigenicity is important for models of tumor immunology in experiments concerned with the host's immunologic reactivity to its own primary tumor, where the questions of "immune escape" and immunoselective pressures are to be evaluated. On a random basis, mutations that affect antigenicity are to be expected; thus, studies of factors that influence tumor antigenicity either qualitatively or quantitatively and studies of the immune response of the host may form the basis for knowledge of how antigenic neoplastic cells escape the host defense mechanism.

Operationally, the information that is available has been and will continue to be utilized in attempts to augment the host response to achieve abatement of the neoplastic process. The potential methods of specific and nonspecific tumor immunotherapy and their history have recently been reviewed (15). Clinically these procedures have been problematic, especially when attempts have been made to increase immunologic reactivity in a nonspecific manner with biologic agents known to stimulate the reticuloendothelial system. In individuals with established tumors, the success of this mode of therapy depends on the stage, type and location of the tumor, the level of antigenicity of the target cells, the status of the host's immune response to the tumor, and the particular immunostimulant used. Thus, investigations of relevant carcinogenesis and immunotherapy models are still needed, so that progressive tumor growth can be correlated with the interaction of these immunologic factors.

This article describes our recent attempts to characterize the balance between host immunologic factors and progressive tumor growth in hamsters treated with chemical carcinogens (16, 17) and in inbred guinea pigs treated first with a transplantable syngeneic hepatocarcinoma and then with Mycobacterium bovis (BCG) as an immunostimulant capable of producing tumor regression (18-22). Although these models have their limitations, they include a number of the variables required for an adequate evaluation of the question of immunologic status and tumor progression. The results, while incomplete and possibly fragmentary, indicate the complexities of the overall problem and provide an impetus for further experimentation, with the eventual aim of translation to cancer patients.

IMMUNOLOGIC REACTIVITY OF HAMSTERS TO ALLOANTIGENS AND TUMOR ANTIGENS OF ISOLOGOUS AND AUTOCHTHONOUS ORIGIN DURING CHEMICAL CARCINOGENESIS

Male Syrian Cr:RGH hamsters (Sprague-Dawley) 4 to 5 weeks old were used for these studies. Animals were treated with 7,12-dimethylbenz(a)anthracene (DMBA) on approximately a 2-mm^2 area of skin posterior to the right shoulder after the hair had been clipped. The chronic DMBA treatment consisted of topical application of 250 µg of DMBA in 25 µl of acetone twice weekly for 86 days. Treatment with acetone alone did not produce tumors or any detectable changes in the skin. The total number of treatments was 25 unless otherwise indicated.

Correlation of Tumor Incidence and Immune Suppression

Regional and systemic humoral immune competence were assayed by subcutaneous (s.c.) and intraperitoneal (i.p.) injection of sheep erythrocytes (SRBC) in

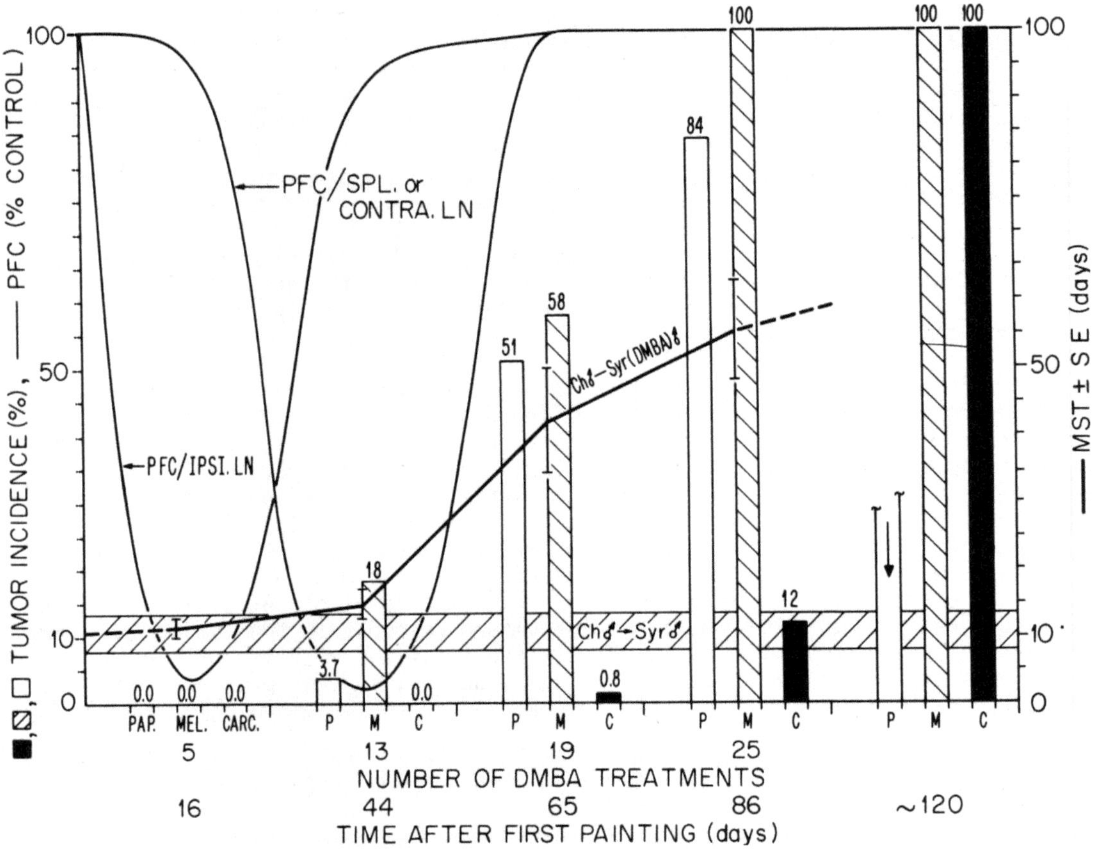

Fig. 1. Correlation of the sequential depression of regional and systemic humoral immunity with allograft mean survival time (±S. E.) and the latency and incidence of papillomas, melanotic lesions, and carcinomas in DMBA-treated hamsters. IPSI: ipsilateral (DMBA-treated side); CONTRA: contralateral (untreated side); SPL: spleen; LN: lymph node; Ch: Chinese hamster donor; Syr: Syrian hamster recipients; P(PAP): papilloma; M(MEL): melanotic lesion; and C(CARC): carcinoma

Fig. 2. Micrographs illustrating DMBA-mediated changes in the cellularity ➔ of the splenic white pulp and the simultaneous pathologic changes in DMBA-treated skin. (a) Reduced white pulp after disappearance of germinal center (5 DMBA treatments). X 150. (b) Remnants of white pulp at maximal depression of anti-SRBC PFC response (13 DMBA treatments). X 25. (c) White pulp with germinal centers after recovery of humoral immunocompetence (19 DMBA treatments). X 150. (d) Hyperplastic, hyperkeratinized epidermis with focal lymphocytic infiltration (5 DMBA treatments). X 250. (e) Section of a typical papilloma (13 DMBA treatments). X 25. (f) Part of a typical DMBA-induced squamous cell carcinoma (19 DMBA treatments). X 250

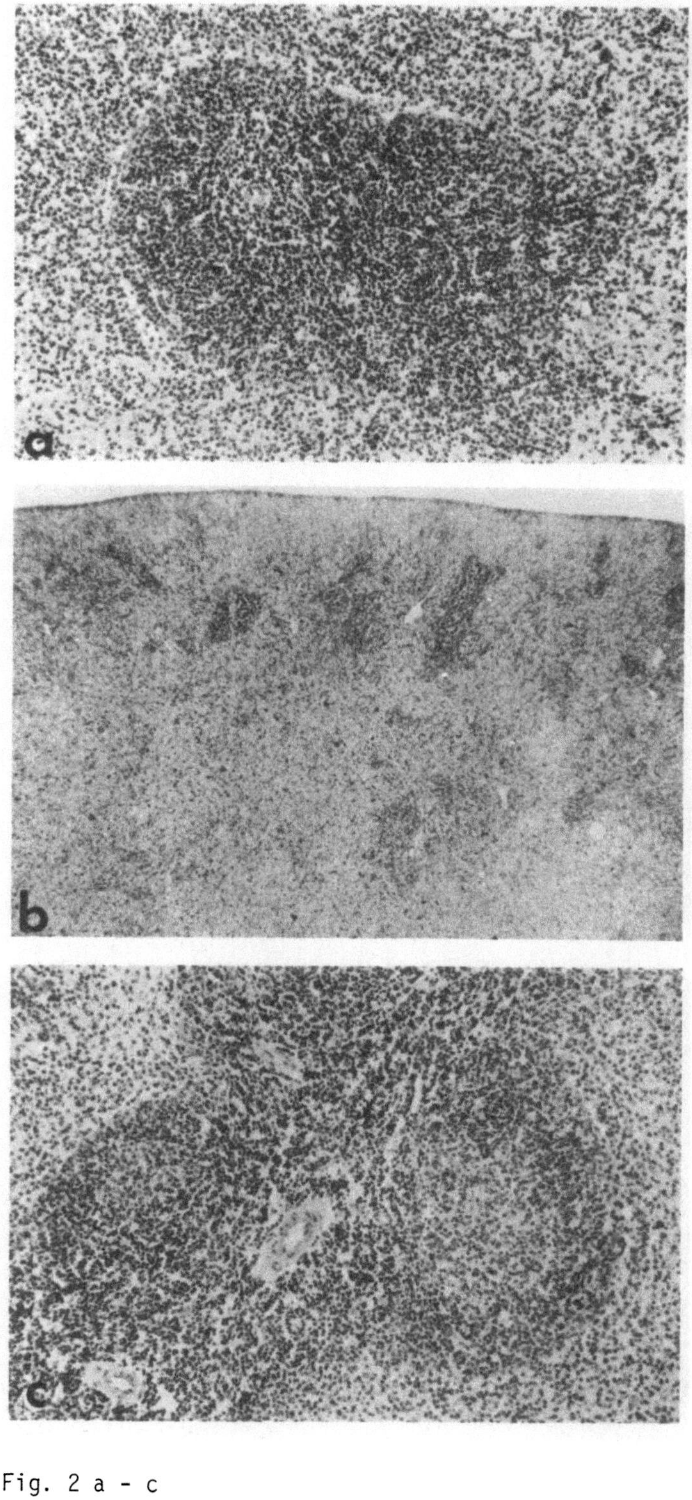

Fig. 2 a - c

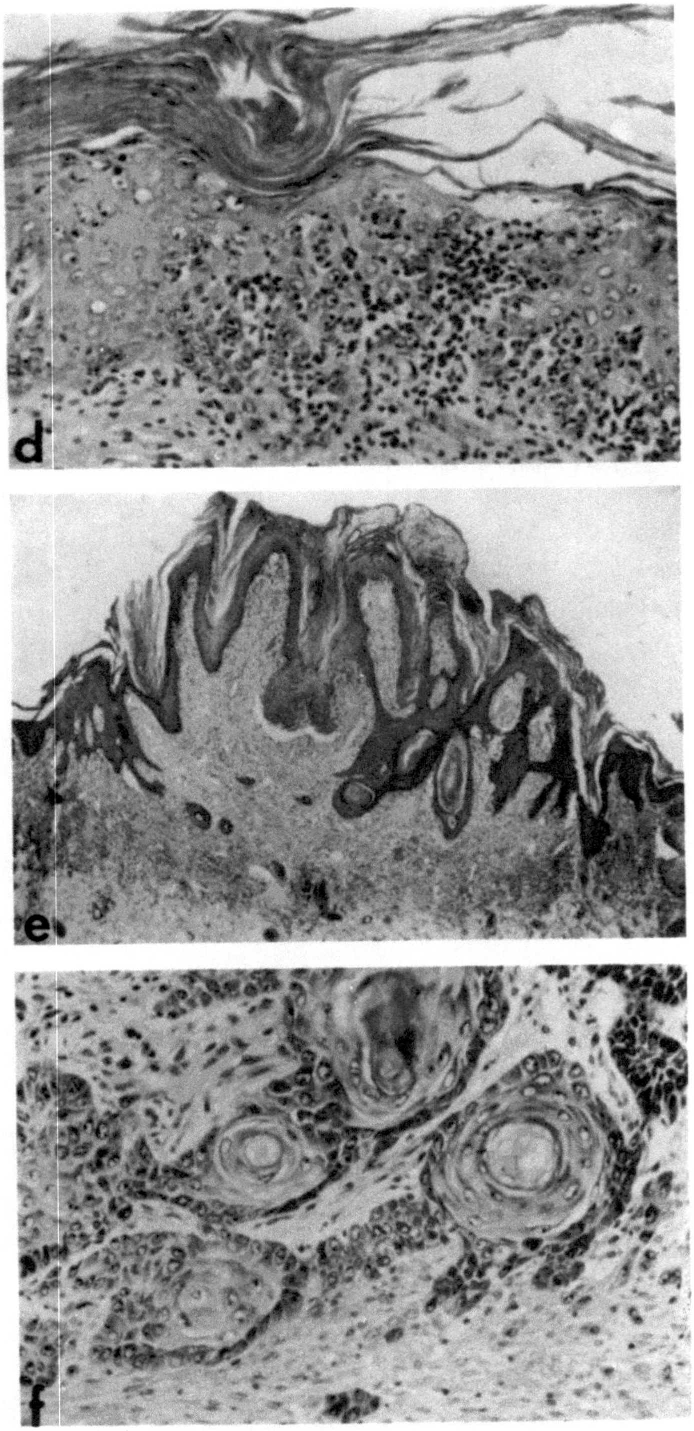

Fig. 2 d - f

animals treated 5, 13, 19, or 25 times with DMBA. Regional and contralateral nodes, and also spleens, were measured for direct plaque-forming cells by the hemolysin plaque-forming assay 5 days after immunization. Cell-mediated immunity was assayed as percentage rejection and mean survival time of Chinese hamster allografts, and the total data for immune competence were compared with the development of tumors in the DMBA-treated hamsters (Fig.1).

Depression of regional humoral immunity in the ipsilateral distal axillary lymph nodes was evident after the fifth DMBA treatment and preceded the appearance of the first skin lesion. Papillomas and melanotic lesions became grossly detectable by the thirteenth DMBA treatment, when depression of humoral immunity in the spleen was maximal. During the recovery phase of systemic humoral immunity (between the thirteenth and nineteenth DMBA treatments), the incidence of papillomas and melanotic lesions increased exponentially. By the nineteenth DMBA treatment, when the development of cellular immunity first became significant, carcinomas were first detected. Carcinoma development paralleled depression of cell-mediated immunity. Thus, a temporal relationship between a transient depression of humoral immunity and papilloma latency, and a direct correlation between the subsequent suppression of cell-mediated immune competence and carcinoma latency were observed in these studies. Histologic changes in the spleen and lymph nodes during the course of DMBA treatment correlated well with the functional assay of immunomodulation in these animals (Fig. 2).

Since cell-mediated immunity is considered to be the more important host response against neoplasia, we further examined its temporal relationship to DMBA treatment and papilloma and carcinoma development. The results of a second experiment, in which allografts were used to study cell-mediated immune competence, again showed that suppression of this component of immunity occurred after papilloma development. To a certain extent the suppression depended on carcinogen dose. However, after the administration of an optimal dose of carcinogen (13 treatments), followed by a considerable period of time without further treatment, suppression of cell-mediated immunity still could be detected (Table 1). The degree of immune suppression was directly proportional to the tumor burden of recipients; it increased with the number of papillomas and was most pronounced in animals with carcinomas.

It appears from these observations that tumor burden, as well as dose of carcinogen, is a decisive factor in the depression of cell-mediated immunity as measured by allograft rejections. Similar conclusions have been considered by other investigators (23, 24). It is also possible that the highly immunogenic allografts used in this study were not suitable for assay of a low-grade, early depression in cell-mediated immunity, which might well be sufficient to support the establishment of induced neoplastic clones. For this reason we tested the cell-mediated immune competence of DMBA-treated recipients of DMBA-pretreated isografts and autografts presumed and known to possess tumor-related antigens.

Carcinogen-Induced Immune Suppression as Measured Against Neoantigens of Isologous and Autochthonous Origin

In these experiments, carcinogen-pretreated skin (19 DMBA treatments) with an average of three papillomas was transplanted onto normal recipients pretreated with antihamster thymocyte serum (ATS) prepared in rabbits, and also onto DMBA-treated (25 treatments) recipients. Three parameters were studied as functions

Table 1. Allograft survival time as a function of time and tumor burden on DMBA-treated hamsters

No. of DMBA treatments of recipients	Day of grafting after the first DMBA treatment of recipients[a]							
	23		52		72		93	
	No. of lesions/group[b]	Survival time[c]	No. of lesions/group[b]	Survival time[c]	No. of. lesions/group[b]	Survival time[c]	No. of lesions/group[b]	Survival time[c]
5	0/5	15 ± 2					0/5	14 ± 2
13			9p/5	13 ± 1			8p/3 1c/1	16 ± 1 46
19					15p/5	23 ± 1	24p/4 1p; 1c/1	35 ± 8 34
25							14p/2 11p; 1c/1 5p; 1c/1	31 ± 2 43 43

[a] Time required for a given number of treatments applied twice weekly plus time between last treatment and grafting.

[b] DMBA-induced lesions present at the time of grafting (p, papilloma; c, carcinoma).

[c] Mean no. of days ± S. E., or actual no. of days.

of immunologic competence of the recipients: (a) number of grafts rejected, (b) graft survival time, and (c) rate of change in mean graft area. The latter is considered to be a reasonable parameter for assessment of carcinogen-mediated toxicity on graft survival, as a reflection of the observable contraction and in some cases early focal ulceration of grafts. For example, if focal ulceration of DMBA-treated skin grafts resulting from carcinogen toxicity, is a major factor in graft rejection, area measurements of grafts on immunologically depressed and normal recipients should be comparable. The immunologic competence of the recipients was further monitored with Chinese hamster skin allografts. The results are shown in Table 2 and Fig. 3. The increased allograft survival times indicated a 2- to 3-fold decrease in cell-mediated immune competence of ATS- and DMBA-treated recipients. The increased percentage and time of survival of DMBA-treated, papilloma-bearing isografts on these immunologically depressed recipients support the role of immunity in the rejection of the grafts. This conclusion was further substantiated by the significant difference in the rate of reduction of mean graft area between the immunologically competent groups and those in which the immune response was depressed (Fig. 3). Although the decline in mean graft area followed the same pattern in ATS- and DMBA-treated groups, it was delayed in the DMBA-treated animals during the period of graft healing (day 0 to day 10). This may have been due to the longer pretreatment of recipients with DMBA than with ATS. In addition, surviving grafts in both groups had a tendency to develop carcinomas after longer time intervals. Furthermore, since DMBA-pretreated isografts were always grafted at least 1 week after the last carcinogen treatment, and since the shortest mean survival times exceeded 30 days, the role of toxicity in the chronic rejection of the isografts was apparently minimal.

Table 2. Effects of immunosuppressive pretreatment of Syrian hamster recipients on the survival of skin grafts from Chinese hamsters (allografts) and Syrian hamsters (isografts)

Grafts		Recipients		Graft rejection	
Type	Pretreatment	No.	Pretreatment	%	Survival time[a]
Allograft	None	12[b]	None	100	13 ± 3
Allograft	None	5	ATS	100	28 ± 3
Allograft	None	5	DMBA (25X)	100	37 ± 4
Isograft	None	25[c]	None	0	200
Isograft	DMBA (19X)	5	None	100	44 ± 6
Isograft	DMBA (19X)	5	ATS	60	70 ± 15
Isograft	DMBA (19X)	5	DMBA (25X)	40	58 ± 3
Isograft	DMBA (19X)	8	DMBA (25X)	20	65 ± 5

[a]Mean no. of days ±S. E.

[b]Data pooled from three experiments.

[c]Data pooled from five experiments.

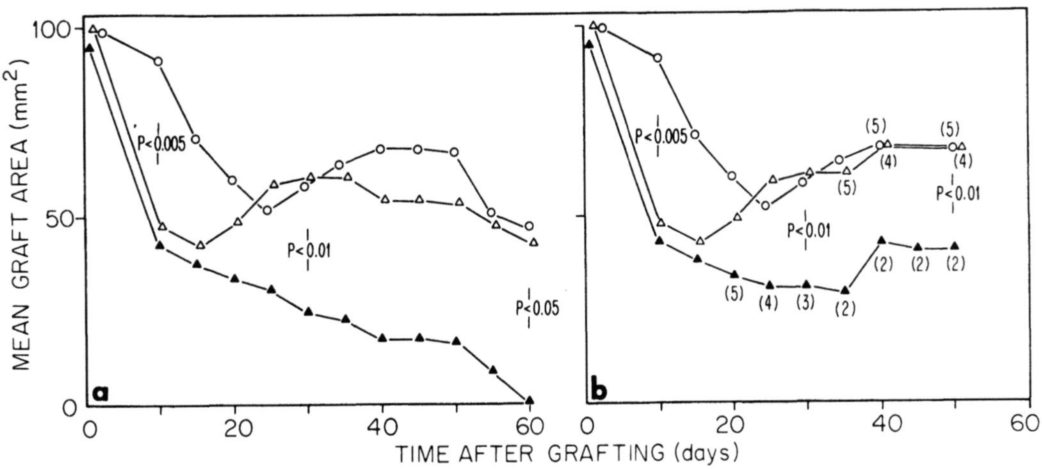

Fig. 3. Decline in surface area of papilloma-bearing (after 19 DMBA pretreatments) isografts on normal and immunosuppressed Syrian hamster recipients. (The efficacy of immunosuppressive treatments was tested with Chinese hamster allografts, and histocompatibility was tested with untreated isografts (Table 2).) ▲: no treatment of recipients; △: ATS pretreatment; ○: 25 DBMA pretreatments (see the corresponding groups in Table 2). Reduction in mean graft area was plotted with (a) and without (b) consideration of rejected grafts. Significance was calculated according to the Student's t-test

Table 3. Fate of DMBA-pretreated contralateral autografts[a]

No. of DMBA treatments of animals	No. of animals per group	Graft rejection %	Survival time[b]	Tumor incidence of grafts[c] p	c
5	5	0		0	0
11	6	50	35 ± 3	0	0
13	5	60	84 ± 3	80	20
19	7	57	72 ± 10	72	43
25	17[d]	76	57 ± 10	59	24

[a]Skin from animals pretreated 5 to 11 times was hyperplastic, and skin pretreated 13, 19, or 25 times had an average of 2, 3, and 4 papillomas, respectively, at the time of grafting.

[b]Mean no. of days ± S. E.

[c]p, papilloma; c, carcinoma.

[d]Data pooled from three experiments.

To study the immune response of carcinogen-pretreated hamsters to autologous neoantigens of DMBA-induced neoplastic clones, skin from the central area of carcinogen treatment was transplanted contralaterally. The immune responses to hyperplastic skin (5 to 11 DMBA pretreatments) and papilloma-bearing skin (13 to 25 DMBA pretreatments) were also evaluated in terms of rejection and tumor incidence of autografts (Table 3).

There was a direct correlation between the percentage of autograft rejection and the increasing immunogenicity of the skin (i.e. increase in the number of papillomas). However, the expected increase in the number of surviving autografts as a function of the number of carcinogen treatments, which was characteristic of pretreated isografts, was not observed in these autograft experiments. From the percentages of allograft and isograft rejection, as well as the mean survival time of the grafts, the cell-mediated immune competence of recipients treated 19 to 25 times with DMBA was expected to be approximately 30 to 40% of normal; yet 76% of the treated, papilloma-bearing autografts were rejected. These discrepant results indicate that prolonged DMBA treatment, while appreciably affecting cell-mediated immune response to isografts and allografts, did not have as appreciable an effect on cell-mediated immune competence in hamsters against DMBA-induced autologous neoantigens.

We recognize that these data are not entirely unique, and that suppression of humoral and cell-mediated immunity to alloantigens during chemical carcinogenesis in experimental models is a well-described phenomenon. We would only emphasize that rather than generalized immune suppression we have detected immunomodulation exemplified by a transient suppression of local and systemic humoral immunity, followed by a more persistent suppression of cell-mediated immunity. In addition, our data suggest that while the depression of cell-mediated immunity, as measured by allograft survival, correlates with carcinogen dose, it is also influenced by the primary tumor mass, i.e., when allografts are performed 20 to 40 days after the last carcinogen treatment, there is a tendency for survival times to be longer in animals with increased tumor burden.

DMBA-pretreated hyperplastic or papilloma-bearing skin grafts had different fates on isologous and autologous recipients. In general, a larger proportion of isografts survived for a longer period of time than similar autografts. When the number of DMBA pretreatments and the tumor incidence of the recipients were increased, the survival and tumor incidence of isografts also increased. Thus, as for allografts, the fate of isografts may be influenced by the tumor burden of the recipients. The survival and tumor incidence of autografts was, however, inversely proportional to the number of DMBA pretreatments of the host. The main difference between these groups was that in the case of isografts the recipients responded to neoantigens to which the recipient had not been exposed, while in the case of autografts the response was to autochthonous neoantigens. From the difference in host response to these grafts, it follows that the available pool of immunologically committed cells may be a limiting factor in the response against isologous neoantigens. In the situation where primary tumor burden of the recipient influences survival time of allografts, competition for uncommitted immunologically competent cells may also be involved.

The specific host response to autochthonous tumors and the competition between emerging neoplastic clones of different antigenicities, interpreted in the light of these experiments, indicates an active rather than a passive role of host immunity in chemical carcinogenesis. An active immunologic response is compatible with the demonstrated phenomenon of concomitant and sincomitant immunity. The depressed immune response of carcinogen-treated recipients to non-tumor-related test antigens and to induced neoantigens and isografts is apparently a function not only of carcinogen-mediated immune suppression but also of antigenic competition with induced neoantigens of the host.

Conclusion

These studies indicate that DMBA-treated animals are able to recognize and reject autochthonous DMBA-treated skin during the early hyperplastic and/or papilloma stage. From the results of studies by MARIANI et al. (25) on the rejection of syngeneic skin grafts containing tumor cells by animals with leukemia, one could assume that the skin is rejected as an "innocent bystander" and that the emerging neoplastic clones are the prime target in the rejection mechanism. Certainly the only equation of the rejection of the treated skin graft to the in situ primary tumor is that there is recognition of and cell-mediated immune reactivity to the emerging neoplastic clones.

We performed further in vitro lymphocyte cytotoxicity tests, using tissue from autochthonous induced carcinomas as target cells and host lymphocytes as effector cells. The data indicate that lymphocyte toxicity existed in animals with small established carcinomas but diminished as the tumors enlarged. These results are compatible with studies demonstrating a reduced lymphocyte response in the presence of increased tumor antigenicity (26) and "blocking factors" in the form of antigen-antibody complexes (27); nevertheless, during some period of tumor development and establishment in the host, a functional, specific immunity exists. The major question that remains is the "success" of the developing tumor in the light of this specific immunocompetence. Certainly one reason for the escape of the in-situ tumor may be a quantitative limitation of the immune competence to the tumor. It is possible that tumor growth normally precedes the development of specific cell-mediated immunity to a degree that constantly favors the tumor system. In addition, it has been pointed out by others that the success of antigenic tumors may be a result of anatomic factors which limit the full expression of the effector arms of the immune system (28).

Experimental models suggest that quantitative and/or anatomic limitations of immune responsiveness to developing tumors can be overcome by treatment with nonspecific immunostimulants. Mycobacterium bovis (BCG), a potent immunostimulant, has been shown to improve host immune response to a variety of antigens. Single BCG vaccinations in experimental animals have resulted in enhanced humoral immunity (29), increased antigen clearance and degradation by phagocytosis (30), heightened resistance to bacterial and viral infections (31), and accelerated homograft reactivity (32, 33). With respect to the latter, there is an extensive literature relevant to the use of BCG or fractions thereof as a nonspecific stimulant of resistance to isogeneic and autochthonous tumors (for review see reference 34). Also, recent studies of a transplantable syngeneic hepatocarcinoma in inbred guinea pigs have shown that intralesional injection with BCG produces regression of established tumors of limited size and of regional lymph node metastases. As a result, "systemic adjuvant therapy" protocols have been initiated to enhance the host response to cancer in man by repeated dermal scarification with BCG (35-38). Also, some attempts at intralesional injection or topical challenge with BCG have been performed, mainly for a limited variety of skin cancers and for some dermal metastatic tumors (39-41). Some of our preliminary studies are relevant and pertinent to this investigational mode of immunotherapy.

MODULATION OF THE IMMUNOCOMPETENCE OF GUINEA PIGS BY REPEATED DERMAL SCARIFICATION WITH BCG[1]

It was felt that it was important to determine what alterations in immune competence would be induced by repeated BCG scarification in outbred and inbred guinea pigs. Most of the earlier studies with immunostimulants have been performed in mice and have usually involved single immunization by intravenous, intraperitoneal, subcutaneous, or intradermal routes. Our studies were performed primarily to determine whether repeated scarification of guinea pigs would result in functional alterations of immunity similar to those demonstrated by single challenges through conventional routes of administration.

Both random-bred male Carworth Farm Duncan-Hartley (CFDH) and inbred guinea pigs (Sewall-Wright strain 2) were used in our studies. The BCG was Tice strain vaccine, lyophilized and reconstituted in water to 1 ml. Viable counts determined by surface growth demonstrated that there were 2 to 4 X 10^8 viable organisms per ml. The scarifications were performed on areas clipped free of hair, cleansed with acetone, and air-dried. Five parallel and five perpendicular scratches approximately 1.5 cm in length were made onto the skin with a 19-gauge needle, with sufficient pressure to cause slight oozing of blood. Dilutions of the BCG were prepared so that approximately 5 X 10^7 viable organisms were applied in 0.1 ml over the freshly scratched areas. One scarification per week for 6 or 8 weeks was performed posterior to the right and left shoulder and anterior to the left and right hip, in that order.

Humoral Immune Capacity to SRBC

Three random-bred guinea pigs were injected i.p. with 1 ml of a 10% suspension of SRBC 24 hours after each scarification and were bled from the foot vein 6 days after scarification. Results of hemagglutinin titers are shown in Table 4. After the second scarification a slight increase in antibody and after the fourth scarification a significant decrease in mean hemagglutinin titer were detected. The mean hemagglutinin titer after the sixth scarification was less than 25% of normal.

Similar studies were performed in inbred strain-2 guinea pigs (Table 4). After the second and fifth scarification with BCG, hemagglutinin titers were compared to those of sham-scarified guinea pigs. The strain-2 guinea pigs demonstrated a lower humoral immune capacity to the 10% SRBC suspension than that of the CFDH random-bred guinea pigs. A mean peak titer measured in the sham-scarified strain-2 controls was 3 $\log_2$ units, achieved at 11 days after immunization, compared to a mean peak titer of 5.4 $\log_2$ units, achieved 6 days after immunization, in the random-bred guinea pigs. However, the most interesting indication that humoral immune competence was suppressed as a result of BCG scarification was detected in the strain-2 guinea pigs. Eleven days after immunization, six out of six control animals showed a response, compared to only one out of six after the second BCG scarification. After five BCG scarifications no responders were detected, whereas six out of six responders with normal antibody levels were detected in the control group. These

[1] These studies were performed in collaboration with Drs. J. Gutterman and E. M. Hersh of the M. D. Anderson Hospital and Tumor Institute, Houston, Texas.

results demonstrate that routine scarification with Tice BCG preparations under some circumstances suppresses humoral immune competence to alloantigens.

Table 4. Humoral and cell-mediated immune competence after repeated dermal scarification with BCG

Number of BCG scarifications	Mean hemagglutinin titer to SRBC in CFDH guinea pigs	SRBC responders/ total no. of strain-2 guinea pigs	Rejection time of strain-2 skin grafts (Mean no. days ± S.E.)
1	4.8 ± 0.7		13.3 ± 0.7
2	6.3 ± 0.7	1/6	12.0 ± 0.0
3	6.0 ± 0		
4	3.3 ± 0.7		9.0 ± 1.0
5	2.7 ± 1.2	0/6	
6	4.0 ± 0		8.8 ± 0.7
7			
8			8.0 ± 0.7
Control	5.4 ± 0.6	6/6	13.3 ± 0.41

Rejection of Allografts and Syngeneic Tumors

The results of strain-2 full-body skin allografts on CFDH guinea pigs after one, two, four, six, and eight scarifications are also shown in Table 4. The mean rejection time in the controls was 13.3 days; in BCG-scarified guinea pigs the rejection time decreased to 9.5 days after the fourth scarification and was approximately 8 days after the sixth and eighth scarifications. The scarification resulted in a 30% decrease in allograft survival time.

A further test of cell-mediated immune competence after BCG scarification was the measurement of survival times and papule sizes of intradermally transplanted syngeneic line-1 hepatocarcinomas in strain-2 guinea pigs. As shown in Table 5, the mean papule size was approximately 50 mm^2 at 13 days both in the controls and in animals that received two BCG scarifications, but in animals that received six scarifications the papules were significantly smaller. It must also be pointed out that in the latter group detectable intradermal tumors developed in only three of the six challenged animals. Thus it is clear that antigenic line-1 hepatocarcinoma is rejected more rapidly in strain-2 guinea pigs that have received six BCG scarifications.

Conclusion

Our immune assays indicate that humoral immune competence to SRBC alloantigens, which requires B- and T-cell cooperation, is suppressed in guinea pigs under-

Table 5. Papule size[a] after intradermal transplantation of line-1 hepatocarcinomas

Days after transplantation	Treatment		
	Sham scarification	2 BCG scarifications	6 BCG scarifications
9	17.0 ± 2.5 (6/6)	12.6 ± 2.3 (6/6)	10.8 ± 5.6 (3/6)
11			5.0 ± 2.4
13	42.3 ± 4.3	51.4 ± 4.2	1.0 ± 1.0
17	10.2 ± 6.1	14.7 ± 9.4	0
21	0	0	0

[a] Mean size (mm^2) ± S. E.

going repeated BCG dermal scarification. Although there have been many reports of enhanced humoral immunity as a function of a single BCG challenge, MATHÉ et al. (42) have indicated that this response is variable during adjuvant therapy in mice. Antigenic competition is one likely explanation for a suppressive effect resulting from repeated dermal scarification with viable BCG organisms. Antigenic competition is readily achieved in experimental systems with respect to humoral immunity, and some limited data suggest that antigenic competition can affect cell-mediated immunity (43). It is interesting to note, however, that in our guinea pig model, allograft reactivity and syngeneic tumor rejection (generally associated with T-cell activity) were enhanced as a function of systemic BCG scarification in both random-bred and inbred animals. Thus, while systemic BCG challenge may have a passive or even a depressive effect on humoral immune competence in this guinea pig model, it is also capable of enhancing cell-mediated immunity as measured by homograft rejection and syngeneic tumor rejection. A possibility of immunomodulation in nonspecific adjuvant therapy has recently been suggested (42). Factors which may preferentially affect one or another component of the immune system are the dose, the ratio of viable to nonviable BCG organisms, and the source and mode of administration of BCG. Certainly several reports have demonstrated that this type of therapy is not unequivocally beneficial in terms of tumor immunoprophylaxis or therapy; in some cases it has even had a positive effect on tumor growth (42). A plausible explanation is that in such cases humoral rather than cell-mediated immunity was stimulated, resulting in the production of blocking factors that protected tumor cells against cytotoxic lymphocytes.

An ideal therapeutic condition would be that described above, where humoral immunity is suppressed while cell-mediated is heightened. The conditions which contribute to this pattern of immune modulation as a result of repeated BCG challenge warrant further investigation. However, keeping in mind that in the previous section of this report we demonstrated a suppressed immunologic responsiveness to extraneous antigen as a function of carcinogenesis and tumor burden, the present results of BCG scarification in normal animals may or may not be pertinent to similar treatment of animals with established tumors.

THE ROLE OF ANTI-BCG AND TUMOR IMMUNITY DURING TUMOR REGRESSION AFTER INTRALESIONAL INJECTION OF BCG[2]

Evidence from several systems indicates that inhibition of tumor growth by the granulomagenic agent BCG requires the development of specific bacterial immunity: in mice (44) and guinea pigs (45), host immune reactivity to BCG is necessary to prevent the growth of tumor cells injected in a mixture with BCG. More importantly, it has been shown that intradermal injection of BCG in anergic patients does not eradicate intradermal metastases in malignant melanoma (36).

Recent results of our investigations of the mechanism of BCG-mediated therapy of established tumors with regional lymph node metastases in inbred guinea pigs suggest that activated cells of the macrophage-histiocyte compartment play a primary and essential role in the destruction of tumor cells (20, 22). In this immunotherapy model, which utilizes a transplantable syngeneic hepatocarcinoma and intralesional injection of BCG (18), it is not unreasonable to assume that tumor inhibition may not require the development of tumor-specific immunity; there is no evidence to substantiate that the activated histiocytes are sensitized to the tumor cells. The destruction of established tumor both in the intradermal transplantation site and in the regional lymph nodes could in part be attributed to the detrimental environment created by the BCG-mediated granulomatous response, since this reaction is quantitatively and qualitatively similar in tumor-bearing and tumor-free animals. Although these arguments relate to local reactivity, an important consideration is control of any metastases that may exist beyond the regional lymph nodes.

We felt it would be particularly important to find out more about the role of specific immunity either to BCG or to tumor cells, and to determine whether lymphocyte cooperation with effector cells of the macrophage-histiocyte compartment is a requirement in this tumor immunotherapy model in guinea pigs, where BCG treatment is administered to established syngeneic tumors with regional metastases. Inbred male guinea pigs (Sewall-Wright strain 2) were used in these studies. Induction of primary hepatomas in strain-2 guinea pigs given the water-soluble diethylnitrosamine by mouth has been described elsewhere (46). The antigenic and biologic properties of the transplantable ascites tumor developed from the primary hepatomas have also been described (47). Guinea pigs were inoculated intradermally in the upper right dorsal quadrant with 0.1 ml or 1 X 10^6 line-10 tumor cells. This tumor grows progressively when 10^6 cells are injected intradermally, and metastasizes to the draining lymph nodes 7 days after inoculation and onset of tumor growth. Guinea pigs die as a consequence of metastases 60 to 90 days after the inoculation.

BCG (Phipps strain TNC 1029) was obtained from the Trudeau Institute. The preparations, frozen and stored at -70°C until just before use, were rapidly thawed in a 37°C water bath and diluted to proper concentrations in a 1% gelatin phosphate-buffered saline solution. Guinea pigs received 40 X 10^6 living BCG organisms in a total volume of 0.4 ml in the tumor site 7 days after implantation.

---

[2] These studies have been performed in collaboration with Drs. B. ZBAR and H. RAPP of the Biology Branch, National Cancer Institute, Bethesda, Maryland.

The Role of Lymphocyte Reactivity and Specific Immunity to BCG Antigens

Experiments using antilymphocyte serum (ALS) were designed to find whether BCG-mediated regression of established tumors could be accomplished in animals that were deficient in lymphocytes but had relatively intact macrophage-histiocyte compartments. Thus, ALS generated in rabbits against nonadherent cells from suspensions of strain-2 guinea pig lymph nodes was used as the lymphocyte-depleting agent. The success of selective lymphocyte depletion was determined histologically and hematologically.

The effects of intralesional BCG injection on tumor growth in guinea pigs receiving a regimen of ALS or normal rabbit serum (NRS) are shown in Fig. 4.

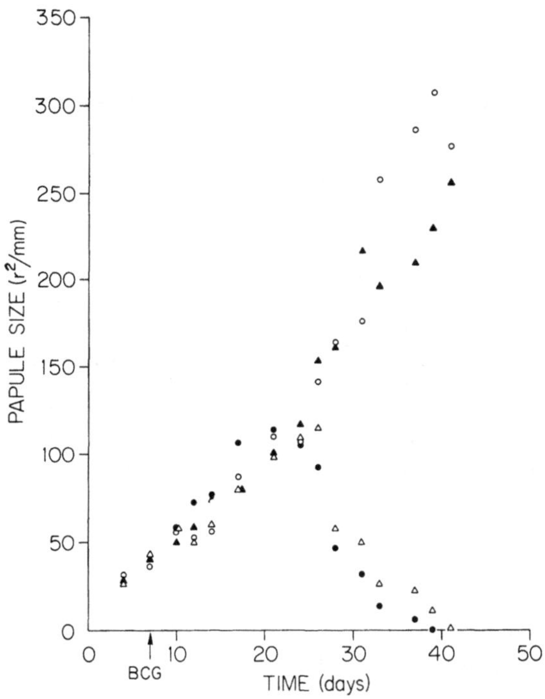

Fig. 4. Effects of antilymphocyte serum (ALS) and normal rabbit serum (NRS) on BCG-mediated tumor regression: ○: tumor alone; ●: tumor + BCG intralesional injection; △ : NRS, tumor + BCG intralesional injections; ▲: ALS, tumor + BCG intralesional injection

Eighteen to twenty days after intralesional injection of BCG (25 to 27 days after tumor) into normal or NRS-treated animals the tumors began to regress, and the skin was tumor-free in both groups at 40 days. In animals treated in both these groups, PPD skin tests were positive at 1 and 2 weeks after BCG. Intralesional injection of BCG into tumor-bearing animals that received a regimen of ALS was ineffective in retarding tumor growth. Tumor growth in ALS-treated animals was essentially the same as that detected in guinea pigs that received tumor cells only. The ALS-treated guinea pigs also had negative skin tests to PPD at 1 and 2 weeks after intralesional injection of BCG, as did the tumor-bearing animals not treated with BCG. Thus an immediate requirement for

for BCG-mediated tumor regression after intralesional injection of a critical number of viable organisms is a specific reactivity of the host to BCG antigens.

These results, as well as the demonstration that intradermal injection of BCG in anergic patients does not eradicate intradermal metastases in malignant melanoma (36), indicate that the effectiveness of BCG therapy in patients with established and incipient tumors will depend on the ability of the host to respond immunologically to the extraneous antigen.

Tumor-Specific Humoral and Cell-Mediated Immunity in BCG-Treated Guinea Pigs

In the syngeneic hepatocarcinoma system in inbred guinea pigs, the effective regression of established tumor after a single intralesional injection of BCG is limited by tumor size (19). The best therapeutic effect is achieved when an intralesional injection is administered 6 to 7 days after tumor transplantation, at which time the tumor papule is approximately 1 cm in diameter and metastases are detected histologically only in the regional lymph node. Since the granulomatous reaction elicited by BCG is restricted primarily to areas infiltrated with the microorganism (tumor site and regional lymph node), the question of control of metastases beyond the regional lymph node is of critical importance. We have demonstrated that during the course of BCG-mediated tumor regression animals develop systemic humoral and cell-mediated immunity (48). A positive reactivity of 32-day plasma from BCG-treated tumor-bearing guinea pigs, detected by immunofluorescence and by complement fixation and transfer tests (49), is evidence for antibody with specificity to line-10 tumor antigens. The development of systemic cell-mediated immunity (Fig. 5) is ultimately demonstrated by the rapid rejection of a second challenge with 1 X 10^6 line-10 tumor cells on the contralateral side of guinea pigs having undergone a BCG-mediated line-10 tumor regression. Histologically, the reaction at the challenge site was essentially like the homograft reaction described by GORER (50) for tumor rejection in actively immunized animals (Fig. 6).

Conclusion

These results, as well as previous studies by others with the BCG-mediated tumor therapy model in inbred guinea pigs (19, 51), have led to the conclusion that the regression of the primary tumor and regional metastases involves several steps. The first step requires specific immunity to the antigenic BCG and is immediately dependent on the immunologic competence of the tumor-bearing host to respond to extraneous antigens. The second step involves the accumulation of histiocytes in the tumor and regional lymph nodes, with the histiocytes being the major effector cells; previous studies of the tuberculous response have suggested that lymphocyte cooperation is required for this reaction (52). The third step is the ultimate development of specific tumor immunity.

This guinea pig immunotherapy model, while establishing several facts, has posed several important questions. One concerns the limitation of tumor size necessary for effective regression after intralesional injection of BCG. Certainly in part this can be attributed to the physical limitations of achieving an adequate tumoricidal granulomatous reaction with a single intralesional injection. However, the possibility of either a systemic or a localized immunologic hyporesponsiveness to the microorganism as a function of tumor mass

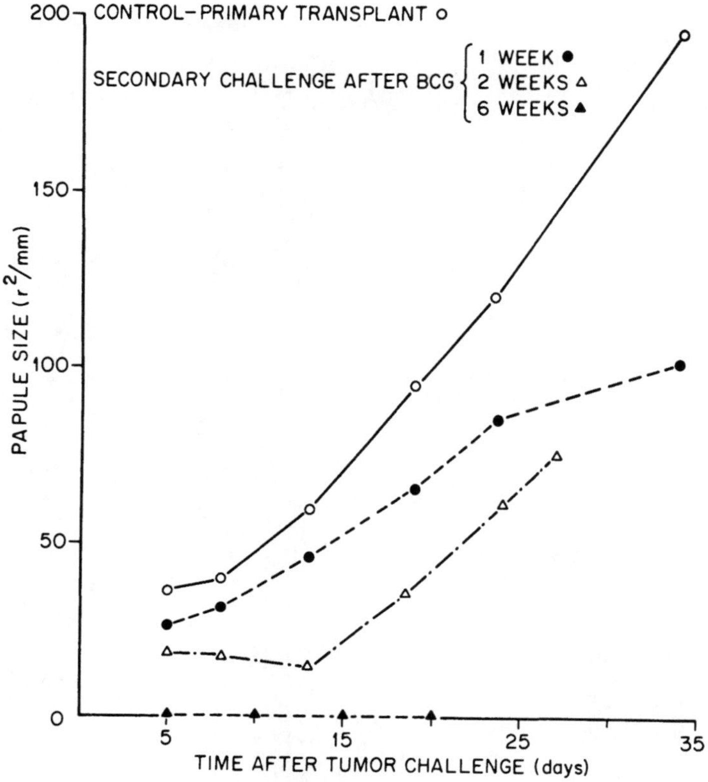

Fig. 5. Development of line-10 tumor-specific immunity after intralesional BCG injection. Papule sizes of tumor growth at the contralateral site when challenged with 1 X 10^6 line-10 cells. ○: tumor growth of primary transplants untreated; ●: secondary challenge 1 week after BCG; △: secondary challenge 2 weeks after BCG; ▲: secondary challenge 6 weeks after BCG

cannot be excluded. The influence of tumor mass on the development of the numerous soluble factors required for cell-mediated immunity must certainly be considered as well as lymphocyte hyporesponsiveness. It has been demonstrated that systemic, tumor-specific humoral and cell-mediated immunity is developed in this model, but the effectiveness of the immune reactivity in controlling distant metastases is an important consideration.

It is not unlikely that, during BCG-mediated regression of tumor in the skin, if metastasis does occur beyond the draining chain of lymph nodes it could be controlled by means of the developing tumor-specific immunity. More importantly, in this particular experimental model it is possible that regression of metastases in the distal lymph nodes (axillary and subcostal) is mediated by tumor-specific immunity. There is still no direct evidence for this conjecture, and one critical experiment argues against this possibility. It has previously been demonstrated that immunization of guinea pigs by intradermal injection of a mixture of BCG and line-10 tumor cells can eradicate by tumor-specific immunity a contralateral challenge with 10^6 tumor cells. However, no therapeutic benefit was derived from contralateral vaccine treatment in animals in which tumors were excised at day 7, and lymph node metastases per-

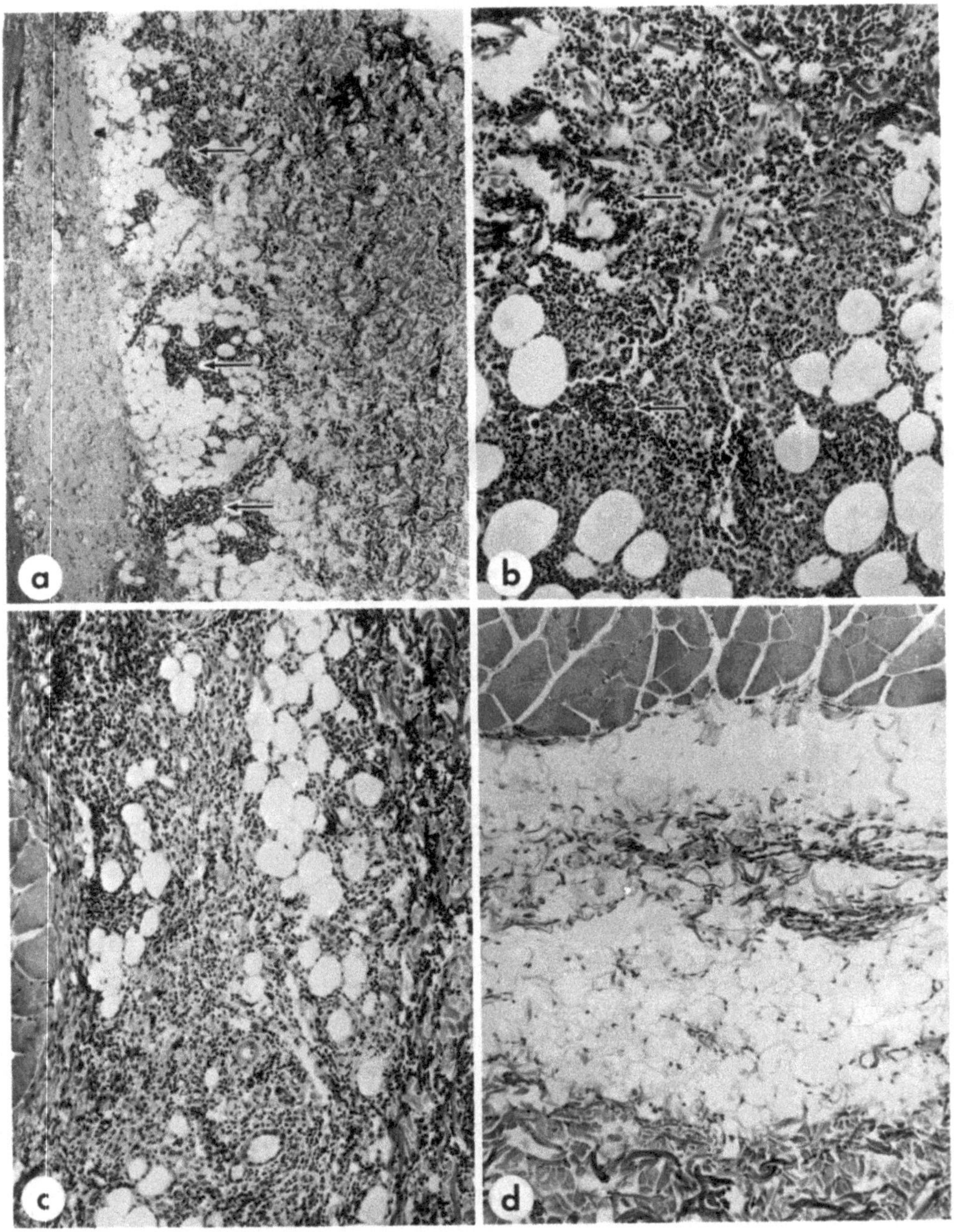

Fig. 6 a - d

sisted (19). The most plausible explanation of this is the failure of BCG to reach axillary and subcostal nodes in a concentration adequate for production of a tumoricidal histiocytosis.

These results further emphasize the need for consideration in immunotherapy of the problems of the immunologic status of the host, the efferent nature of lymph-node reactivity, and anatomic limitations in focusing developing tumor-specific immunity on tumors at different sites. The answers to such questions are being sought in further experiments with this model.

← Fig. 6. Histology of skin site after secondary challenge with 1 X 10^6 line-10 tumor cells in recipients previously having undergone a BCG-mediated tumor regression as a result of intralesional injection. (a) One day after secondary challenge with line-10 tumor cells at the contralateral intradermal site. Note the tumor cells dispersed throughout the dermis and aggregated (arrow) in the panniculus adiposis. Hematoxylin and eosin, X 30. (b) Two days after secondary challenge with line-10 tumor. Tumor mass is surrounded and infiltrated with mononuclear cells (arrow). Hematoxylin and eosin, X 125. (c) Seven days after secondary challenge with line-10 tumor. Hematoxylin and eosin, X 125. (d) Ten days after secondary challenge with line-10 tumor. Hematoxylin and eosin, X 125

REFERENCES

1. BLACK, M. M., SPEER, F. D., OPLER, S. R.: Some components of biologic predeterminism in cancer. Surg. Gynecol. Obst. 102, 223 (1956).
2. BLACK, M. M., SPEER, F. D.: Sinus histiocytosis of lymph nodes in cancer. Surg. Gynecol. Obst. 106, 163 (1958).
3. HAMLIN, I. M. E.: Possible host resistance in carcinoma of the breast. A histological study. Brit. J. Cancer 22, 383 (1968).
4. WOODRUFF, M. E.: Immunological aspects of cancer. Lancet 1964 , 265.
5. STJERSWÄRD, J.: Effect of cancer and its treatment on the immune response. In: Oncology 1970, Vol. 2, p. 322 (Eds R. L. CLARK, R. W. CUMLEY, J. E. MCCAY, M. M. COPELAND). Chicago: Year Book Medical Publishers 1971.
6. ISRAEL, L.: Cell-mediated immunity in lung cancer patients: data, problems, and propositions. Cancer Chemother. Rep. 4, 279 (1973).
7. HERSH, E. M., WHITECAR, J. P., Jr., MCCREDIE, K. B., BODEY, G. P., FREIREICH, E. J.: Chemotherapy, immunocompetence, immunosuppression and progress in acute leukemia. New Engl. J. Med. 285, 1211 (1971).
8. HELLSTRÖM, K. E., HELLSTRÖM, I.: Cellular immunity against tumor antigens. Advanc. Cancer Res. 12, 167 (1969).
9. HELLSTRÖM, I., HELLSTRÖM, K. E., SJÖGREN, H. O., WARNER, G. A.: Demonstration of cell-mediated immunity to human neoplasms of various histological types. Int. J. Cancer 7, 1 (1971).
10. HERBERMAN, R. B., ROSENBERG, E. B., HALTERMAN, R. H., MCCOY, J. L., LEVENTHAL, B. G.: Cellular immune reactions to human leukemia. Nat. Cancer Inst. Monogr. 35, 259 (1972).
11. HERBERMAN, R. B.: Cellular immunity to human tumor-associated antigens. Israel J. Med. Sci. 9, 300 (1973).
12. U. S. House of Representatives: H. R. Hearings, 92nd Congress, Stock Number 5270-1144, p. 8. 1971.
13. JOHNSON, S.: The effect of thymectomy and the dose of 3-methylcholanthrene on the induction and antigenic properties of sarcomas in C57BL mice. Brit. J. Cancer 22, 93 (1968).
14. BARTLETT, G. L.: Effect of host immunity on the antigenic strength of primary tumors. J. Nat. Cancer Inst. 49, 493 (1972).

15. CURRIE, G. A.: Eighty years of immunotherapy: A review of immunological methods used for the treatment of human cancer. Brit. J. Cancer 26, 141 (1972).
16. SZAKAL, A. K., HANNA, M. G., Jr.: Immune suppression and carcinogenesis in hamsters during topical application of 7,12-dimethylbenz(a)anthracene. Nat. Cancer Inst. Monogr. 35, 173 (1972).
17. SZAKAL, A. K., HANNA, M. G., Jr.: Cell-mediated immune response of hamsters to alloantigens and tumor antigens of isologous and autochthonous origin during chemical carcinogenesis. Cancer Res. 34, 138 (1974).
18. ZBAR, B., TANAKA, T.: Immunotherapy of cancer: Regression of tumors after intralesional injection of Mycobacterium bovis. Science 172, 271 (1971).
19. ZBAR, B., BERNSTEIN, I. D., BARTLETT, G. L., HANNA, M. G., Jr., RAPP, H. J.: Immunotherapy of cancer: Regression of intradermal tumors and prevention of growth of lymph node metastases after intralesional injection of Mycobacterium bovis (Bacillus Calmette-Guerin). J. Nat. Cancer Inst. 49, 119 (1972).
20. HANNA, M. G., Jr., ZBAR, B., RAPP, H. J.: Histopathology of tumor regression after intralesional injection of Mycobacterium bovis. I. Tumor growth and metastasis. J. Nat. Cancer Inst. 48, 1441 (1972).
21. HANNA, M. G., Jr., ZBAR, B., RAPP, H. J.: Histopathology of tumor regression after intralesional injection of Mycobacterium bovis. II. Comparative effects of vaccinia virus, oxazolone, and turpentine. J. Nat. Cancer Inst. 48, 1697 (1972).
22. SNODGRASS, M. J., HANNA, M. G., Jr.: Ultrastructural studies of histiocyte-tumor cell interactions during tumor regression mediated by intralesional injection of Mycobacterium bovis. Cancer Res. 33, 701 (1973).
23. LINDER, O. E. A.: Survival of skin homografts in methylcholanthrene-treated mice and mice with spontaneous mammary cancers. Cancer Res. 22, 380 (1962).
24. ROWLAND, G. F., EDWARDS, A. J., HURD, C. M., SUMNER, M. R.: Changes in lymphoreticular tissues during growth of a murine adenocarcinoma. III. Plaque-forming cell response in lymph nodes and spleen. J. Nat. Cancer Inst. 47, 32 (1971).
25. MARIANI, T., MARUYAMA, Y., GOOD, R. A.: Tumor cell-related syngeneic skin graft rejection in Gross leukemia. Nat. Cancer Inst. Monogr. 35, 309 (1972).
26. BLACK, M. M.: Cell-mediated response in mammary cancer. In: Immunology of Breast Cancer (Ed. B. A. STAHL). London: Heinemann Medical Books 1973.
27. SJÖGREN, H. O., HELLSTRÖM, I., BANSAL, S. C., HELLSTRÖM, K. E.: Suggestive evidence that the "blocking antibodies" of tumor bearing individuals may be antigen-antibody complexes. Proc. Nat. Acad. Sci. (Wash.) 68, 1372 (1971).
28. GORER, P. A.: The antigenic structure of tumors. Advanc. Immunol. 1, 345 (1961).
29. STJERNSWÄRD, J.: Effect of Bacillus Calmette-Guerin and/or methylcholanthrene on the antibody-forming cells measured at the cellular level by a hemolytic plaque test. Cancer Res. 26, 1591 (1966).
30. BIOZZI, G., STIFFEL, C., HALPERN, B. N., MOUTON, D.: Recherches sur le mécanisme de l'immunité nonspecifique produit par les mycobacteries. Rev. franc. Étud. Clin. Biol. 5, 876 (1960).
31. MACKANESS, G. B.: The immunological basis of acquired resistance: J. Exp. Med. 120, 105 (1964).
32. BALNER, H., OLD, L. J., CLARKE, D. A.: Accelerated rejection of male skin isografts by female C57BL mice infected with Bacillus Calmette-Guerin. Proc. Soc. Exp. Biol. (N. Y.) 109, 58 (1962).
33. VITALE, B., ALLEGRETTI, N.: Influence of Bacillus Calmette-Guerin infection on intensity of homograft rejection in rats. Nature (Lond.) 199, 507 (1963).

34. YASHPHE, D. J.: Immunological factors in nonspecific stimulation of host resistance to syngeneic tumors. A review. In: Immunological Parameters of Host-Tumor Relationship (Ed. D. W. WEISS), p. 90. New York: Academic Press 1971.
35. MATHÉ, G., POUILLART, P., SCHWARZENBERG, L., AMIEL, S. L. SCHNEIDER, M., HAYAT, M., DEVASSAL, F., JASMIN, C., ROSENFELD, C., WEINER, R., RAPPAPORT, H.: Attempts at immunotherapy of 100 patients with acute lymphoid leukemia: Some factors influencing results. Nat. Cancer Inst. Monogr. 35, 361 (1972).
36. MORTON, D. L., EILBER, F. R., MALMGREN, R. A., WOOD, W. C.: Immunological factors which influence response to immunotherapy in malignant melanoma. Surgery 68, 158 (1970).
37. GUTTERMANN, J. U., MCBRIDE, C., FREIREICH, E. J., MAVLIGIT, G., FREI, E. III, HERSH, E. M.: Active immunotherapy with BCG for recurrent malignant melanoma. Lancet 1973 , 1208.
38. GUTTERMANN, J., MAVLIGIT, G., MCBRIDE, G., FREI, E. III, HERSH, E. M.: BCG stimulation of immune responsiveness in patients with malignant melanoma. Cancer 32, 321 (1973).
39. MORTON, D. L.: Immunotherapy of human melanomas and sarcomas. Nat. Cancer Inst. Monogr. 35, 375 (1972).
40. MASTRANGELO, M. J., KIM, Y. H., BORNSTEIN, R. S., CHEE, D. O., SULIT, H. L., YARBRO, J. W.: Clinico-pathological correlation of BCG induced melanoma regression. Proc. Amer. Ass. Cancer Res. 14, 65 (1973).
41. KLEIN, E.: Immunotherapeutic approaches to the management of neoplasms. Nat. Cancer Inst. Monogr. 35, 379 (1972).
42. MATHÉ, G., KAMEL, M., DEZFULIAN, M., HALLE-PENNENKO, O., BOURUT, C.: An experimental screening for "Sytemic adjuvants of immunity" applicable to cancer immunotherapy. Cancer Res. 33, 1907 (1973).
43. LIACOPOULOS, P.: Suppression of immunological responses during the induction of immune paralysis with unrelated antigens. Tex. Rep. Biol. Med. 23, 63 (1965).
44. BARTLETT, G. L., ZBAR, B.: Tumor-specific vaccine containing Mycobacterium bovis and tumor cells: Safety and efficacy. J. Nat. Cancer Inst. 48, 1709 (1972).
45. ZBAR, B., BERNSTEIN, I. D., RAPP, H. J.: Suppression of tumor growth at the site of infection with living bacillus Calmette-Guerin. J. Nat. Cancer Inst. 46, 831 (1971).
46. RAPP, H. J., CHURCHILL, W. H., Jr., KRONMAN, B. S., ROLLEY, R. T., HAMMOND, W. G., BORSOS, T.: Antigenicity of a new diethylnitrosamine-induced transplantable guinea pig hepatoma: Pathology and formation of ascites variant. J. Nat. Cancer Inst. 41, 1 (1968).
47. ZBAR, B., WEPSIC, H. T., RAPP, H. J., BORSOS, T., KRONMAN, B. S., CHURCHILL, W. H., Jr.: Antigenic specificity of hepatomas induced in strain-2 guinea pigs by diethylnitrosamine. J. Nat. Cancer Inst. 43, 833 (1969).
48. HANNA, M. G., Jr., SNODGRASS, M. J., ZBAR, B., RAPP, H. J.: Histopathology of tumor regression after intralesional injection of Mycobacterium bovis. IV. Development of immunity to tumor cells and to BCG. J. Nat. Cancer Inst. 51, 1897 (1973).
49. RAPP, H. J., BORSOS, T.: Molecular Basis of Complement Action, p. 105. New York: Appleton-Century-Croft 1970.
50. GORER, P. A.: Some recent work in tumor immunity. Advanc. Cancer Res. 4, 149 (1956).
51. ZBAR, B., WEPSIC, H. T., BORSOS, T., RAPP, H. J.: Tumor graft rejection in syngeneic guinea pigs: Evidence for a two-step mechanism. J. Nat. Cancer Inst. 44, 473 (1970).
52. ANDO, M., DANNENBERG, A. M., SHIMA, K.: Macrophage accumulation, division, maturation and digestive and microbicidal capacities in tuberculous le-

sions. II. Rate at which mononuclear cells enter and divide in primary BCG lesions and those of reinfection. J. Immunol. 109, 8 (1972).
53. BLACK, M. M.: Human breast cancer. A model for cancer immunology. Israel J. Med. Sci. 9, 284 (1973).
54. SOKAL, J. E., AUNGST, C. W., HAN, T.: Effect of BCG on delayed hypersensitivity response of patients with neoplastic disease. Int. J. Cancer 12, 242 (1973).

Tumor Induction in Immunologically Privileged Sites

M. Vandeputte and H. Sobis

This paper deals with tumor induction in two immunologically privileged sites, the brain and the pregnant uterus.

In transplant patients receiving long-term treatment with immunosuppressive drugs, a high incidence of lymphoreticular neoplasms with cerebral localization is observed (1). This unusual predilection of lymphomas for the brain may indicate that the brain is an immunologically privileged site in which antigenic tumor cells may continue to develop by escaping the immune surveillance of the host (2). This is also in line with the observation that the recurrence of Burkitt's lymphoma, a tumor in which immunological defences are thought to play a role in containing tumor progression (3), is often due to cerebral involvement (4). A similar observation has been made in the case of patients suffering relapses in acute leukemia (5). Interestingly enough, an experimental model using polyoma virus in immunosuppressed rats treated with antilymphocytic serum or subjected to thymectomy at birth leads to the conclusion that the tumors appearing in the brains of these rats (cerebral hemangiomas) are less sensitive to immune surveillance than are the visceral polyoma tumors (6, 7).

Another, experimentally more interesting, immunologically privileged site for tumor induction is the pregnant uterus. Since in all pregnancies resulting from heterospecific matings the fetus is an allogeneic graft in the uterus of the mother, some particular mechanism(s) must be operative to allow its normal development. Whatever the mechanism(s) involved, it is possible that because of the special immunological relationship existing during pregnancy one could induce tumors in the uterus by inoculating a virus which normally does not provoke neoplasms in adult immunologically competent rodents. That this is indeed the case has now been shown with mouse sarcoma virus (MSV-MLV), which regularly induces yolk sac carcinoma in rats fetectomized at day 12 of their pregnancy and injected with the virus (8, 9). Various observations indicate the fetal origin of tumors obtained by this method; they never grow out when the fetus is a hybrid to the mother. This is also to be expected, as apart from the tumor-associated transplantation antigens (TSTA), the tumor contains the histocompatibility antigens of the father, and the presence of these will lead to their rejection by the host; histologically, the tumor can easily be classified as a yolk-sac carcinoma probably derived from parietal yolk sac; one of the important biochemical characteristics of these tumors is their capacity to secrete α-fetoprotein.

Apart from yolk-sac carcinomas, two cases of teratocarcinomas were recorded in this study. This observation led us to investigate the possibility that these teratocarcinomas might also be derived from the yolk sac, a fetal membranous structure lined with cells that have the potential to differentiate into various tissues. To test this hypothesis, laparotomy was performed (as in the previous experiment) twelve days after mating in pregnant primiparous rats. The fetuses were removed from both horns. In one horn the fetal membranes were left outside the uterus horn. In the contralateral horn the fetal membranes were removed together with the fetuses. All placentas were left in situ. No virus was inoculated. Six weeks later, all R-female rats mated with an R-male developed extrauterine tumors in the horn in which the fetal membranes were left outside the uterus horn. In the contralateral horn a small tumor was recorded only very occasionally. None of the R-female rats mated with BN males (hybrid fetuses) developed tumors. Histologically, the tumors were benign teratomas with a variety of tissues such as epithelial cysts, skeletal tissues with cartilage and bone, endodermal tissue and glandular tissue. This operative procedure, which is quite simple and permits the development of teratomas in nearly all the rats treated in this way, may be of great value in the further study of the pathogenesis of teratomas and of the expression of fetal antigens during cell differentiation.

REFERENCES

1. PENN, I., STARZL, T. E.: Malignant tumors arising de novo in immunosuppressed organ transplant recipients. Transplantation 14, 407 (1972).
2. MEDAWAR, P. B.: Immunity to homologous grafted skin. III. Fate of skin homografts transplanted to brain, to subcutaneous tissue and to anterior chamber of the eye. Brit. J. exp. Path. 29, 58 (1948).
3. KLEIN, G.: Immunological studies on Burkitt's lymphomas. Postgrad. med. J. 47, 141 (1971).
4. CLIFFORD, P., SINGH, S., STJERNSWÄRD, J., KLEIN, G.: Long-term survival of patients with Burkitt's lymphoma: an assessment of treatment and other factors which may relate to survival. Cancer Res. 27, 2578 (1967).
5. MATHE, G.: Immunological approaches of leukemia treatment. Ann. Inst. Pasteur 122, 855 (1972).
6. VANDEPUTTE, M., DENYS, P., LEYTEN, R., DE SOMER, P.: The oncogenic activity of the polyoma virus in thymectomized rats. Life Sci. 2, 475 (1963).
7. VANDEPUTTE, M.: The effect of heterologous antilymphocytic serum on the oncogenic activity of polyoma virus. Life Sci. 7, 855 (1968).
8. VANDEPUTTE, M., SOBIS, H., BILLIAU, A., VAN DE MAELE, B., LEYTEN, R.: In utero tumor induction by murine sarcoma virus (Moloney) in the rat. I. Biological characteristics. Int. J. Cancer 11, 536 (1973).
9. SOBIS, H., VANDEPUTTE, M.: In utero tumor induction by murine sarcoma virus (Moloney) in the rat. II. Histological and ultrastructural characteristics. Int. J. Cancer 11, 543 (1973).

Patterns of Neoplastic and Nonneoplastic Diseases of Praomys (Mastomys) Natalensis

H. L. Stewart and K. C. Snell

We wish to introduce a unique animal, the mastomys, which is not well known to the scientific coummunity. Mastomys develop certain diseases that constitute suitable animal models for study and experimentation on 1) chemotherapy of immunological disorders, and 2) tumorigenesis in such immunological disorders.

A particular reason for introducing this animal is that its immunology has not been worked out, and certainly some of its diseases and possibly its tumors may result from reduced immunologic surveillance. There are certain unusual conditions that need study by experts, that we have observed in necropsy and histologic examination of some 600 mastomys.

Mastomys are a distinct subgenus of rodent, intermediate in size between the mouse and the rat. They are native to South Africa. Formerly designated Rattus (Mastomys) natalensis, they were later reclassified as Praomys (Mastomys) natalensis, and the animals are still referred to as mastomys. They differ in their disease pattern from other rodents by the development of spontaneous neoplastic and nonneoplastic diseases far in excess in number per animal, variety and rarity of those commonly encountered in mice and rats. Some of these are unique to mastomys, and others have been seen only rarely in other rodents. The converse of this is that certain diseases common to other rodents rarely or never occur in mastomys.

DEGENERATIVE JOINT DISEASE

Severe degenerative joint disease of diarthroses and intervertebral disks develops regularly during the second year of life (13). Virtually all peripheral articulations, with the exception of the hips, shoulders, and sacro-iliacs are affected, but the elbows and the knees are most severely involved.

In the diarthrodial joints, there is extensive erosion of articular cartilage and sclerosis of epiphyseal bone, and in some animals proliferative synovitis and periarticular mucoid cystic change are prominent.

Fibrillation of the costal joints is frequent at both the sternal and the vertebral ends of the ribs. The cartilage is disrupted, leaving round islands of necrotic chondrocytes within amorphous and hyaline material.

The subchondral portions of the vertebral bodies become deformed in advance of the lesions; erosion and eburnation extend into the epiphyses, sometimes penetrating to a considerable depth. A mild degree of marginal osteophyte formation is frequently present on both the ventral and the dorsal edges. Aseptic necrosis of the secondary centers of ossification of the vertebrae is a common finding. Degeneration of intervertebral disks results in gross narrowing of the spaces between the vertrebral bodies. Portions of degenerated disks protrude dorsally into the spinal canal in multiple segments of the spine. This usually elevates and occasionally disrupts the dura mater and exerts pressure leading to degeneration in different segments of the spinal cord and the cauda equina. Massive myelomalacia occasionally follows; more often, focal areas of demyelination, infiltration by Gitter cells, and clusters of cholesterol crystal clefts are present in the cauda equina. Clinically, after 2 years of age, most mastomys are disinclined to use the hind legs and about 10% show overt paraplegia.

In man, rheumatoid arthritis is the most prevalent connective tissue disease and is considered to be related to an abnormal autoimmune state. On the other hand, osteoarthritis is not considered a connective tissue disease. This seems to agree with the findings in mastomys, since the few tests we have conducted failed to demonstrate abnormal globulins in the blood. The subject, however, has been inadequately explored, and before autoimmunity is ruled out as a cause of the arthritis, more elaborate and sophisticated studies must be performed.

GLOMERULONEPHRITIS

Approximately 80% of mastomys of our colony develop one or more of three forms of glomerulonephritis, i.e. membranous, proliferative, and severe chronic forms (11).

The severe chronic form has been diagnosed in a few young animals, but is largely found in animals aged 18-36 months. Grossly, the kidneys appear unremarkable in some cases, while in others the surface has a finely or coarsely granular appearance and the tissue is pale or grayish tan. Histologically, all portions of the nephron and the interstitial tissue are involved, while the extraglomerular blood vessels remain normal. Within the tuft, however, the capillaries become thickened and the lumen reduced, and some may appear telangiectatic. Adhesions and crescents are often present, and many glomerular tufts contain inflammatory cells. Occasional glomeruli are obliterated. Tubular segments of the nephron show progressive alterations of hypertrophy, atrophy and flattening of the lining cells, desquamation of epithelial cells and casts. The interstitial tissue becomes thickened, hyperemic and infiltrated with lymphocytes, plasma cells and granulocytes.

We think transition stages and progression can be traced from early membranous glomerulonephritis to the proliferative form and from either or both of these lesions to the severe chronic form. In membranous glomerulonephritis, 10% or more of glomeruli may be involved, while the tubules, interstitial tissue, and extraglomerular vascular system remain virtually intact. Later, nearly all the capillary tufts show hyaline thickening of the glomerular loops and basement membrane of Bowman's capsule, producing the wire-loop appearance. With the lesion of proliferative glomerulonephritis, in addition to these changes, the glomeruli show the feature of hypercellularity. In a few specimens an occasional glomerulus shows an acute degenerative lesion characterized by intracapillary hyaline thrombi, narrowing sometimes to the point of occlusion of the capillaries, and swelling and thickening of their walls by fibrinoid. This phenomenon is reminiscent of the glomeruli of patients with disseminated lupus erythematosus, which is thought to reflect an autoimmune disease or hypersensitivity mechanism.

The development of the glomerular alterations in mastomys as revealed by electron microscopy has been described elsewhere (17). The earliest alterations consist of diffuse thickening of the basement membrane of the peripheral capillary loops, loss of the three-layered structure and the appearance of small nodules on the epithelial aspect of the membrane. Subsequently, swollen visceral epithelial cells with bizarrely formed nuclei appear, and the glomerular basement membrane shows diffuse thickening with subepithelial nodules. In many, the mesangial region is expanded with a striking increase of cellularity. Collagen fibrils are commonly observed in the mesangial matrix, as are lipofuscin bodies in the cytoplasm and inclusions in the nuclei of mesangial cells. Free cells and many microvilli originating in the visceral epithelial cells are commonly seen in Bowman's space. The capillaries occasionally contain polymorphonuclear leukocytes and aggregates of thrombocytes. Immunofluorescence studies using rabbit antimastomys immunoglobulins have initially shown fluorescence in the mesangial region. With aging, the fluorescence increases and a granular deposition of the globulins becomes evident along the peripheral capillary loops. This suggests that the renal disease that mastomys develop is a type of immune-complex glomerulonephritis (10, 9).

MYASTHENIA GRAVIS

Myositis and atrophy of skeletal muscle are present in approximately one fifth of the animals with thymoma. Other lesions that seem to be associated are severe myocarditis and chronic inflammation, often with degeneration and atrophy of the extraorbital and intraorbital lacrimal glands and the lingual, harderian, and one or more of the salivary glands. In one 17-month-old female mastomys with the combination of thymoma, polymyositis and myocarditis, serum-globulin reactivity, presumably autoantibody against striated muscle, was found in a high titer (15). The sera from thirteen mastomys used as age- and sex-matched controls all reacted to produce striational staining in low titer (up to 1/10), whereas sera from younger animals failed to react. There is a possibility that the myositis, myocarditis, inflammatory lesions of other sites, thymomas, and thymic hyperplasias of mastomys may have some relationship to myasthenia gravis of man, which is believed by some to be associated with autoimmunity. Tests of muscle tone before and after the use of neostigmine would be of assistance in establishing a diagnosis of myasthenia gravis.

UBIQUITY OF THE PLASMA CELL

When mastomys are well under one year of age, plasma cells begin to populate the spleen, lymph nodes, and lymph nodules of the intestine, and thereafter they may account for a high proportion of the cells at these sites. Plasma-cell and lymphocytic thyroiditis is exceedingly common, and collections of plasma cells in the salivary and orbital glands in other viscera, including the heart, and in the mesenteries are by no means infrequent. This suggests a relationship to the tissue changes associated with Sjögren's syndrome. We have applied the term "pseudolymphoma" to an unusual disease in one mastomys, mentioned later, using this term in the same sense as TALAL and associates (16) for tumor-like aggregates of lymphoid cells of dubious malignancy found in various organs of patients with Sjögren's syndrome. The association of polymyositis and autoantibodies with striated muscle in mastomys with thymomas and the development of membranous glomerulonephritis suggestive of an immune-complex disease adds weight to the possibility that the hematopoietic diseases also have an autoimmune basis. A body of information has been built up from studies in man and animals, including NZB/BL mice (8, 1), that may shed light on interrelationships between neoplasia and hypergammaglobulinemia, dysproteinemia, and autoimmune diseases.

THYMOMA

About one third of our mastomys develop thymic hyperplasia or thymoma by the time they are two years old, and many more when they are older (14). The male-female ratio is 2 to 1. The thymomas may attain a width of 3 cm, compromising the space in the thoracic cavity. The histologic pattern of the thymoma corresponds closely to that in man, in whom the normal relationship of cortex to medulla is effaced and the different thymic cellular and structural components appear in abnormal relationship to each other. In the hyperplastic thymus, the pattern of cortical and medullary markings is reproduced, although the regularity seen in the noninvoluted thymus of young animals is much less pronounced.

It should be noted that thymomas and the hyperplastic lesions arise from the involuted thymus. In some mastomys a remnant of involuted thymus is attached to a globular nodule of hyperplastic thymic tissue. To us this indicates that the usual process of thymic involution proceeds uninterrupted until late in life, when something happens that induces a new formation of thymic tissue. The reasons for this phenomenon are a mystery. One might suspect that this thymic overgrowth is a response to a slowly developing cellular immune defectiveness that requires immune surveillance. Perhaps it is more than coincidental that there is a close correlation between the age distribution of the animals with thymic hyperplasia and thymoma and chronic glomerulonephritis.

HEMATOPOIETIC NEOPLASMS

Interrelated neoplastic, reactive, and inflammatory diseases of the hematopoietic tissues are found in about 10% of our necropsy series of nearly 600 mastomys, most of which were old. We have classified about a quarter of the cases as either nodular-follicular lymphosarcoma or diffuse lymphosarcoma. Slightly more than one-half of the cases are reticulum cell sarcomas, well-differentiated, anaplastic or mixtures of well-differentiated and anaplastic reticulum cell sarcoma with lymphosarcoma. There is one example each of solitary plasma-cell myeloma of the cervical spine and pseudolymphoma (mentioned above). The other fraction of the cases is made up by atypical reticulum cell hyperplasia and inflammation. None of the animals has had leukemic blood. No hematopoietic neoplasm originated in the thymus. The plasma cell myeloma was readily transplanted, but attempts to transplant 3 other neoplasms were unsuccessful. All the reticulum-cell sarcomas were classifiable as the Type B neoplasm of DUNN (3). We have speculated whether, in mastomys, there is a relationship between an autoimmune state and the occurrence of the reticulum cell sarcomas, hyperplastic lesions and inflammatory processes so often associated with an abundance of plasma cells, some of which contain intracytoplasmic and intranuclear PAS-positive inclusions.

GASTRIC CARCINOIDS

Argyrophilic carcinoid tumors of the glandular stomach develop in approximately two-thirds of old male and one-third of old female mastomys (12). The Sevier-Munger and Azzopardi silver methods applied to formalin-fixed tissues reveal the diagnostic coal-black granules in the cytoplasm of the carcinoid cells. The neoplasm originates as proliferations of argyrophil cells within the gastric glandular mucosa in the body or fundus. The foci enlarge, coalesce, and infiltrate the muscularis mucosa and submucosa. The submucosal deposit comes to constitute the main mass of the neoplasm. There is early invasion of lymphatic and blood vessels followed by metastasis to regional lymph nodes, pancreas, liver and lungs.

Some carcinoids have been successfully transplanted to the thigh muscles of other mastomys and have been carried for several generations. They retain the identical histologic pattern and reaction to silver salts as the primary tumors. Many host animals in which the transplant has attained a diameter of 1.0 cm or more develop multiple ulcers of the stomach, duodenum, and upper jejunum. The animals die of intestinal hemorrhage, perforating ulcers or peritonitis.

Chemical examination of such transplantable argyrophilic gastric carcinoids revealed that they contained appreciable amounts of histamine, and that the dialyzed microsome-free supernatant of the tumor tissue produced significant amounts of histamine in the presence of L-histidine and pyridoxal phosphate (6). These findings evidently account for hypersecretion of gastric acid and the alimentary tract ulcers. The transplanted carcinoids contain appreciable activities of specific histidine decarboxylase and aromatic L-amino acid decarboxylase, which may relate to the inherent properties of the cell of origin, the histamine-containing argyrophilic cell distributed in the gastric mucosa (7).

From their ultrastructural observations, CAPELLA and co-workers attributed the histamine-dependent hyperchlorhydria of tumor-bearing animals to the function of the carcinoid cells, which resemble the enterochromaffin-like cells and the round granule cells of the acid-secreting portion of the glandular stomach (2). To our knowledge, mastomys are the only animals other than man to develop argyrophilic carcinoid tumors of the stomach. We have not seen the characteristic right-sided cardiac fibrosis that occurs in some patients with massive carcinoid deposits in the liver, because the carcinoids of mastomys do not elaborate 5-hydroxyindoles.

MISCELLANEOUS

Other neoplasms relatively commonly encountered in mastomys are hepatomas, metastasizing granulosa cell tumors of the ovaries, adenomas of the adrenal gland cortex, pituitary gland, pancreatic islets and parotid gland, adenomatous polyps of the ileocecal junction, and hemangiomas of many different sites. Neoplasms that are seen in mastomys and are rarely, and in one or two instances have never been, encountered in mice or rats are chordomas, synovial sarcomas, carcinoma of the nasopharyngeal tube, papillomas of the lacrimal sac, carcinoma of the extrahepatic bile duct, teratoma of the mediastinum, carcinoma of the female prostate, granular cell myoblastoma of the uterine horn, seminomas of the testis, carcinomas of the rete testis and carcinosarcomas of the seminal vesicles. Conversely, tumors that are common in mice but rare in mastomys are leukemia, alveologenic tumors of the lung, osteosarcoma and mammary gland tumors.

In conclusion, evidence has been presented that the mastomys develops diseases of an immunologic nature. Some of these animal models of disease suggest a combination of a defective or overactive immunological responsiveness with autoimmune disorders and neoplasia. The mastomys is unique among rodents in the patterns of diseases that it develops or does not develop. Some model systems of disease of the mastomys could be used for experimental immunosuppression and chemotherapy.

REFERENCES

1. BARNES, R. D., TUFFREY, M. A., BERRY, C. L.: J. pathol. Bact. 95, 391 (1968).
2. CAPELLA, C., SOLCIA, E., SNELL, K. C.: J. nat. Cancer Inst. 50, 1471 (1973).
3. DUNN, T. B., DERINGER, M. K.: J. nat. Cancer Inst. 40, 771 (1968).
4. DUTCHER, T. F., FAHEY, J. L.: J. nat. Cancer Inst. 22, 887 (1959).
5. FUDENBERG, H. H.: Amer. J. Med. 51, 295 (1971).
6. HOSODA, S., NAKAMURA, W., SNELL, K. C., STEWART, H. L.: Science 170, 454 (1970).
7. HOSODA, S., NAKAMURA, W., SNELL, K. C., STEWART, H. L.: Biochem. Pharmacol. 20, 2671 (1971).
8. MCINTIRE, K. R., LAW, L. W.: J. nat. Cancer Inst. 39, 1197 (1967).
9. NOTKINS, A. L.: J. exp. Med. 134, 41s (1971).
10. OLDSTONE, M. B. A., DIXON, F. T.: J. exp. Med. 134, 32s (1971).
11. SNELL, K. C., STEWART, H. L.: J. nat. Cancer Inst. 39, 95 (1967).
12. SNELL, K. C., STEWART, H. L.: Gann 8, 39 (1969).
13. SOKOLOFF, L., SNELL, K. C., STEWART, H. L.: Ann. rheum. Dis. 26, 146 (1967).
14. STEWART, H. L., SNELL, K. C.: J. nat. Cancer Inst. 40,1135 (1968).
15. STRAUSS, A. J. L., SNELL, K. C., DUNTLEY, B. J., SOBAN, E. J., STEWART, H. L.: Lancet I, 1126 (1968).
16. TALAL, N., SOKOLOFF, L., BARTH, W. F.: Amer. J. Med. 43, 50 (1967).
17. VAN NOORD, M. J., VAN PELT, F. G., HOLLANDER, C. F., DAEMS, W. T.: Lab. Invest. 26, 364 (1972).
18. WALDENSTRÖM, J.: Harvey Lect. 56, 211 (1961).

Summary

E. Grundmann

It appears that only two experimental methods of immunosuppression have a clear-cut effect on carcinogenesis: antilymphocytic serum (or antilymphocyte globulin) and neonatal thymectomy. ALS and ALG are most effective if applied just before the initiating phase of carcinogenesis. This seems to be a decisive factor. In particular, continuous application of ALS will shorten the latent period. The type of ALS (rabbit, horse etc.) has no influence on the result. Neonatal thymectomy has the same effect. Experience with immunosuppressive drugs such as Azathioprine and Cortisol, and with carcino-chemotherapeutics like Actinomycin D, Vinblastine and Cyclophosphamide has so far been very restricted. They do not seem to induce an increased tumor incidence. Special experiments performed by R. KROES, J. W. WEISS and coll. (Bilthoven) on 300 male rats confirm the above mentioned results with ALG. Relatively low doses of the liver carcinogen N-hydroxy-fluorinylacetamide induced tumors more frequently in ALG-treated rats than in controls after a 20-week observation period. But after 26 weeks, the incidence of these tumors was again the same in test animals as in saline or NRG controls, indicating that ALG pretreatment had only shortened the period of latency. Azoxymethane, a compound inducing intestinal tumors, gives a high rate of liver angiosarcomas when combined with ALG. In a test with this combination the rats died even before the normal induction period for intestinal tumors had elapsed. It is not quite clear why azoxymethane together with NRG also induces such anaplastic angiosarcomas, though in a substantially lower rate.

Studies on the immunosuppressive effect of numerous typical chemical carcinogens made by G. R. SCHERF and D. SCHMÄHL (Heidelberg) revealed no convincing correlation between carcinogenic and immunosuppressive properties of these compounds. Testing methods were the hemagglutination test and the enumeration of plaque-forming spleen cells. The authors examined 16 compounds which induce cancer in rats and which are also able to reduce the activity of the immune system, especially after continuous application. Cyclophosphamide, Natulan and Thio-Tepa, which are experimentally carcinogenic, depress only the hemagglutination. Sanamycin (= Actinomycin C) has the same immunosuppressive activity, but no carcinogenic activity. The influence of the highly carcinogenic N-nitroso compounds on the immune system was of a very different intensity, even though the compounds were administered in a comparable toxic dosage and with comparable increments. Doses that do not influence the immune system are nevertheless carcinogenic. Other well-known carcinogenic agents, such as 3-methyl-cholanthrene, 3,4-benz(a)pyrene, fail to show suppressive effects on the immune response in rats, as measured by the hemagglutination test and by the plaque technique.

Experimental observations indicate that immunosuppression has a strong tendency to induce lymphomas. The investigations by G. KRUEGER (Cologne) demonstrate that concomitant and persistent stimulation of mice with antigens provokes lymphomas. He used Azathioprine, Methotrexate, and Cyclophosphamide. Without antigen stimulation the lymphoma incidence was significantly lowered. Methotrexate without antigen stimulation induced no lymphomas at all. Triethylenemelamine provoked lymphomas neither with nor without antigen stimulation. Up to 12% of DBA mice receiving azathioprine were found to have malignant lymphomas, and up to 10% of BALB/c mice treated with Cyclophosphamide had malignant tumors without immune stimulation. It was concluded that the effects of both stimulatory and inhibitory influences on the immune system have separate modes of interference with cell proliferation and with cell differentiation. The intensity of interference may be different for both systems, clinically resulting in chronic infections or sepsis. If the interference of functional inhibitors is chiefly focused on cell differentiation, a progressive cell proliferation is provoked, eventually resulting in the growth of tumor cells. A defective cellular immune response may be more dangerous than an impaired humoral immune response. Defective cellular immune surveillance may be a pacemaker for lymphoreticular malignancy.

Long-term studies on renal homograft recipients are described by I. PENN (Denver). The incidence of de-novo malignancies following transplantation is 5 - 6%, i.e. 100 times that in the general population of the same age range. The Denver Tumor Registry records 184 patients with de-novo cancer; 181 recipients of kidney transplants and 3 of cardiac homografts. Of these patients, 68% had epithelial cancers and 32% mesenchymal tumors, mostly lymphomas with a predilection for the central nervous system. The most common sites of the epithelial tumors were the skin, lip, and cervix uteri. The average induction time (after transplantation) was 31 months in the case of epithelial neoplasms and 21 months in that of mesenchymal malignancies. Azathioprine, prednisone, ALG and Actinomycin C were the main immunosuppressive agents used in the therapy of organ transplant recipients. Other immunosuppressive measures included local irradiation of the transplant and splenectomy. Patients with epithelial tumors had a relatively good prognosis; 87% of these patients are still living, as opposed to 19% of those with mesenchymal malignancies. The possibility that malignant cells might be accidentally transplanted from donors with cancer cannot be excluded. Such cancer cells might grow within the transplanted organ after immunosuppression. In patients from whom preexisting cancers have been removed the risk of recurrence or metastases of the original tumor is 36% after organ transplantation and immunosuppression. It appears significant that malignancies also develop in some cases in which immunosuppressive agents are used in the treatment of nonmalignant diseases such as psoriasis, chronic renal diseases, rheumatoid arthritis, systemic lupus erythematosis, dermatomyositis etc. The agents most commonly used were Methotrexate, Azathioprine, and Cyclophosphamide. The number of patients at risk is not known.

The above results, not yet fully evaluated as to their possible significance, are underlined by the investigations of M. WINNEWISSER and her co-workers (Munich). A few days after clinical administration of cytostatic agents, a marked immunosuppressive effect becomes obvious. It is caused by selective damage to the PHA-sensitive T-lymphocytes. Several days after maximal depression of this lymphocyte response all patients showed an overshoot reaction to PHA in vitro. This "rebound" phenomenon is interpreted as an increase in immunological surveillance. The patients received a massive dose of combination therapy, consisting of vinblastine sulfate (5 - 10 mg), Cyclophosphamide (500 mg) and Amethopterin (20-50 mg). This single massed dose was repeated at intervals of 10 to 21 days. The PHA stimulation is depressed only for a short time. The "rebound phenomenon" may be caused by an ineffectiveness of immunological blocking factors. Clinical treatment has to be adapted to the periodicity of this "rebound phenomenon" when the timing of high doses is chosen. Intervals of three weeks seem to be most advantageous and in the same sense, immunotherapeutic treatment appears indicated only after a similar delay.

M. G. HANNA and his co-workers (Oak Ridge) discuss the balance existing in each patient between the aggressive potential of tumor cells and the degree of retardation by specific immune mechanisms. Their experiments comprised several models aimed at evaluation of the pattern of host immunity during carcinogenesis and so-called nonspecific immunotherapy of transplanted and established tumors. Most of the previously published experience and the special experiments of the authors suggest that the host's immune system plays an active rather than a passive role during chemical carcinogenesis. The development of a specific immunity lags behind tumor growth because the sensitization by tumor antigens is a consequence of the development of tumor cells. Anatomical factors may limit the expression of the immunity. There are also antagonistic actions between various tumor-specific immune components. Thus, the balance between tumor and host is, in most cases, inclined in favor of the tumor. Repeated percutaneous applications after skin scarification ultimately produce modulation of the immune competence in animals, and especially suppression of the humoral immune competence in normal guinea pigs. At the same time, allograft reactivity and isogenic tumor rejection are enhanced. The conditions that contribute to this pattern are still undetermined. BCG has a stepwise reaction on the immune system that involves histiocytes and lymphocytes. Immunotherapy may prove helpful in conditions of minimal cancers or cancer residuals. For these, immunotherapy could be attempted in malignant diseases diagnosed early, as a primary rather than a secondary therapeutic measure. Another, more conservative, possibility lies in combined application of surgery, irradiation chemotherapy and immunotherapy with the purpose of destroying the famous "last malignant cell."

A remarkable example for physiological and locally defined depression of antitumor immunity is the central nervous system, as demonstrated by N. VANDEPUTTE and H. SOBIS (Leuven). Tumors appear to be somehow "protected" in this localization. Another similarly privileged site is the pregnant uterus. It is possible to induce tumors in the uterus by inoculation of a virus which does not provoke neoplasms in other organs in adult rodents. The mouse-sarcoma virus (MSV-MLV) was cited as an example: this virus regularly induced yolk-sac carcinomas in rats fetectomized at day 12 of their pregnancy and injected with the virus. The tumors were of fetal origin. In another experiment the authors removed fetuses of pregnant primiparous rats 12 days after mating. In one horn of the uterus the fetal membranes were left outside. Six weeks later, all rats developed extrauterine tumors in the horn where the fetal membranes had been left outside. Histologically, these tumors were benign teratomas. The method seems to present a promising model for further studies on the pathogenesis of teratomas.

An animal that is apparently eminently suitable for immunological cancer research is discussed by H. L. STEWART and K. C. SNELL (Bethesda). This animal, the mastomys, differs in its disease pattern from other rodents by the frequent development of spontaneous diseases that occur only rarely in other species. During the second year of life, mastomys start to suffer from severe diseases of the joints, similar to human rheumatic arthritis. A large proportion, 80%, of all mastomys develop a certain form of immune-complex glomerulonephritis, and 30% of them develop thymoma, myositis and atrophy of skeletal muscles. There may be a parallel to myasthenia gravis in humans. Quite a number of lymphoreticular tumors are found: reticulosarcoma, lymphosarcoma, and plasma cell myeloma. The most remarkable feature of mastomys is the high incidence of carcinoids such as have never been observed in other animals. The immunological connection between the so-called immune diseases of mastomys and their tumors is still obscure.

General discussion of all the experimental and clinical observations leads to the following conclusions: it cannot be denied that the use of immunosuppressive drugs favors an elevated incidence of malignant tumors. The typical carcinogenic compounds have only a limited immunosuppressive effect. The possibility cannot be excluded, however, that cytostatic agents given for the purpose of immunosuppression will provoke malignant tumors or, at least, favor their development. The mutual interactions have not yet been adequately explained. It is certain, however, that the balance of host immune competence is impaired by chemical carcinogenic and cytostatic agents. The use of immunosuppressive drugs should be restricted solely to cases that cannot receive any other treatment. Secondary malignancies observed after long-term immunosuppression are a warning signal. Careful investigation into all these cases is essential. It will supplement the animal experiments which have provided extensive information about the involvement of the immune systems in malignant growth.

The Cell Cycle in Cancer Chemotherapy*

R. Baserga

A somewhat simplified view, surgery and radiotherapy have been remarkably successful in dealing with primary cancers. In most anatomically localized cancers, with few exceptions surgery or radiotherapy can achieve effective removal of the primary lesion with quite a low rate of recurrence at the site of the initial tumor. The major problem in the therapy of the cancer patient is presented by disseminated neoplastic lesions, either primary (e.g. leukemia) or secondary (metastases from primary tumors). Once tumors are disseminated, surgery and radiotherapy become impotent and the only remaining effective way of dealing with widespread cancer is chemotherapy, where the term is used rather loosely to mean any kind of generalized treatment. It should be stressed at this point that I see chemotherapy as a form of treatment of disseminated cancer, i.e. leukemias, lymphomas and metastases from primary tumors. Thus, although chemotherapy has had some measure of success against a few primary tumors (choriocarcinoma, Wilms' tumor, etc.), it surprises me that in the 20 years since I became interested in oncology, most of the chemotherapeutic trials have been slanted toward the treatment of primary tumors. The size and complexity of primary tumors make them unsuitable as experimental tools for the study and evaluation of chemotherapy, a finely tuned methodology based on small differences between cancerous tissues and normal tissues. To use chemotherapy for the treatment of primary tumors is like using a thoroughbred to plow a field; one ruins both the thoroughbred and the field. The present discussion is therefore written with the basic assumption that the most effective and, especially, the most promising area of chemotherapy is the handling of disseminated tumors like lymphomas and metastases from primary tumors.

One obvious approach to the chemotherapy of disseminated cancer is the immunological one, and immunotherapy is certainly an exceedingly promising avenue which already has important practical applications. The present paper does not deal with this approach to chemotherapy, since immunotherapists are also contributing to this volume. A second approach is the judicious use of the cell cycle, both from a kinetic and from a biochemical point of view, which is my own special interest. The rest of this discussion therefore centers on how our knowledge of the cell cycle can help us to plan a more rational chemotherapy. For the relation of the cell cycle to radiotherapy, the reader is referred to the work of TUBIANA (28).

*This work was supported by U. S. P. H. S. research grant CA 12923 from the National Cancer Institute.

A brief review of the currently accepted meaning of "cell cycle" seems appropriate. In modern terms we can divide the cell populations of the adult animal into three categories, i.e. (1) continuously dividing cells, which continuously move through the cell cycle from one mitosis to the next, (2) nondividing cells, which leave the cell cycle and die without dividing again, and (3) G_0-cells, which in ordinary circumstances neither synthesize DNA nor divide, but can be stimulated to do so by an appropriate stimulus. Extensive reviews of the cell cycle, the kinetics of cellular proliferation and the methodology for studying the cell cycle have been published by a number of investigators (18, 13, 9, 3, 15, 10), and the reader is referred to these articles for further details. The classification of cells into three types applies to populations of different cells, as well as to individual cells within homogeneous clonal populations. Thus, in many tissues of the adult animal there are populations of similar cells that contain continuously dividing cells, quiescent cells that can go back to the cell cycle, and nondividing cells. This is true also of tumors, which may contain cells that divide continuously, other cells that do not participate in the proliferating process but can be brought back to the cell cycle by an immunological stimulus, and dying cells (23). This makes it easy to understand that the growth of any cell population depends on three factors, namely (1) the length of the cell cycle, (2) the fraction of dying cells and (3) the fraction of G_0 cells momentarily out of the cell cycle but capable of returning to it under appropriate circumstances (BASERGA, passim).

At the time when the cell cycle was discovered (11), most textbooks still described cancer as an uncontrolled, wild growth, although careful observers had already noticed from chemotherapeutic trials that normal cells were as sensitive as cancer cells to the effect of drugs that inhibited cell proliferation. There was still hope that normal and tumor cells could be distinguished on the basis of kinetics and it was therefore disappointing, in 1962, to find that the cell cycle of continuously dividing normal cells of mice was shorter than the cell cycle of some of the fastest growing mouse tumors (2). It was pointed out at the time that the growth of tumors in vivo does not necessarily depend on an increased speed of cellular proliferation, i.e. on the shortening of the cell cycle, but may depend on other factors, e.g. the growth fraction (16) and the rate of cell loss. These results have been confirmed by abundant data subsequently gathered in experimental animals, in man, and even in in-vitro situations (17). It must be borne in mind that the important point is not whether the cell cycle of normal cells is shorter than the cell cycle in tumors originating from similar cells. In fact, in most cases, the length of the cell cycle is longer in normal cells than in their neoplastic counterparts, but since we are dealing with chemotherapy as a systemic treatment, the real question is whether there are normal cells in the adult animal whose cell cycle is shorter than that of tumor cells. If this is so, chemotherapy aimed at the destruction of proliferating cells will have a very toxic effect on the host. This is what actually happens, as is well known, in terms of both cell kinetics and chemotherapy. The cell cycle of the cells of the lining epithelium of the small intestine and of some bone-marrow cells is actually shorter than the cell cycle of many tumors (10). These data therefore explain retrospectively some of the failures of chemotherapy aimed at the destruction of proliferating cells.

There is still another approach, and this has been the dream of cancer researchers for the past 50 years, i.e. to find some differences between normal and tumor cells at the biochemical level. The best place to look is, of course, the cell cycle itself. The rest of this discussion will be devoted to our understanding of the molecular basis of cellular proliferation and the question of whether any differences can be detected between normal and tumor cells at the molecular level.

Several reviews have been written already on the subject of the molecular basis of cellular proliferation and the reader is referred to those reviews for detailed information (4, 5). The available evidence can be summarized as follows: The biochemical events occurring between one mitosis and the next proceed in an orderly fashion, and are programmed in roughly the same way as they are in the cell cycle of bacterial cells. Although gene products are certainly involved in the regulation of the flow of cells through the cell cycle, the best evidence for activation of the genome comes from G_0 cells stimulated to proliferate. The events that occur in G_0 cells stimulated to proliferate are common to most models of stimulated DNA synthesis and involve a "ping-pong" mechanism in which rounds of RNA and protein synthesis alternate until DNA and histones are replicated and, finally, the cell divides. The events upon which we would like to focus are the activation of the genome and the synthesis of nonhistone chromosomal proteins, which seem to play a major role in the control of cell proliferation in mammalian cells. As a model we shall take WI-38 human diploid fibroblasts, which grow to form confluent monolayers within 5 to 7 days after plating if the medium is not changed. At this time, labeling of the cells with thymidine-^{3}H shows that about 8/1000 of the cells are labeled over a labeling period of 12 hours. However, when these quiescent confluent monolayers of WI-38 are stimulated to proliferate by a change of medium containing 10% fresh serum, marked stimulation of cell proliferation occurs, and under optimal circumstances as many as 80% of the cells are stimulated to synthesize DNA and divide. The sequence of events in the prereplicative phase of these cells stimulated to proliferate is essentially the same as that described above. We will concentrate here on the increase in chromatin template activity and the synthesis of the nonhistone chromosomal proteins that accompany the stimulation of WI-38 cells.

Within 1 hour after stimulation of cell proliferation there is an increase in template activity of the chromatin isolated from WI-38 cells. The increase probably represents an activation of the genome since in essence, chromatin template activity is a measure of the in-vitro ability of a population of cells to synthesize RNA. Data obtained in collaboration with other workers have indicated that the increase in chromatin template activity occurring at 1 hour is not inhibited by actinomycin D but is inhibited by cycloheximide, which is an inhibitor of protein synthesis (8, 20). Since the data indicated that the synthesis of new proteins was necessary for the increase in chromatin template activity, and since it seemed that the increase in chromatin template activity was directly correlated to the stimulation of cell proliferation (22), we looked for the proteins or protein that could regulate the increase in chromatin template activity and thus represent the initial trigger for the stimulation of cell proliferation. Chromatin has essentially two protein components, histones and nonhistones, and since histones are not synthesized until the time of DNA replication we looked at nonhistone chromosomal proteins as the possible regulators of gene activation and, therefore, of cell proliferation in WI-38 cells.

In fact, the synthesis of nonhistone chromosomal proteins in WI-38 cells increases within 30 minutes after stimulation of cell proliferation (19). The stimulation of nonhistone chromosomal protein synthesis is selective, as shown in my laboratory by TSUBOI, who found that only the synthesis of a certain class of nonhistone chromosomal proteins was increased when WI-38 human diploid fibroblasts were stimulated to proliferate (27).

There are now several examples of increased synthesis of nonhistone chromosomal proteins in a variety of models of stimulated DNA synthesis, including the estrogen-stimulated uterus (26), the isoproterenol-stimulated salivary gland (24), the hamster embryo fibroblasts, in which DNA synthesis is stimulated by SV-40 infection (21), quiescent hamster fibroblasts stimulated to proliferate by a nutritional change (6), and, finally, phytohemagglutinin-stimulated lymphocytes (14).

We thought that it would be possible to define the role of nonhistone chromosomal proteins in the control of chromatin template activity and cell proliferation more closely if the chromatin were separated into its different components and reconstituted with components of our choice. Chromatin from either stimulated or unstimulated WI-38 cells was isolated and DNA dissociated from proteins. The DNA was discarded, histones and nonhistones were separated and then new hybrid chromatins were reconstituted by gradient dialysis, in one case with HeLa DNA, a mixture of histones from both stimulated and unstimulated cells, and the nonhistone chromosomal proteins of nonstimulated cells. In the other case the chromatin was exactly similar except that the nonhistone chromosomal proteins came from the stimulated cells. When the template activity of the hybrid chromatins was measured, the hybrid chromatin containing the nonhistone chromosomal proteins from stimulated cells had a higher template activity than the hybrid chromatin with nonhistone chromosomal proteins from quiescent cells (25). When the DNA and the nonhistone chromosomal proteins are pooled and the hybrid chromatins differ only in the histone component, there is no difference in chromatin template activity. Thus these experiments indicate that the chromatin component responsible for the increased chromatin template activity when cells are stimulated to proliferate are the nonhistone chromosomal proteins, and that these proteins very probably regulate cell proliferation in WI-38 human diploid fibroblasts, and possibly in other mammalian cells.

The possibility of distinguishing nonhistone chromosomal proteins of normal diploid cells and their SV-40 transformed counterparts was also examined.

The transformed cells used were 2RA cells.[1] They are SV-40 transformed WI-38, rather stable and hypertetraploid. They also go through a stationary phase, but their saturation density is about twice that of WI-38 in terms of cell number, and four times in terms of DNA (7). The results indicated the presence in stationary 2RA cells of certain low-molecular-weight nonhistone chromosomal proteins that are absent in quiescent WI-38 human diploid fibroblasts (LIN and BASERGA, unpublished results). Incidentally, this difference in gel-electrophoretic profile of nonhistone chromosomal proteins in WI-38 and 2RA has also been confirmed in another laboratory (STUDZINSKI, pers. comm.).

We have also compared the nonhistone chromosomal proteins of WI-38 and 2RA cells by immunologic methods. In these experiments chromatin was isolated from WI-38 cells and used to immunize either rabbits or chickens. These antibodies anti-WI-38 chromatin were then reacted with different antigens in a complement fixation test.

The antibodies anti-WI-38 chromatin can recognize the difference between WI-38 and 2RA chromatin, and give a much more pronounced reaction with WI-38 chromatin used for immunization of the rabbit than with the chromatin of 2RA cells.

---

[1] 2RA cells kindly donated by Dr. VINCENT CRISTOFALO, Wistar Institute, Philadelphia

The complement-fixing activity of antibodies anti-WI-38 chromatin was then tested, using not chromatin but the nonhistone chromosomal proteins isolated from either WI-38 or 2RA cells. Again, the antibodies anti-WI-38 chromatin recognized the difference between the two sets of nonhistone chromosomal proteins and reacted much more intensely with the nonhistone chromosomal proteins of WI-38 than with those of 2RA (31). When histones from either WI-38 or 2RA are reacted with anti-WI-38 chromatin, however, there is no difference in the extent of complement fixation, indicating that these anti-WI-38 chromatin antibodies do not recognize differences between histones of the two cell types (31). It therefore seems that both from a biochemical and from an immunological point of view there are certain differences between the nonhistone chromosomal protein components of normal diploid cells and their SV-40 transformed counterparts.

Similar reports indicating that there are differences in the gel-electrophoretic profile of nonhistone chromosomal proteins of certain normal tissues, e.g. liver, and tumorous tissues, e.g. hepatomas, have already appeared in the literature (29, 1, 12, 30). In all these studies, however, the tissues chosen for the extraction of nonhistone chromosomal proteins consisted of a mixture of cells, and some of the differences could be ascribed to the fact that the cellular composition of hepatoma, in terms of blood vessels, bile canaliculi, stroma etc., is somewhat different than the cell composition of a normal liver. However, even when pure populations of cells are used, as in our present experiments, differences in nonhistone chromosomal proteins are apparent both at the biochemical and at the normal immunological levels.

We think that these findings are of considerable importance because they suggest a possible difference in biochemical composition between normal and neoplastic cells. It is not surprising that differences may be more significant at the level of chromatin than at the phenotypic level. It is reasonable to assume that the expression of a single protein, say in the cytoplasm or in the membrane, depends on a multicistron effect which, in turn, is regulated not by one single protein but by a group of proteins, so that it is not unlikely that a single phenotypic difference at the membrane level could correspond to differences in 3 or 4 proteins at the level of chromatin. In other words, chromatin could amplify subtle biochemical immunological differences between normal and neoplastic cells.

In conclusion, there is a considerable amount of evidence indicating that nonhistone chromosomal proteins regulate gene activity, and specifically cell proliferation, in mammalian cells. Evidence that the control is exerted by a protein, or a class of proteins with a molecular weight of approximately 35,000 and that there are some substantial differences between the non-histone chromosomal proteins of tumor cells and their normal counterparts is rapidly increasing. Although attempts to detect biochemical differences between normal and cancer cells have been a source of disappointment for the past 50 years, it is possible that this time we may have finally reached the molecular structures that show the most consistent differences; they are the same structures that control cell proliferation, which is obviously altered in cancer cells.

REFERENCES

1. ARNOLD, E. A., BUKSAS, M. M., YOUNG, K. E.: A comparative study of some properties of chromatin from two "Minimal Deviation" hepatomas. Cancer Res. 33, 1169 (1972).
2. BASERGA, R., KISIELESKI, W. E.: Comparative study of the kinetics of cellular proliferation of normal and tumorous tissue with the use of tritiated thymidine. J. nat. Cancer Inst. 28, 331 (1962).
3. BASERGA, R., MALAMUD, D.: Autoradiography: Techniques and Application. New York: Harper and Row (1969).
4. BASERGA, R. (Ed.). Biochemistry of Cell Division. Springfield, Ill.: Thomas 1969.
5. BASERGA, R. (Ed.): The Cell Cycle and Cancer, Vol. 1. In: The Biochemistry of Disease. New York: Marcel Dekker 1971.
6. BECKER, K., STANNERS, C. P.: Control of macromolecular synthesis in proliferating and resting Syrian hamster cells in monolayer culture. J. cell. Physiol. 80, 51 (1972).
7. COSTLOW, M., BASERGA, R.: Changes in membrane transport function in G_0 and G_1 cells. J. cell. Physiol. (in press).
8. FARBER, J., ROVERA, G., BASERGA, R.: Template activity of chromatin during stimulation of cellular proliferation in human diploid fibroblasts. Biochem. J. 122, 189 (1971).
9. FEINENDEGEN, L. E.: Tritium-labeled Molecules in Biology and Medicine. New York: Academic Press 1967.
10. GAVOSTO, F., PILERI, A.: In: The Cell Cycle and Cancer (Ed. R. BASERGA), p. 99. New York: Marcel Dekker 1971.
11. HOWARD, A., PELC, S. R.: Nuclear incorporation of P 32 as demonstrated by autoradiographs. Exp. Cell. Res. 2, 178 (1951).
12. KADOHMA, N., TURKINGTON, R. W.: Altered populations of acidic chromatin proteins in breast cancer cells. Cancer Res. 33, 1194 (1973).
13. LAMERTON, L. F., FRY, R. J. M. (Eds): Cell Proliferation. Oxford: Blackwell 1962.
14. LEVY, R., LEVY, S., ROSENBERG, S. A., SIMPSON, R. T.: Selective stimulation of nonhistone chromosomal protein syntheis in lymphoid cells by photohemagglutinin. Biochemistry 12, 224 (1973).
15. LIPKIN, M. In: The Cell Cycle and Cancer (Ed. R. BASERGA), p. 6. New York: Marcel Dekker 1971.
16. MENDELSOHN, M. L.: Autoradiographic analysis of cell proliferation in spontaneous cancer of C3H mouse. III. The growth fraction. J. nat. Cancer Inst. 28, 1015 (1962).
17. NORRBY, K.: Population kinetics of normal, transforming and neoplastic cell lines. Acta path. microbiol. scand. 78, Suppl. 214, 3 (1970).
18. QUASTLER, H., SHERMAN, F. G.: Cell population kinetics in the intestinal epithelium of the mouse. Exp. Cell. Res. 17, 420 (1959).
19. ROVERA, G., BASERGA, R.: Early changes in the synthesis of acidic nuclear proteins in human diploid fibroblasts stimulated to synthesize DNA by changing the medium. J. cell. Physiol. 77, 201 (1971).
20. ROVERA, G., FARBER, J., BASERGA, R.: Gene activation in WI-38 fibroblasts stimulated to proliferate: Requirement for protein synthesis. Proc. nat. Acad. Sci. (Wash.) 68, 1725 (1971).
21. ROVERA, G., BASERGA, R., DEFENDI, V.: Early increase in nuclear acidic protein synthesis after SV-40 infection. Nature New Biol. 237, 240 (1972).
22. ROVERA, G., BASERGA, R.: Effect of nutritional changes in chromatin template activity and nonhistone chromosomal protein synthesis in WI-38 and 3T6cells. Exp. Cell Res. 78, 118 (1973).

23. STEEL, G. G., ADAMS, K., BARRETT, J. C.: Analysis of the cell population kinetics of transplanted tumors of widely differing growth rate. Brit. J. Cancer 20, 784 (1966).
24. STEIN, G., BASERGA, R.: The synthesis of acidic nuclear proteins in the prereplicative phase of the isoproterenol-stimulated salivary gland. J. biol. Chem. 245, 6097 (1970).
25. STEIN, G., CHAUDHURI, S., BASERGA, R.: Gene activation in WI-38 fibroblasts stimulated to proliferate: Role of nonhistone chromosomal proteins. J. biol. Chem. 247, 3918 (1972).
26. TENG, C. S., HAMILTON, T. H.: Role of chromatin in estrogen action in the uterus. II. Hormone-induced synthesis of nonhistone acidic proteins which restore histone-inhibited DNA dependent RNA synthesis. Proc. Nat. Acad. Sci. (Wash.) 63, 465 (1969).
27. TSUBOI, A., BASERGA, R.: Synthesis of nuclear acidic proteins in density inhibited fibroblasts stimulated to proliferate. J. cell. Physiol. 80, 107 (1972).
28. TUBIANA, M.: The kinetics of tumor cell proliferation and radiotherapy. Brit. J. Radiol. 44, 325 (1971).
29. WAKABAYASHI, K., HNILICA, L. S.: The immunospecificity of nonhistone protein complexes with DNA. Nature New Biol. 242, 153 (1973).
30. YEOMAN, L. C., TAYLOR, C. W., JORDAN, J. J., BUSCH, H.: Two dimensional polyacrylamide gel electrophoresis of chromatin proteins of normal rat livers and Novikoff hepatoma ascites cells. Biochem. biophys. Res. Commun. 53, 1067 (1973).
31. ZARDI, L., LIN, J., BASERGA, R.: Immunospecificity to nonhistone chromosomal proteins of antichromatin antibodies. Nature (in press).

Proliferative Parameters Relevant to Cancer Therapy*

M. F. Rajewsky

It is becoming increasingly widely accepted that besides a better knowledge of the in-vivo pharmacokinetics and of the effective tissue concentrations of therapeutic agents, reliable data on the proliferative properties of both neoplastic tissues and critical normal cell systems (i.e. stem cells of the bone marrow and intestinal epithelium, and the cell populations involved in the immune response) may be indispensable for the design of more rational schemes of tumor therapy. The steady growth of the body of information on the proliferative characteristics of mammalian cell systems during past years has supported and given direction to this trend. However, the initial rapid advances in this field have also uncovered new and unexpected difficulties, whose solution will require new efforts on both the conceptual and the methodological side (6, 13-15, 21, 25).

Much of the interest in a "cell cycle-oriented" approach to cancer therapy can be attributed to the observation that many of the cytocidal agents presently used preferentially affect proliferating cells (P-cells, i.e. cells that proceed through the cell cycle with its constituent phases G_1, S (DNA replication), G_2 and M (mitosis; see Fig.1). In general, cell systems with a high proportion of rapidly proliferating cells appear to be more sensitive to such proliferation-dependent agents than cell populations containing more slowly proliferating cells and/or larger fractions of cells in a nonproliferative state (Q-cells).

In many instances, maximum cytocidal effects are observed when proliferating cells are treated during specific phases of the cell cycle (cell cycle phase-specificity; see 7, 9, 13, 15). In other words, the sensitivity of P-cells to the cytocidal effects of phase-specific agents varies as a function of their position (age) in the cell cycle at the time of exposure (age sensitivity). As in the case of compounds specifically inhibiting DNA replication (e.g. cytosine-arabinoside, hydroxyurea), which at appropriate concentrations selectively kill cells during the S-phase of the cell cycle, phase specificity is usually attributed to an interference with molecular processes characteristic of the cell cycle phase concerned. However, for many phase-specific cytocidal agents the precise nature of the critical molecular interaction is still unknown. Furthermore, it is important to note that the cell cycle phase of maximum sensitivity, in terms of the cytocidal effect of a given agent, is not necessarily identical with the phase during which the

*Supported by the Deutsche Forschungsgemeinschaft as part of the research programme of the Forschergruppe "Biochemische und Immunologische Grundlagen der Leukämie- und Tumortherapie" (Tübingen).

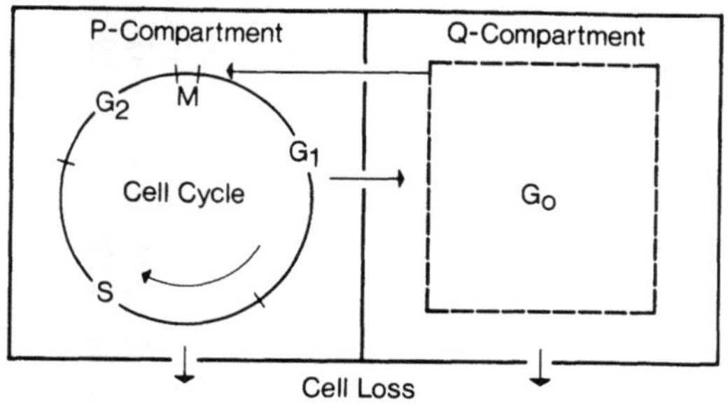

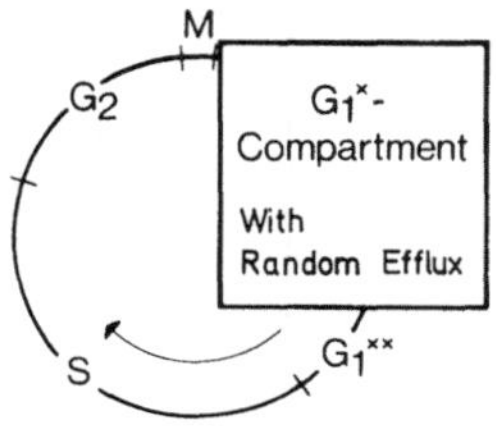

Fig. 1. Above. Diagrammatic representation of a cell system containing proliferating cells (P-cells) and nonproliferating cells (Q-cells). The Q-compartment contains a subcompartment of cells (G_0-cells) with the capacity to reenter the P-compartment under certain conditions. Below. An alternative model (1, 13) in which, after mitosis, P-cells enter a subcompartment of G_1 (G_1^x), from which the cells are released at random into a second G_1-compartment (G_1^{xx}), and the S-G_2-M sequence of the cell cycle

progression of cells through the cell cycle may subsequently be blocked, or during which cell death finally occurs. Indeed, in certain cases, cells may even complete one or several cycles after a lethal interaction with a phase-specific agent. The phase specificity of the cytocidal effect is, of course, a concentration-dependent phenomenon, in the sense that for a given agent it will be maximally expressed within a certain concentration range, but become masked at excesssive concentrations of high toxicity. The list of cytocidal agents demonstrated to be mono- or multi-phase-specific is growing steadily, and includes not only chemical substances, ionizing radiation, and shifts in temperature, but apparently also biological processes such as antibody-mediated immune cytolysis (8, 9, 13, 15; Table 1).

There are a number of proliferative parameters of malignant (and normal) cell systems that have particular relevance in view of the therapeutic application of proliferation-dependent and phase-specific agents (Table 2).

Table 1. Cell cycle-phase specificity of various cytocidal agents in cultured mammalian cells (from RAJEWSKY, M. F. (13); see (13) for literature references)

Agents:	Maximum cytocidal effect resulting from exposure of cells in: G_1	G_1-S	S	G_2	M	Cell type:	References:
Inhibitors of DNA synthesis							
Hydroxyurea, Cytosinearabinoside			▼			HeLa S 3, Mouse L Chin.Hamst. V 79 Chin.Hamst. DON-C Mouse Lymphoma	MAURO and MADOC-JONES (1970), BACCHETTI and WHITMORE (1969), KIM et al. (1967), SINCLAIR (1965, 1967), KARON and SHIRAKAWA (1969), GRAHAM and WHITMORE (1970), KIM et al. (1968), LOZZIO (1969)
Pederine, Daunomycin			▼				
FUDR	▼		▼	▼			
Inhibitors of RNA synthesis							
Chromomycin succinate			▼			HeLa S 3, Mouse L Chin.Hamst. V 79	FUJIWARA (1967), MAURO and MADOC-JONES (1970), BACCHETTI and WHITMORE (1967, 1969), DJORDJEVIC and KIM (1968), ELKIND et al. (1968)
Actinomycin D, Nogalamycin		▼			▼		
Inhibitors of protein synthesis							
Cycloheximide, Puromycin		▼				HeLa S 3	MAURO and MADOC-JONES (1970)
Streptovitacin A		▼					
Antimitotics							
Colchicine, Demecolcin			▼			HeLa S 3 Chin.Hamst. V 79 Mouse Lymphoma	MAURO and MADOC-JONES (1970)
Griseofulvin			▼				
Vincristine sulfate			▼				
Vinblastine sulfate	▼		▼		▼		

Monofunctional alkylating agents							
Ethylmethanesulfonate Methylmethanesulfonate	▼ ▼				▼ ▼	HeLa S 3 Chin.Hamst. V 79	HAHN, pers. comm. quoted by MAURO and MADOC-JONES (1970), NIAS <u>et al</u>.(1970)
Difunctional alkylating agents							
Nitrogen mustard Uracil mustard Mitomycin C Sulfur mustard	 ▼ 	▼ ▼ 			▼ ▼ ▼ ▼	HeLa S 3, Mouse L Chin.Hamst. V 79	MAURO and MADOC-JONES (1970), DJORDJEVIC and KIM (1968), MAURO and ELKIND (1968), WALKER (1966), WALKER and HELLEINER (1963)
Radiation							
X-rays		▼			▼	HeLa S 3 Chin.Hamst. V 79	TERASIMA and TOLMACH (1963), SINCLAIR (1968), MAURO and MADOC-JONES (1970)
Temperature							
High (+ 42°C) Low (- 196°C)				▼ ▼		L 1210 leukemia HeLa S 3 Chin.Hamst. V 79	GIOVANELLA <u>et al</u>. (1969), PALZER and HEIDELBERGER (1973), KOCH <u>et al</u>. (1970)
Immune reactions							
Antibody-mediated, Complement-dependent Cytolysis	▼			▼(?)		Mouse Lymphoma Chin.Hamst. V 79	CIKES (1970), LERNER <u>et al</u>. (1971), SHIPLEY (1971)

Table 2. Parameters and symbols currently in use to characterize the proliferative properties of cells and cell populations (from RAJEWSKY, M. F. (16))

Parameters	(Symbols)	Description
Proliferative State of a Cell	P	Describes cells which can be demonstrated to proceed through the different phases of the cell cycle, i.e. replicate their DNA and divide (P-cells).
Non-proliferative State of a Cell (General)	Q	Describes cells which cannot, during the period of observation, be demonstrated to proceed through the cell cycle and divide (Q-cells).
Reversible non-proliferative State of a Cell Retaining the Potential for Proliferation	G_0	Describes Q-cells which can be shown to (temporarily) resume proliferation upon appropriate stimulation (G_0-cells), e.g. parenchymal cells of the adult liver after elimination of part of the population by partial hepatectomy.
Non-proliferative "End State" of a Cell (Irreversible)	E	Describes Q-cells which - according to present knowledge - have irreversibly lost the potential for proliferation, e.g. mature granulocytes, adult neurons or myocytes ("E-cells").
Cell number	n	Total number of cells of a given cell population.
Proliferative Fraction (P. F.)	n_p/n	Ratio of the number of P-cells, n_p, to the total cell number, n, in a given cell population.
Cell Cycle Time (Intermitotic Time)	t_C	Mean (median) duration of the cell cycle (C) of the P-cells of a cell population.
Duration of G_1, S, G_2, and M	t_{G_1}, t_S, t_{G_2}, t_M	Mean (median) duration of the cell cycle phases G_1, S, G_2, and M of the P-cells of a cell population. Equivalent to the mean (median) transit (or: residence) times of P-cells through (in) the G_1, S, G_2, and M "subcompartments" of the cell cycle.

Flux	$F_{(fg)}$	Fraction of a cell population passing the border line between two adjacent (sub)compartments f and g (of the cell cycle) per unit time.
Mitotic Index (M. I.)	n_M/n	Ratio of the number of cells in mitosis (M-cells), n_M, to the total cell number, n, of a given cell population.
^3H- (^{14}C-) Thymidine Labeling Index	n_{S*}/n	Ratio of the number of cells in the S-phase of the cell cycle (S-cells) labeled with radioactive thymidine, n_{S*}, to the total number of cells, n, in a given cell population.
Fraction of ^3H- (^{14}C-) Labeled Mitotic Cells (F. L. M.)	n_{M*}/n_M	Ratio of the number of M-cells labeled with radioactive thymidine during a preceding S-phase, n_{M*}, to the total number of M-cells in a given cell population.
Population Doubling Time	t_{Deff}	Time effectively required for the doubling of the total cell number of a cell population. In tumors, t_{Deff} is equal to the Volume Doubling Time as long as necrosis, or changes in cell volume or amount of extracellular fluid are insignificant during tumor growth.
Potential Doubling Time	$t_{Dpot} = \lambda \cdot \frac{t_S}{L.I.} = \frac{\ln 2 \cdot t_C}{\ln(1 + P.F.)}$	Time theoretically required for the total cell number to double on the basis of cell production rate, in the absence of cell loss. The coefficient λ depends on the position of the S-period within the cell cycle and on the age distribution of the P-cells (22).
Rate of Cell Production, "Cell Birth Rate" (Fraction of n per Unit Time)	$k_{pr} = \frac{M.I.}{t_M}$	This relationship holds for both "steady state" and exponential growth. If M.I. and t_M are not known, k_{pr} for a cell population composed of both P- and Q-cells can also be derived from $(n_P/n)/t_C$ for "steady state" conditions, or $\ln(1 + n_P/n)/t_C$ ($= \frac{\ln 2}{t_{Dpot}}$) for exponential growth.

Table 2 (Continued)

Parameters (Symbols)		Description
Rate of Cell Loss (Fraction of n per Unit Time)	$k_1 = \frac{\ln 2}{t_{Dpot}} - \frac{\ln 2}{t_{Deff}}$	Rate of cell loss in the case of an expanding (growing) cell population (tumor) (22).
Cell Loss Factor (C. L. F.)	$\Phi = \frac{k_1}{k_{pr}} = 1 - \frac{t_{Dpot}}{t_{Deff}}$	Rate of cell loss as a fraction of the rate at which cells are added to the cell population by mitosis (20). For a "steady state" condition where the rate of cell loss equals the rate of cell production, $\Phi = 1.0$.

(i) The proliferative fraction (10), i.e. the ratio of the number of actually proliferating cells of a population to the total cell number.

Although of considerable operational value, the concept of a proliferative fraction suffers from the difficulty of defining a truly nonproliferating cell (Q-cell). Present methods do not allow us to distinguish with complete certainty between nonproliferating and slowly or discontinuously proliferating cells. In a number of normal cell systems, some of the nonproliferating cells can be "triggered back" into a proliferative state according to functional or reparative requirements (G_0-cells; see 13). A variety of observations (6, 25) suggest that in malignant cell systems, too, depending on environmental conditions, some of the Q-cells may re-enter the cell cycle (or, if previously slowly proliferating, begin to proceed through the cell cycle at an increased speed).

(ii) The mean (median) duration of the cell cycle (intermitotic time; t_C) of the P-cells of a population, and the durations of the different cell cycle phases (t_{G1}, t_S, t_{G2+M}).

The classic method for the estimation of these parameters is the fraction of labeled mitoses (FLM) technique (11, 23; see also Fig. 2a). Due to its sensitivity to the spread in cell-cycle time of the individual P-cells, this technique can also be used to obtain information on another parameter, namely

(iii) the distribution of cell cycle times of the proliferating cells in a given population (see Fig. 2b)

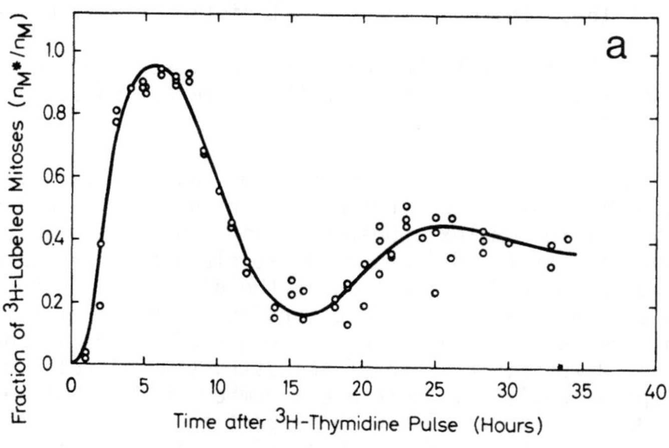

Fig. 2 a. Fraction of labeled mitoses (F.L.M.). Curve for solid BICR/M1R_k tumors grown subcutaneously in rats of the Marshall strain (from RAJEWSKY, M. F., and GRÜNEISEN, A. (17)). o: Mean values for single tumors. Optimized curve computed by the method of STEEL, G. G., and HANES, S. (24)

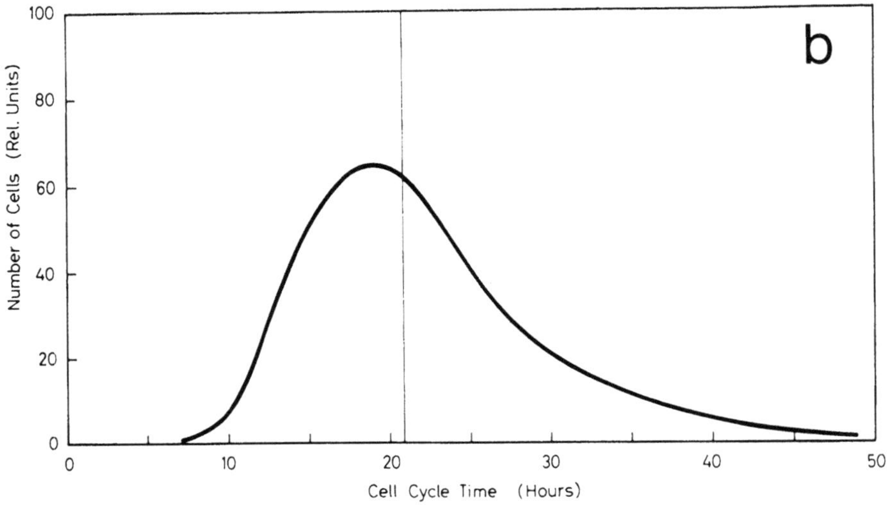

Fig. 2 b. Distribution of cell cycle times (t_C) in solid BICR/M1R_k-tumors, as computed from the F.L.M. data shown in Fig. 2 a by the method of STEEL, G. G., and HANES, S. (24). The vertical bar indicates the median value for t_C (from RAJEWSKY, M. F. and GRÜNEISEN, A. (17))

On the other hand, the difficulty of obtaining estimates of cell-cycle parameters representative of the majority of the proliferating cells in a population by the FLM technique increases with the spread in cell-cycle times of the P-cells (23). Furthermore, the technique is not sufficiently sensitive to detect differences in the cell cycle parameters of multiple phenotypically indistinguishable subpopulations of cells. Unfortunately, to varying extents, both these features are characteristic of many primary tumors.

(iv) The age-distribution of the proliferating cells of a population, i.e. the proportions of cells in the different phases of the cell cycle at a given time (Figs. 3 and 4).

Although age-distribution diagrams based on mean values (i.e. ignoring spread) are often used, the true age distribution of the P-cells in a primary tumor has a more complex appearance due to the spread in cell-cycle time and in the duration of the different cell-cycle phases. An interesting experimental approach to the determination of the distribution of cells in the different phases of the cell cycle according to their relative DNA content is provided by the recently developed technique of pulse cytophotometry (Fig. 4; 14, 15, 18). However, in spite of the attraction of pulse cytophotometry for this type of analysis, there are a number of difficulties that must be acknowledged, in particular with respect to its application in the study of neoplastic tissues and leukemia. First, the techniques presently available for the conversion of solid tissues into single cell suspensions are open to the criticism that a preferential loss or enrichment of specific classes of cells can be difficult to exclude. In addition, the majority of nonproliferative cells possess a G_1-DNA content and a smaller proportion a (G_2 -M)-DNA content, i.e. these cells cannot easily be distinguished from cycling G_1- or G_2 -cells, respectively. While these problems can be overcome (the latter e.g. by the use of appropriately designed block-release schemes for the separation of nonproliferative cells with a G_1-DNA content from true G_1-cells), it is be-

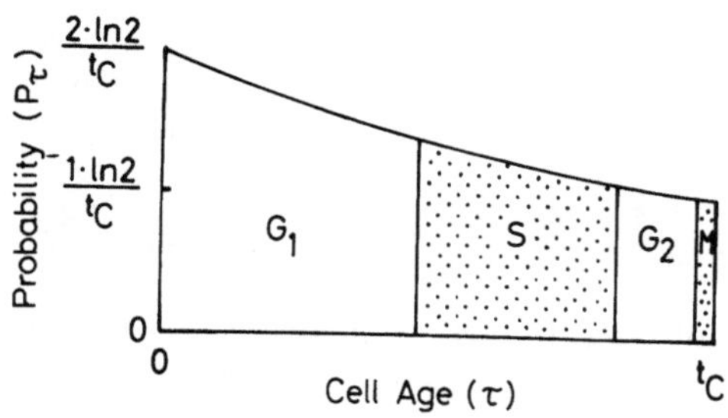

Fig. 3. Diagrammatic representation (ignoring the spread in the duration of the cell cycle, t_C, and its constituent phases) of the age distribution of an asynchronously proliferating cell population in exponential growth (from RAJEWSKY, M. F., GRÜNEISEN, A. and REMMER, I. (18)). Cell age (τ) given in units of t_C

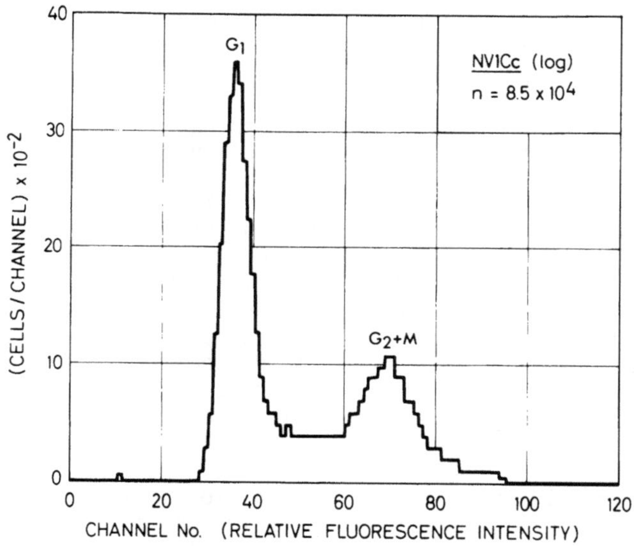

Fig. 4. Pulse-cytophotometric analysis of the cell cycle phase distribution of cultured log phase NV1Cc-rat neurinoma cells, according to their relative DNA content (from HANKE, K. and RAJEWSKY, M. F. (4)). Sample size: 8.5 x 10^4 cells. Ethidium bromide-stained DNA. Pulse cytophotometer ICP 11 PHYWE AG, Göttingen. See (14) for preparative procedures. The first peak (on the left) represents cells with a G_1-DNA content, the second peak is due to cells with a G_2-M-DNA content. S-cells give relative fluorescence values between these maxima

yond the resolving power of the technique to recognize very small subpopulations of cycling cells against the background of large fractions of nonproliferative cells (4). This may be the case, for example, if analysis of a small proportion of proliferating leukemic blasts is attempted in peripheral blood. Furthermore, unlike autoradiography, pulse cytophotometry cannot provide data for individual subpopulations of heterogeneous cell systems containing proliferating cells with differing phenotypes and proliferative properties unless the cells vary significantly in their relative DNA content (4).

The age distribution and knowledge of t_C and the duration of the different cell-cycle phases can yield another parameter of considerable importance in phase-specific therapy, namely

(v) the fraction of a proliferating cell population reaching (or entering) a given cell-cycle phase per unit time (21).

In estimating this parameter, however, it would be dangerous to rely entirely on theoretical values derived for intact cell systems, since proliferative parameters can be subjected to significant changes under the influence of therapy or other factors.

Besides attempts to use proliferative parameters of cell populations as a basis for the construction of therapeutic schemes i.e. by deriving optimum time intervals between therapeutic doses, optimum durations for the maintenance of effective drug concentrations, and suitable combinations of agents with differing phase specificities there have been attempts to investigate possible ways of modifying the age distribution of proliferating cells in both malignant and normal cell systems prior to phase-specific therapy (5, 7, 12, 15, 18, 19).

If, under in-vivo conditions, the age distribution of the (asynchronously) proliferating cells of a population could be manipulated in such a way that an increased proportion of neoplastic cells would temporarily be accumulated in (or pass through) a defined cell cycle phase (partial synchronization), the subsequent application of a cytocidal agent directed specifically against cells in the phase concerned would presumably be more effective than under normal conditions. Furthermore, as the cell cycle parameters of the critical normal cell systems and neoplastic cell populations are unlikely to be identical, the periods of maximum sensitivity for normal and malignant cell populations would tend to become dissociated as a function of time after partial synchronization. This, in turn, could permit a relative "protection" of normal cells from the cytocidal effects of a phase-specific drug if it were applied at a time of increased sensitivity of a neoplastic cell population.

Evidently, the basic conditions for this kind of "processing" of cell populations for subsequent "cell cycle-adapted" therapy are (a) knowledge of the proliferative parameters of the cell systems involved, and (b) techniques permitting a controlled modification of the age distribution and prediction of the subsequent proliferation kinetics of these cell populations in vivo.

The distribution of the P-cells of a population over the cell cycle, for example, can be modified by temporarily slowing down or blocking the progression of cells through the cell cycle at a specific stage, e.g. DNA synthesis or mitosis. Cells in phases not affected by the block will then continue their passage through the cell cycle and accumulate to a degree depending on the duration of the block at the beginning of the blocked phase. After block reversion, these cells will proceed through the cell cycle in a partially synchronized manner. As cell populations are characterized by varying degrees of spread in cell-cycle time, the degree of synchrony will become progressively "damped" as a function of time after block reversion.

The cell cycle kinetics of cell populations after temporary specific inhibition of DNA synthesis (e.g. by hydroxyurea), or of mitosis (e.g. by vinblastine) can be monitored by sequential determinations of both the fraction of cells in the S-period of the cell cycle (after pulse labeling of S-cells with

^{3}H-thymidine and autoradiography) and the mitotic index (i.e. the fraction of cells in mitosis). Less time-consuming and more elegant, but still confined to suitable model cell systems, is the recording of the sequential changes in the distribution of cells in the different phases of the cell cycle by pulse-cytophotometric analysis (Fig. 5). By this means the time intervals can be determined where maximum or minimum fractions of a population of cycling cells are found in defined subcompartments of the cell cycle, and estimates can be obtained of the fraction of cells entering or leaving a specific subcompartment of the cell cycle. This information is required for precisely timed application of phase-specific cytocidal agents.

The impression that techniques such as those described may make it possible to modify the distribution of proliferating cells in the cell cycle in a controlled and predictable manner under in-vivo conditions, prior to phase-specific therapy, should not divert us from the fact that various unfavorable properties of autochthonous tumors will in many instances reduce a therapeutic advantage over conventional schemes of treatment.

It has already been mentioned that many primary tumors are characterized by broad overall distributions of cell cycle time. In such cases it will be difficult to accumulate appreciable proportions of cells in sensitive phases of the cell cycle, unless very protracted blocks are used for partial synchronization (15, 26).

Many tumors in clinically detectable stages of growth apparently possess relatively large fractions of nonproliferative cells (Table 3). Although in part endowed with the capacity to re-initiate DNA replication and cell division, these cells will tend to escape the cytocidal effects of agents directed primarily against P-cells. Unfortunately, clinical and experimental studies indicate that so-called clonogenic tumor cells recruited from the nonproliferative compartment may contribute substantially to tumor regrowth after exhaustive therapeutic elimination of the proliferative compartment (6, 25). Consequently, it might be advantageous, although perhaps paradoxical at first sight, to search for methods of "triggering back" into cycle the potentially clonogenic tumor cells that are temporarily hidden in the Q-compartment. The observations suggesting that temporarily nonproliferative tumor cells may re-enter the cell cycle e.g. after therapeutic elimination of part of the cell population (25) and possibly also in a state of depressed immune reactivity of the host (3, 17) imply that quiescent tumor cells are probably not activated by preprogrammed cellular mechanisms. It seems more likely that microenvironmental conditions and extracellular factors are involved, which are open to investigation and may eventually be exploited in the context of therapy.

It has been suggested that in primary tumors (analogous to normal multicompartment renewal cell systems) a small fraction of cells with stem cell properties (tumor stem cells) are responsible for growth, whereas the majority of cells do not possess an unlimited capacity for division, i.e. are not clonogenic (6, 23). Support for this hypothesis is derived from observations that (a) primary tumors are often characterized by relatively low proliferative fractions combined with high rates of cell loss, and (b) only a small proportion of cells from such tumors give rise to cell clones in the few in-vitro and in-vivo assay systems presently available. There is, however, reason to doubt the general existence of a specific class of tumor cells with the predetermined biological rôle of stem cells. It may be that many cells in a malignant cell system are potentially capable of giving rise to cell clones, and that the probability of this occurring depends on a complex combination

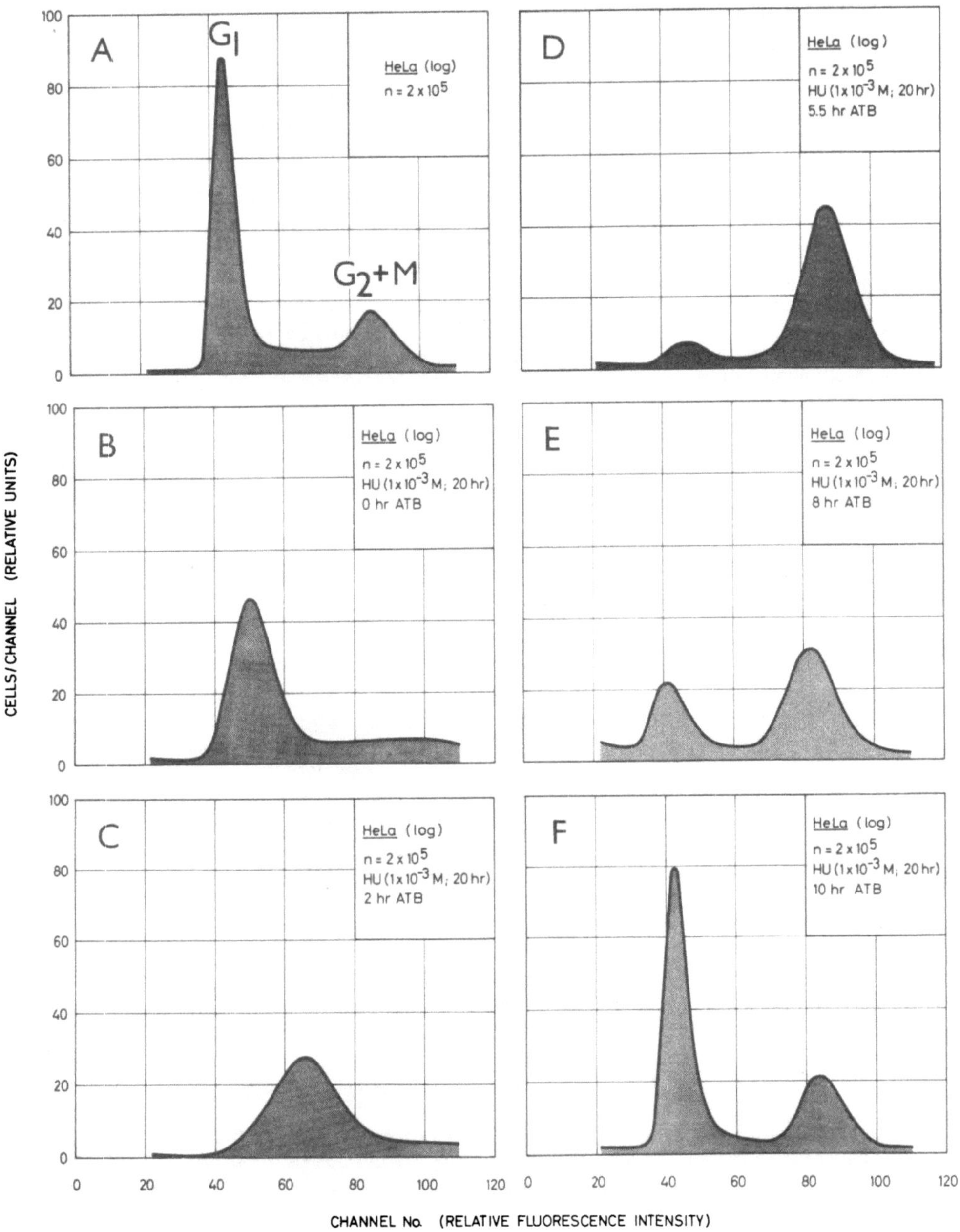

Fig. 5. Pulse-cytophotometric analysis of log phase HeLa cells, as a function of time after the termination of a 20 h block of DNA synthesis with hydroxyurea (10^{-3} M) (from RAJEWSKY, M. F., GRÜNEISEN, A., and REMMER, I. (18)). (A) Untreated control (asynchronous population) (B) 0 h after termination of block (ATB) (C) 2 h ATB (D) 5.5 h ATB (E) 8 h ATB (F) 10 h ATB

Table 3. Proliferative parameters of malignant tumors (mainly based on data compiled by STEEL, G. G. (23))

Parameter	Frequently-passaged animal tumors (n=13)	Transplanted animal tumors (≦ 4 passages) (n=9)	Primary animal tumors (n=5)	Human tumors (n=4)	Human malignant melanoma[c] (n=1)
t_D (h)	50	233	253	1392[a] (median)	1000
t_C (h) median	22	32	17	52	72
t_D/t_C	2	7	15	27[a]	14
t_S (h) median	8	12	8	17	21
$(t_{G1}+t_{G2})/t_C$	0.64	0.61	0.57	0.56	0.58
Proliferative Fraction	0.60	0.27	0.49	0.45	0.18
Cell Loss Factor	0.31	0.49	0.85	~0.70 -0.95[b]	0.70

a (2)

b (25)

c (20)

of factors, among which the immune response of the host and the spatial arrangement and density of malignant cells in relation to the blood capillaries play an important part. However, irrespective of the definition of tumor stem cells, it would of course be most important in the context of therapy if the clonogenicity of tumor cells were also due to (or favored by) specific proliferative parameters differing from those of the majority of cells in the population. Besides the development of reliable assays for clonogenic tumor cells, this would require methods allowing discriminative determination of the proliferative parameters of the clonogenic cells in tumors, i.e. of a small, phenotypically undefined fraction of the population. Such techniques are presently not available.

Finally, one of our most important objectives is still the development of methods for the protection of the critical normal cell systems during cancer therapy with proliferation-dependent cytocidal agents. Before differences in the proliferative characteristics of normal versus malignant cell populations can be effectively exploited, the corresponding proliferative parameters of each must be known. Unfortunately, our knowledge, for example of the proliferative properties of the stem cells of bone marrow or intestinal epithelium in man, is still inadequate, and techniques allowing quick and reliable estimates of the proliferative parameters of individual malignant tumors have not yet been developed.

REFERENCES

1. BURNS, F. J., TANNOCK, I. F.: Cell Tiss. Kinet. 3, 321 (1970).
2. CHARBIT, A., MALAISE, E. P., TUBIANA, M.: Europ. J. Cancer 7, 307 (1971).
3. DECOSSE, J., GELFANT, S.: Science 162, 698 (1968).
4. HANKE, K., RAJEWSKY, M. F.: Pulse-Cytophotometry (Eds. C. A. M. HAANEN et al.). Ghent: European Press-Medikon 1975, in press.
5. KLEIN, H. O., LENNARTZ, K. J., GROSS, R., EDER, M., FISCHER, R.: Dtsch. med. Wschr. 97, 1273 (1972).
6. LAMERTON, L. F.: Brit. med. Bull. 29, 23 (1973).
7. MADOC-JONES, H., MAURO, F.: J. nat. Cancer Inst. 45, 1131 (1970).
8. MADOC-JONES, H., MAURO, F.: In: Handbook of Exp. Pharmacology (Eds. O. EICHLER et al.), p. 206. Berlin, Heidelberg, New York: Springer 1974.
9. MAURO, F., MADOC-JONES, H.: Cancer Res. 30, 1397 (1970).
10. MENDELSOHN, M. L.: J. nat. Cancer Inst. 28, 1015 (1962).
11. QUASTLER, H., SHERMAN, F. G.: Exp. Cell Pres. 17, 420 (1959).
12. RAJEWSKY, M. F.: Exp. Cell Res. 60, 269 (1970).
13. RAJEWSKY, M. F.: Z. Krebsforsch. 78, 12 (1972).
14. RAJEWSKY, M. F.: Proliferative parameters of cell populations and cancer therapy. In: Erythrocytes, Thrombocytes, Leukocytes; Recent Advances in Membrane and Metabolic Research (Eds. E. GERLACH et al.) p. 460. Stuttgart: Thieme 1973.
15. RAJEWSKY, M. F.: Bull. Cancer 60, 143 (1973).
16. RAJEWSKY, M. F.: Proliferative parameters of malignant cell systems. In: Handbuch der allgemeinen Pathologie (Eds H.-W. ALTMANN et al.), Vol. VI. 5-6, p. 289. Berlin, Heidelberg, New York: Springer 1974.
17. RAJEWSKY, M. F., GRÜNEISEN, A.: Europ. J. Immunol. 2, 445 (1972).
18. RAJEWSKY, M. F., GRÜNEISEN, A., REMMER, I.: Studia Biophysica 31/32, 367 (1972).
19. RAJEWSKY, M. F., HÜLSER, D. F., FABRICIUS, E.: Z. Krebsforsch. 76, 266 (1971).

20. SHIRAKAWA, S., LUCE, J. K., TANNOCK, I. F., FREI III, E.: J. clin. Invest. 49, 1188 (1970).
21. SKIPPER, H. E.: The cell cycle and chemotherapy of cancer. In: The Cell Cycle and Cancer (Ed. R. BASERGA), p. 358. New York: Marcel Dekker 1971.
22. STEEL, G. G.: Cell Tiss. Kinet. 1, 193 (1968).
23. STEEL, G. G.: Cell Tiss. Kinet. 5, 87 (1972).
24. STEEL, G. G., HANES, S.: Cell Tiss. Kinet. 4, 93 (1971).
25. TUBIANA, M.: Brit. J. Radiol. 44, 325 (1971).
26. WILMANNS, W., WILMS, K., RAJEWSKY, M. F.: Biochemische Grundlagen der Behandlung von Leukosen. In: Leukämie (Eds R. GROSS, J. VAN DE LOO), p. 459. Berlin, Heidelberg, New York: Springer 1972.

Different Types of DNA-Synthesis and Their Importance in Cancer Growth and Therapy

A. Caputo

A review of the present state of knowledge about the mechanisms by which DNA replicates shows that we have definite knowledge that replication begins at a well-defined point (initiation time) in a specific region of DNA (initiation site), and that the cycle of replication hardly ever begins at a random position or at any other than the programmed time.

In considering the fundamental events which regulate, or promote, the initiation process, I have identified three main types of DNA replication: spontaneous, stimulated and induced synthesis.

The normal semiconservative synthesis by which DNA spontaneously replicates requires, in addition to the building blocks assembled by a series of enzymes, a pre-existing DNA chain, which acts both as template regulating the unidirectional elongation of the assembly, and as a primer, by means of its terminal group for the new growing pieces.

At present, the general pattern of DNA replication involves three main concatenate steps: the synthesis of a short RNA chain by an early RNA polymerase, followed by the use of the end of the RNA chain as a primer for DNA growth, and, lastly the erasure of the RNA nucleases. The role of RNA as starter at a specific place on DNA provides the natural facility of a message for translating, which is soon discarded.

This normal pattern, operatively completed during the S-phase of the cycle, is strictly dependent on the structural integrity of the DNA, a condition which in the cell provokes the signal for initiation.

Evidence has been accumulated which conclusively suggests that the initial event is the unbalancing of energy levels, which causes the initiation process.

There is a close correlation between the modified energy that is the critical factor in initiation and the appropriate, and so far elevated, concentration of the precursors in the pool. It is well known that the enzymes required for activation of the precursors are present in small amounts in G_0-cells, which are quiescent, do not synthesize DNA and do not divide. As well as the spontaneous, semiconservative replication, we must also consider the so-called "stimulated DNA synthesis" which occurs only in G_0-cells and after appropriate stimulation. Although the information on this subject is still limited, there are obviously features that are common to both types of synthesis and differences that have been detected by biochemical examination. Both spontaneous and stimulated DNA synthesis occur at a defined time in the cycle, during the S-phase. More precisely, it should be emphasized that the operative schedule for DNA replication is initiated at different points of the G_1-phase, but is absolutely completed by the end of the S-phase.

The stimulus itself plays the role of the initiator system and therefore the subsequent operative schedule includes the same enzyme machinery as is employed in spontaneous synthesis. Another common denominator of spontaneous and stimulated synthesis is that both are strcitly dependent on the integrity of the native DNA molecule, and in both cases nicks must be produced in one or both strands of the duplex to promote the action of DNA polymerase.

The mechanism by which the genome of the quiescent cell is activated has been the subject of extensive studies over the past decade, but no definite model scheme can yet be drawn up, and its generalization may pose many problems. Nevertheless, there are biochemical events that occur and have been constantly recognized over the whole range of different model systems, and their importance can be stressed in principle. First of all, it has been observed that there is always a lapse of several hours between the application of the stimulus and the origin of the S-phase of the cycle. This latency, which is necessary for DNA replication, is characterized by the increase of different molecular species of RNA, and among them a pre-existing RNA is used as template for translation of early proteins independently of the activation of the gene. Even when the occurrence of specific RNA molecules is a prominent event of the prereplicative phase of non-continuously-dividing cell systems, additional macromolecular events have sometimes been recognized. An increase in protein synthesis has been observed and studies with inhibitors specific for protein synthesis suggest that the newly synthesized proteins are essential for the subsequent onset of DNA replication.

Spontaneous DNA synthesis and stimulated DNA synthesis have a common pattern involving an identical enzymic machinery. The schedules are differently programmed in their initial steps, however, the role of the spontaneous initiator (time- and space-specific) in continuously-dividing-cells having as its counterpart the application of the stimulus, which is independent of time and requires molecular changes for its own specificity. In non-continuously-dividing cells the inability of DNA to undergo replication is thus determined by the absence of the initiation process.

The patterns of spontaneous and stimulated DNA synthesis are strictly dependent on the integrity of the native DNA molecule. However, in some circumstances of normal cell evolution, and frequently in cancer transformation, several types of structural changes in the DNA molecule have been documented. The events when chemicals, radiations or viruses modify the helical conformation and subsequently alter DNA functionality are particularly open to speculation.

The mechanism which operates at the molecular level for restoration of the function is an "induced DNA synthesis" with the specific role of repairing the altered regions of the molecule. The model of repair replication has been discovered and studied in essence by radiobiologists, but it should be emphasized at this point that induced syntheses generally occur at any site where chemicals, viruses and physical agents affect the integrity of the native DNA molecule. It might be said that in induced synthesis the signal for initiation is provided by the energy coming from the rupture of the chemical bonds at the site(s) where the inducer has affected the single- or double-stranded conformation. Insofar as the synthesis takes place for the purpose of repairing the points altered in the DNA molecule, the early prerequisite is the localization and then the excision of the damage. This is accomplished by means of nickase enzymes, such as endonuclease and exonuclease. All the specificity of repair synthesis resides in its primary step, where enzymes able to recognize only specific chemical groups have been identified.

In the patterns of spontaneous, stimulated and induced synthesis, it is obvious that the different substrates (initiation site, stimulation area, and disrupted regions) need to be specifically recognized, and therefore it is essentially that they differentiate the three types of DNA synthesis.

Although DNA is a target upon which several inducers act to produce damage, the nature of repairable lesions is quite different, according to the specificity of the agents.

The next important question is whether there is only one mechanism of induced synthesis or whether the specific lesions require separate, corresponding mechanisms. What has experimentally achieved seems clearly enough to indicate that the removal of a pyrimidine dimer for its own chemical nature ought to be different from that of the alkylated guanine or from the insertion of a short or large piece of viral genome. Nevertheless, it must be clearly pointed out that only one basic mechanism does occur, and that the only variable is confined to the first step, where a very specific enzyme (endonuclease) recognizes the peculiarity of the altered conformation and ruptures the bonds linking the damaged sequence to the adjacent normal ones. Chemically speaking, endonuclease recognizes the nature and extent of intrastrand and/or interstrand linkage very accurately. Although highly purified preparations of endonuclease have not yet been obtained, there is much experimental evidence demonstrating that even the crude enzyme preparation is active only on their specific substrates.

One might wonder how a virus, which obviously represents a completely different type of inducer, can have a similar effect on DNA. The specificity of viral endonuclease has been convincingly demonstrated and the enzyme acts next to the base pairs guanine-cytosine on sequences rich in thymine-adenine. This indicates that the integrational event depends on some preferential sequences of the virions, and other preferential counterparted sequences may also be necessary; these would be supplied by the host-cell chromosomal DNA to cause the arrangements appropriate to the carcinogenic effect or to the infection.

Tumor growth results from the heterogeneous aggregation of different cell populations, even if all of them derive ultimately from a single element. The consequence is that the mitosis activity is not set at a constant range and the proliferation of malignant cells is therefore unregulated and unrestrained. At a molecular level, this lack of hierarchy is most probably determined by the overlapping of different types of DNA replication, and is especially related to the types of synthesis induced by different endogenous and/or exogenous effectors.

Even if DNA represents the keystone in normal evolution and cancer transformation, the complexity of its molecular organization requires an adjacent system to finalize the process, which depends on normal or abnormal information. Thus, before DNA replication, a pre-existing system makes available DNA with a new specific function. Otherwise, it would be impossible to understand how any effectors, whether chemicals, radiation, virions, or hormones etc., can play both oncogenic and antiblastic roles. It is of interest to recall the operative role of stimulated and induced DNA synthesis. As in any case DNA is the target molecule, I should briefly mention the interest of those special structures called "repeated sequences." The repeated DNAs are made up by sequences of various length (down to 300 nucleotides) repeated up to several thousand times. Very recently, BECKER has suggested that the genes which control the synthesis of the cellular DNA and the synthesis of the proteins are situated in an adjacent position to a repeated poly-dG- dC sequence, while all the genes that contain information for the cellular structural proteins are adjacent to poly-dA-dT sequences. Thus, according to the nature of different polynucleotide sequences, the transcription of the two different groups of genes might require different DNA-dependent RNA polymerases which transcribe different classes of messenger RNA at different stages of the cycle. The mRNA molecules which are transcribed from a DNA strand with poly-dC sequences might contain complementary polyguanine sequences (designated Gm RNA), while the poly-dT sequences in the transcribed DNA strand might be transcribed into polyadenine sequences in the mRNA molecules (designated AmRNA). Obviously, such transcriptional control does not occur in the prereplicative phase of the cell cycle, where other activities are in progress, mainly the synthesis of early RNA with priming activity and the synthesis of the enzymes required for DNA replication. In this case "nonrepetitive" RNA polymerases are necessary.

The implications for cancer transformation deriving from an organization such as DNA repeated sequences must also be considered.

Let us first consider the transformation of a cell by a tumorigenic virus. Evidence has been obtained that oncogenic viral DNA, whether circular or linear, resembles the cell genomic DNA in its organization. The presence of cytosine-rich and thymine-rich clusters have well been documented in polyoma and human papilloma virus; in addition, a large number of poly dG-dC sequences have been found. This type of organization is essential for the replication cycle of the virus, and it has been demonstrated that differential areas of viral genome supply two essential types of information, recognized by the presence of an early mRNA and a late mRNA. In viral DNA the poly-dG-dC sequences characterize the genes coding for nonstructural proteins (enzymes for activation of DNA precursors, nucleases, polymerases and polyligases) while the genes for the structural proteins are adjacent to poly dA-dT sequences. The early messenger RNA molecules are transcribed from the genes adjacent to poly-dG-C (early genes), while the late messenger RNA molecules are transcribed from genes adjacent to poly dA-dT sequences (structural genes). The late messenger which transcribes information for capsid protein, viral antigens and the enzyme machinery for the synthesis of the host cell genomic DNA might therefore contain poly-A sequences. It is implied that the cells able to be transformed by oncogenic DNA viruses are those with DNA in a conformation that is suitable for offering the necessary counterparted poly dG-dC sequences.

Although it is very difficult to provide an accurate definition of the molecular events that sustain malignancy, from the preceding discussion one can extrapolate that in cancer causation there is an inversion of the spontaneous DNA replication versus stimulated or induced syntheses.

The problem of reparability is of fundamental importance, and some points need to be carefully considered. Independently of the nature of the indcuer, and according much more to the molecular flexibility of DNA, repair mechanisms may be more or less effective in relation to the phases of cell cycle. With irradiation, the delay of synchronous nuclear division is maximal in the late G_1-phase or in the early S-phase and falls gradually in the middle of the S-phase. The data collected for several cell systems indicate that the extent of unrepaired DNA damage persisting 3-4 hours after irradiation at different stages in the cycle is parallelled by the delay in mitosis: greatest for irradiation in late G_1 and early S, less for that in mid-S and absent after irradiation in G_2. This type of pattern depends on the "fixation" of the damage, which still occurs if the damaged site becomes involved in replication before it can be repaired and/or rejoined. The presence of breaks in parental strands during replication might lead to the insertion of improper bases or to gaps in the newly synthesized strands, which subsequently inhibit the repair. Since repair and/or the rejoining processes require an appropriate length of time, damage produced during the late G_1- or early S-phases has a better chance of entering into the ongoing replication process before they can be repaired. Since the main property of a tumor is the unlimited growth, a derangement of the normal mechanism of cell replication is obviously the operative factor. Cancer transformation is an unreversible phenomenon, and therefore the oncogenic factor directly or indirectly modifies the content and/or the expression of the genomic information which codes for the molecular systems controlling normal cell replication. Owing to the irreversibility of the lesion it can be predicted that any action taken against the abnormal growth might also affect the mechanisms which control and regulate the normal growth, i.e. any anti-oncogenic factor, like the oncogenic agents, might have direct or indirect effects on the content and/or the expression of the genomic DNA from which the stability of neoplastic growth derives. Therefore it does not seem paradoxical that the oncogenic factor can act as an anti-oncogenic and vice versa. Hence, it may be a general rule that the positivity (→ neoplastic transformation) or the negativity (→ inhibition of cancer growth) depends on a series of events which all collectively regulate the "active concentration" of the effector and concomitantly the "exposed state" of genomic DNA.

As far as the active concentration is concerned, the importance of appropriate doses in the realization of the mutagenicity and/or the oncogenicity of chemicals, radiation, viruses, etc., is well documented. In such an intricate framework, any effector can inhibit, block or deviate the standard replication of only some of the cell clones without simultaneously affecting, sometimes even enhancing, the replication of other clones in the same tumor. Since in both oncogenicity and anti-oncogenicity the antagonizing effects can be obtained with a single dose, obviously the reactivity of genomic DNA is the critical factor in the response. The so-called exposed state of DNA reflects a particular conformation of the DNA molecule in which preferential effects are determined to a maximal extent and irreversibly. If an antiblastic effector, regardless of its nature, interacts with DNA in the prereplicative phase of the cycle, the exposed conformation of DNA molecules and the lower repairability of the induced damage will modify the genome more extensively, according to significant alterations of the templating and/or priming activities of DNA. As previously stated, the sensitivity or resistance of cancer cells to biological, physical or chemical agents is the expression of a steady-state equilibrium between the number and/or the extent of damage to DNA molecules and the capacity to be specifically repaired. Thus, by shifting the equilibrium in one direction it should be possible to increase the sensitivity of the cancer cell according to the degree of damage to the DNA molecules, when the development of tumor resistance to antiblastic agents will be accounted for by an increased number of repaired molecules. Obviously, in the cancer cell, apart from the DNA which represents the fundamental target, other constituents regulating the functionality of the target are of relevant interest. Among these, special consideration should be given to RNAs which before and after DNA replication determine the operativity of the system by controlling the fidelity of transcription.

So far, since faulty DNA replication results in stabilized or temporary nonfunctional, or misfunctional, events followed by altered cell replication, the effectiveness of cancer therapy depends also on the appropriate centering of the targets: DNA, repair mechanisms and RNA transcription. Unfortunately, inhibitors that can selectively affect the molecular machinery of cancer cells are not available. Molecular biologists have provided a series of very interesting data which have added much to our knowledge on the mechanisms of control and regulation, rather than offering a useful tool for cancer therapy. Until we have an understanding of the very initial events in cancer causation, based on actual knowledge, it is rather difficult to predict a selective anticancer effect for any single inhibitor. However, as cancer represents the main problem in human pathology and favorable effects are sometimes obtained in therapy by appropriate evaluation and application of the data obtained in experimental models, I should like to conclude with a generalized scheme. The strategy should involve one or all of three main levels, DNA synthesis, transcription and translation. However, at present, information on possible selective effects is limited strictly to a few cases.

1. Abolition, or reduction of the effectiveness of the stimulation acting on the stimulus itself or modifying the specific molecular requirements in the target cells.

2. After the induction of specific damage by chemical or physical effectors on DNA molecule block the initial step (endonucleases incision) which specifically characterizes the repair replication in order to enhance the chemico- or radio-sensitivity, according to the differences of cycle times between normal and neoplastic cells.

3. Inhibition of the enzymes specifically involved in the initial step of insertion of viral genome fragment(s) in order to prevent the integration in host-cell chromosomal DNA.

4. Inhibition of early RNA polymerase to prevent the synthesis of early specific RNAs which interfere with normal primer and/or template RNAs inducing misfunctionality.

5. According to the possibility that in the cancer cell transcriptional processes are particularly controlled, and different types of repetitive RNA polymerase transcribe repetitive sequences of poly dG-dC or poly dA-dT, the inhibition of these enzymes will avoid the molecular arrangement required for malignancy.

6. The juxtaposition of repetitive sequences in the course of transcription may be altered by the action of some inhibitors (e.g. actinomycin, cordycepin, aflatoxin) which affect the elongation process of transcription nonselectively. As a result, differently sized mRNAs will miscode for the abnormal information of neoplastic DNA.

7. Inhibition of initiation or termination processes of translation by means of the use of antibodies which specifically recognize and block initiation or termination codons at the ends of the messenger RNA molecule.

8. Alteration of the translocation process during translation by means of process-selective drugs (fusic acid, cycloheximide, etc.) to modify the polypeptide chain length and thus change the antigenic functionality of newly synthesized proteins.

Investigations on Partial Synchronization in Ascites Tumors of Different Ploidy and in Solid Transplantable Tumors*

K. J. Lennartz, H. O. Klein, and W. Féaux de Lacroix

In contrast to in-vitro studies (3, 4, 11, 20, 21, 27, 28, 30) investigations on in-vivo synchronization of normal and malignant cells are still few in number. One experimental approach to this problem is that of RAJEWSKY (24-26). In his experiments a satisfactory degree of synchrony was obtained in a transplantable mammary carcinoma (rat) following the administration of hydroxyurea, an inhibitor of DNA synthesis.

In our investigations we tried to induce partial synchronization in vivo in different neoplastic cell systems (mouse) by temporary blocking of mitosis (T_M). Like the studies of RAJEWSKY, this approach required a suitable inhibitor with minimum cytotoxicity in a low dose. We used vincristine (VCR), a leurosine-like alkaloid of vinca rosea (10).

After intraperitoneal injection (i.p. inj.) of VCR (0.025 µg/g body weight) it was demonstrated that under in-vivo conditions neoplastic cells of the mouse were reversibly blocked in T_M (13-17). After release of the blocking effect a subpopulation of cells finished T_M and proceeded almost synchronously through the cell cycle.

Other results (2) indicate that the half-life ($t_{1/2}$) of VCR is short, permitting a limited blocking effect. This is a prerequisite for avoidance of cell damage, provided that the inhibiting agent is applied in a low dose. According to an estimation based on supravital staining with lissamin green (9) the dose of VCR used in the synchronization experiments (0.025 µg/g) did not cause an increase of cell damage in diploid Ehrlich ascites tumor (EAT) cells (5th day after inoculation of 18 x 10^6 tumor cells into male NMRI mice). The data were supported by quantitative measurements of cell multiplication. However, a higher dose of VCR had a cytocidal effect and did not lead to synchronization (6; also observed by present authors).

The model cell systems used were ascitic and solid tumors of male mice (NMRI; C3H) with well-known proliferative characteristics: a diploid ($EAT_{dipl.}$) and a tetraploid EAT (ELT), further diploid EAT cells growing in a solid form after subcutaneous transplantation (sc. transpl.) and a partly differentiated transplantable mammary carcinoma (C3H/Tif/Bom; H B, Dr. C. W. Friis, Ry, Denmark).

Analysis of the proliferative characteristics was performed as in previous studies (for experimental techniques, see 5, 18, 19).

*supported by Deutsche Forschungsgemeinschaft.

ASCITIC TUMORS

$EAT_{dipl.}$

Proliferative parameters: The $EAT_{dipl.}$ grows asynchronously, as does the ELT (22). According to the growth curve, there was a constant population doubling time (T_{Deff} = 26 h) up to day 5 after inoculation (18 x 10^6 tumor cells), indicating an exponential growth in this period of cell multiplication. The mean generation time (T_C) determined at day 5 after inoculation by the method of labeled mitoses (LM) (23) was 19 h, the DNA synthesis time (T_S) 11 h and the mean duration of G_2 phase + mitosis = $(T_{G2} + T_M)_m$ was 4 h. Similar results were obtained with the aid of the double-labeling technique (DLT) (8, 18, 19, 29). According to the percentage of labeled cells found after repeated i.p. inj. of ^{3}H-thymidine (^{3}H-TdR; 25 μCi per inj.; specific activity 2Ci/mMol; NEN Chemicals GmbH; over an interval of 5 h) at the time T_C - T_S an approximate value of 0.70 was estimated for the growth fraction (GF). The cell loss factor (ϕ) was 0.10.

Induction of Partial Synchronization (day 5 after inoculation of 18 x 10^6 tumor cells)

After i.p. inj. of VCR (0.025 μg/g), two peaks of the fraction of mitoses (MI) were observed as a function of time. The first mitotic wave (m.w.) lasted from the time of injection (0) to the 25th h and the second one from the 50th to the 65th h. The peaks were found at the 10th and the 60th h respectively. The second peak (MI = 0.06) was relatively low compared with the first one (0.15), but it exceeded the MI of the controls by a factor of 2.3.

Between the two m. w. the MI was in the same range as the controls.

The ^{3}H-TdR-labeling index (LI), i.e. the ratio of cells in T_S to the total number of tumor cells, also varied as a function of time after VCR. A peak of the LI with a value of 0.60 was found between the two m. w. at the 35th h (LI in controls = 0.36 ± 0.05). The data were reproduced in separate experiments (1).

The results were consistent with those obtained by means of cytophotometric measurement of the relative nuclear DNA content after Feulgen staining (13-15) Furthermore, a double-labeling experiment was performed to find out whether the fraction of cells of the second m. w. were the cells previously accumulated in T_M, forming the first m. w., or whether the cells of the second m. w. originated from the nonproliferative compartment (Q-compartment, G_0-cells) and were triggered into the proliferative (p-) compartment. Up to the 15th h after VCR (0.025 μg/g) tumor-bearing mice received 10 μCi ^{3}H-TdR i.p. (specific activity 2 Ci/mMol; NEN Chemicals GmbH) every 5 hours. Between the 35th and 45th h, the interval in which the increase in LI was observed, the ascites tumor cells were labeled every 5 hours with ^{14}C - TdR (4 μCi per inj.; specific activity 25-30 mCi/mMol; NEN Chemicals GmbH). According to this technique, the cells of the second m. w. would be double-labeled with ^{3}H- and ^{14}C - TdR if a synchronized subpopulation had been produced. By autoradiography (G5 emulsion, Ilford London; exposure time 7-10 d) it was established that more than 50% of the ascites tumor cells of the second m. w. were double-labeled.

The data obtained by different experimental techniques allow the conclusion that the $EAT_{dipl.}$ may be partially synchronized in vivo after the application of VCR (0.025 μg/g).

ELT

This tetraploid EAT showed no truly exponential growth. There was an increasing prolongation of T_{Deff} dependent upon the time after inoculation (see also 7, 12). At day 5 after inoculation (18 x 10^6 tumor cells) T_{Deff} was about 60 h (cf. 7). The method of LM, applied at day 5/7 after inoculation, revealed a T_S of 21 h; $(T_{G2} + T_M)_m$ was 5 h. With the aid of the DLT an equal value of T_S was estimated. T_C was 41 h. For GF a value of 0.90 was measured. The factor ϕ was 0.27.

Induction of Partial Synchronization (day 5 after inoculation of 18 x 10^6 tumor cells)

After one i.p. inj. of VCR (0.025 μg/g), two significant mitotic peaks were found. The second peak of MI was again markedly lower than the first one, but it exceeded the MI of the control group by a factor of about 3. The first m. w. lasted from 0 to the 20th h and the second one from the 65th to the 75th h.

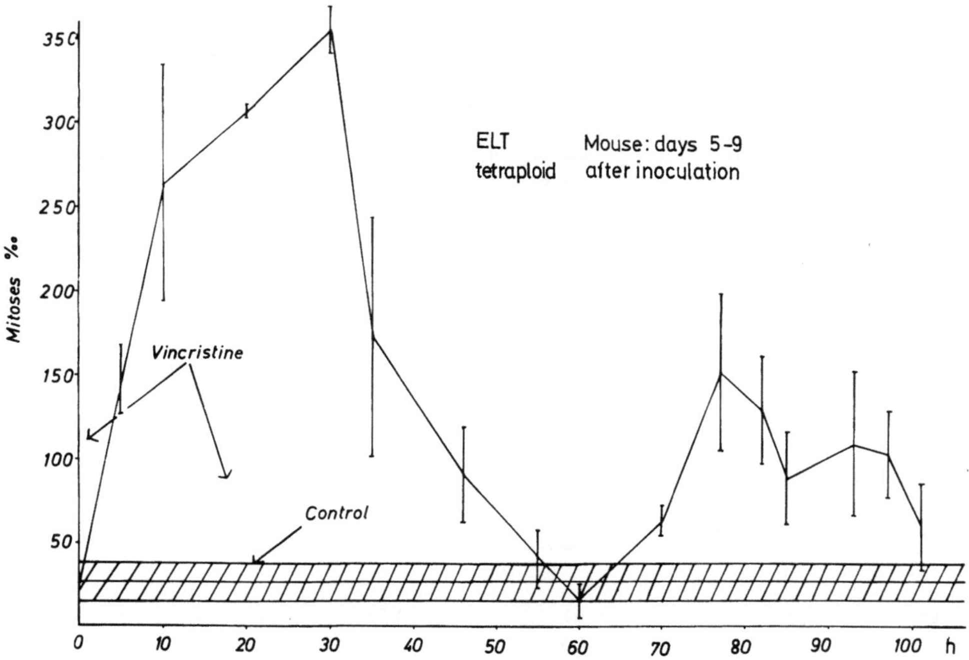

Fig. 1. Fraction of mitoses (MI) as a function of time after two intraperitoneal injections of vincristine (0.025 μg/g per inj.; interval between the two inj. = 12 h) in a tetraploid Ehrlich ascites tumor (ELT; growing in male NMRI mice). Onset of the experiment at day 5 after inoc. (18 x 10^6 tumor cells). (The vertical bars represent the confidence limits of the average)

After two i.p. inj. of VCR (0.025 μg/g per inj.) within 12 h the second m. w. was more prominent, suggesting a higher degree of synchronization (Fig. 1).

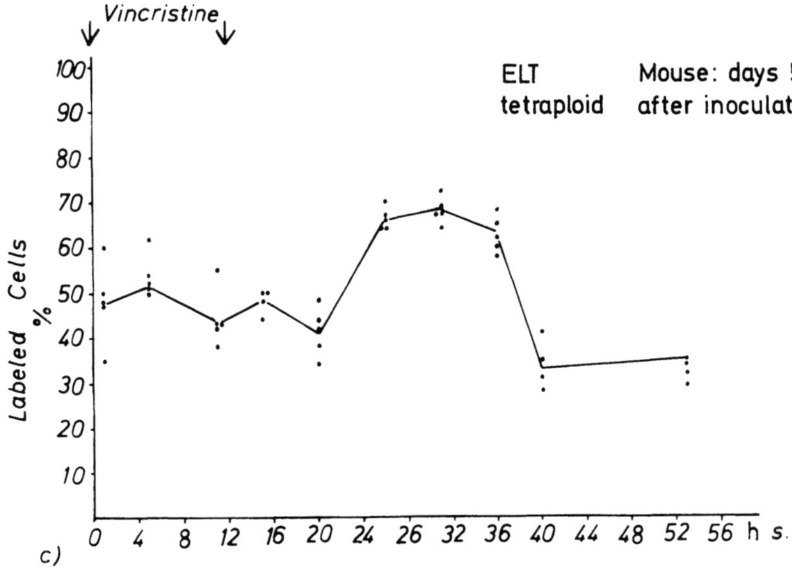

Fig. 2. Fraction of DNA-synthesizing cells (^{3}H-thymidine labeling index = LI) as a function of time after two intraperitoneal (i.p.) injections of vincristine (VCR; 0.025 μg/g per inj.; interval between the two inj. = 12 h) in a tetraploid Ehrlich ascites tumor (ELT; growing in male NMRI mice). Onset of the experiment at day 5 after inoc. (18 x 10^6 tumor cells); i.p. inj. of ^{3}H-TdR (2 μCi/g; 2 Ci/mMol) at different intervals after VCR one hour before sacrifice of the tumor-bearing mouse. (Each point represents one animal test)

Between the 20th and the 40th h after VCR the LI increased to values of about 0.70 (Fig. 2) as against 0.44 ± 0.04 in the controls. The width of the wave of the increased LI corresponded to a relatively long T_S (= 21 h).

The data suggest that the ELT can also be partially synchronized.

SOLID EXPERIMENTAL TUMORS

Diploid EAT Cells Growing in a Solid Form

Proliferative parameters: Like ascitic neoplastic cells, diploid EAT cells growing in a solid form showed no diurnal fluctuation of the MI and LI. At least the cells at the periphery of the solid nodule grow asynchronously.

After sc. transpl. an increase of the tumor volume was found over a period of up to 4 weeks (volume-doubling time = 10-11 days). The cell cycle estimated at the day 21 after transpl. was similar to that of the $EAT_{dipl.}$ determined at the day 5 after inoculation (T_C = 24 h, T_S = 12 h, $(T_{G2} + T_M)m$ = 3 h). For GF a value of about 0.50 was estimated. The factor ϕ was 0.85.

Induction of Partial Synchronization (day 21 after transpl.)

Following the administration of VCR (0.025 μg/g i.p.) two peaks of MI were also found for the diploid EAT cells growing at the periphery of the tumor nodule (Fig. 3). The first peak was observed at the 10th and the second one at the 55th h after VCR, a similar result to that obtained in the ascitic $EAT_{dipl.}$. However, the second mitotic peak was more prominent for the solid form of growth, showing no difference after one or two inj. of VCR (0.025 μg/g pro i.p. inj. with an interval of 10 h). The MI of the second mitotic peak was higher by a factor of about 3.5 than the MI of the controls.

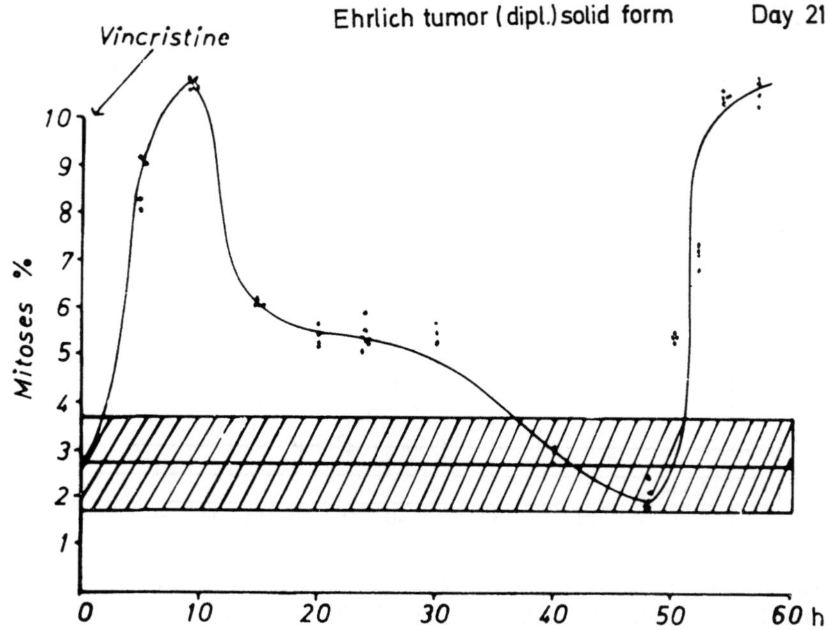

Fig. 3. Fraction of mitoses (MI) as a function of time after one intraperitoneal injection of vincristine (0.025 μg/g) in a diploid Ehrlich ascites tumor (EAT) growing in a solid form in male NMRI mice after subcutaneous transplantation. Onset of the experiment at day 21 after transpl.

Partly Differentiated Mammary Carcinoma (HB)

This experiment was designed to test whether VCR can also lead to a partial synchronization in a transplantable solid mammary carcinoma (HB). The histological features were characterized by differentiation of an adenoid pattern as well as solid epithelial areas (5).

Proliferative parameters: the growth characteristics were analyzed on day 21 after transpl. into the flank of male C3H mice. At this time the solid tumor exhibited rapid growth according to the volume curve (volume-doubling time = about 7 days). The MI showed a moderate diurnal fluctuation, indicating that the growth was not asynchronous. Examination by the method of LM on day 21 after transpl. revealed a T_C of 18.5 h, a T_S of 4.5 h and $(T_{G2} + T_M)_m$ of 2.5 h. GF was 0.52 and the factor ϕ was 0.73.

Induction of Partial Synchronization (day 21 after transpl.)

Fig. 4 shows the course of MI as a function of time after two i.p. inj. of VCR (0.025 µg/g per inj.). The interval between the two injections was 12 h. Two peaks of the MI were found in this case also: the first peak at the 15th and the second at the 65th h after VCR. The second mitotic peak exceeded the MI of the control group by a factor of about 3. The results were consistent with the data obtained with the other neoplastic cell systems tested.

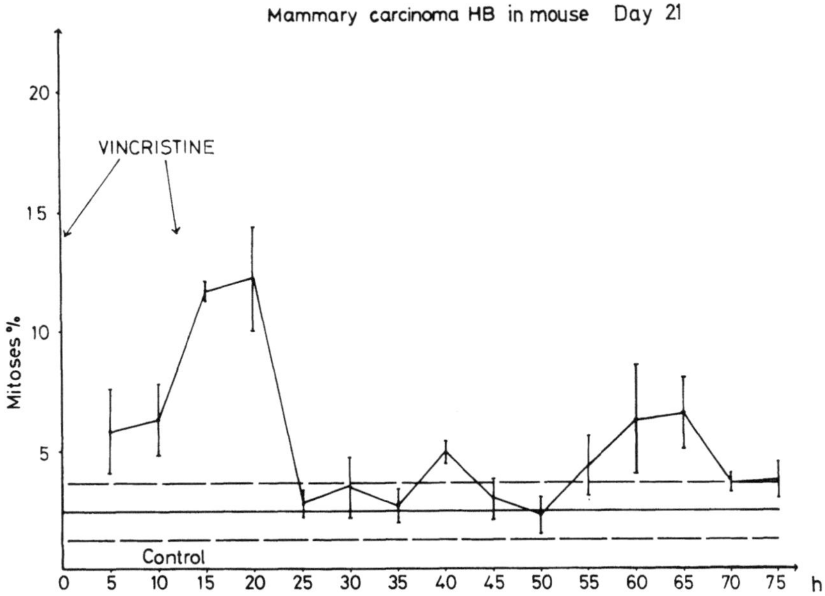

Fig. 4. Fraction of mitoses (MI) as a function of time after two intraperitoneal injections of vincristine (0.025 µg/g per inj.; interval between the two inj. = 12 h) in a partly differentiated mammary carcinoma (HB; growing in male C3H mice). Onset of the experiment on day 21 after transpl. (The vertical bars represent the standard deviation of the mean)

CONCLUSION

The results of the experiments indicate that the neoplastic cell systems tested, i.e. ascitic and solid experimental tumors were partially synchronized in vivo after one or two doses of VCR. In view of the level of the second mitotic peak observed after VCR it must be conceded that in our own experiments only a moderate degree of synchronization was obtained. In this context one must take into account that even well-synchronized cell populations can rapidly lose the synchrony, as was demonstrated in the case of Chinese hamster cells after mitotic selection (4). The decay of synchrony is dependent on the width of the distribution of the generation time of the cell system (27).

The interval between the first and the second mitotic peaks (Figs. 1, 3, 4) after VCR suggests that VCR caused T_C in the synchronized subpopulation to be extended by a factor of 1.5 to 3.0. The data collected in separate experiments with the $EAT_{dipl.}$ suggest that T_{G2} is made longer as well as T_{G1}. No significant change was observed for T_S (1).

After application of VCR in a dose used for the induction of partial synchronization of the neoplastic cells, in mouse the bone-marrow cells (total cell population) also showed marked variation in the fraction of mitoses and DNA-synthesizing cells as a function of time, indicating modified cell proliferation. It was established that the position of the second mitotic peak of the bone-marrow cells was different from that of the neoplastic cell systems tested (13).

These experimental conditions should allow timing of cycle phase-specific agents in antineoplastic treatment of the experimental tumors.

REFERENCES

1. ADLER, D., DÖRING, M., LENNARTZ, K. J.: Unpublished data.
2. BEER, C. T., WILSON, M. L., BELL, J.: A preliminary investigation of the fate ot tritiated vinblastine in rats. Canad. J. Physiol. Pharm. 42, 368 (1964).
3. CAMERON, I. L., PADILLA, G. M. (Ed.): Cell synchrony. Studies in biosynthetic regulation. New York, London: Academic Press 1966.
4. ENGLEBERG, J.: A method of measuring the degree of synchronization of cell population. Exp. Cell Res. 23, 218 (1961).
5. FEAUX DE LACROIX, W., KLEIN, P. J., KLEIN, H. O., LENNARTZ, K. J.: Vergleichende autoradiographische Untersuchungen an einem teils differenzierten und einem anaplastischen transplantablen Mammacarcinom der Maus. Beitr. Path. 150, 287 (1973).
6. HARTENSTEIN, R., ERHART, H., HOFFMANN, K.: Zellkinetische Untersuchungen beim Ehrlich-Aszitestumor unter Vincristin. Z. Krebsforsch. 79, 213 (1973).
7. HAUSCHKA, T. S., GRINNEL, S. T., REVESZ, L., KLEIN, G.: Quantitative studies on the multiplication of neoplastic cells in vivo. J. nat. Cancer Inst. 19, 13 (1957).
8. HILSCHER, W., MAURER, W.: Autoradiographische Bestimmungen der Dauer der DNS-Verdopplung und ihres zeitlichen Verlaufs bei Spermatogonien der Ratte durch Doppelmarkierung mit C-14- und H-3-Thymidin. Naturwissenschaften 49, 352 (1962).
9. HOLMBERG, B.: On the permeability to lissamin green and other dyes in the course of cell injury and cell death. Exp. Cell Res. 22, 406 (1961).
10. JOHNSON, J. S., ARMSTRONG, J. G., GORMAN, M., BURNETT, J. P.: The vinca alkaloid: a new class of oncolytic agents. Cancer Res. 23, 1390 (1963).
11. KIM, H. J., STAMBUK, B. K.: Synchronization of HeLa cells by vinblastine sulfate. Exp. Cell Res. 44, 631 (1966).
12. KLEIN, G., REVESZ, L.: Quantitative studies on the multiplication of neoplastic cells in vivo. J. nat. Cancer Inst. 14, 229 (1953).
13. KLEIN, H. O., LENNARTZ, K. J.: Proliferationskinetische Grundlagen der Behandlung von akuten Leukosen. In: Leukämie (Eds R. GROSS, J. VAN DE LOO). Berlin, Heidelberg, New York: Springer 1972.
14. KLEIN, H. O., LENNARTZ, K. J.: Chemotherapy after synchronization of tumor cells. Seminars in Hematology 11, 203 (1974).

15. KLEIN, H. O., LENNARTZ, K. J., GROSS, R., EDER, M., FISCHER, R.: In vivo- und in in vitro-Untersuchungen zur Zellkinetik und Synchronisation menschlicher Tumorzellen. Ihre Bedeutung für die zytostatische Therapie. Dtsch. med. Wschr. 97, 1273 (1972).
16. KLEIN, H. O., LENNARTZ, K. J., HABICHT, W., EDER, M., GROSS, R.: Synchronisation von Ehrlich-Ascites-Tumorzellen und ihre Bedeutung bei der Anwendung eines alkalierenden Cytostaticum. Klin. Wschr. 48, 1001 (1970).
17. KLEIN, H. O., LENNARTZ, K. J., TEICHMÜLLER, W., GROSS, R.: Cytostatic treatment of partially synchronized tumor cells in animals and men. In: Advances in Antimicrobial and Antineoplastic Chemotherapy (Eds M. HEJZLAR, M. SEMONSKY, S. MAZAK) Munich, Berlin, Vienna: Urban & Schwarzenberg 1972.
18. LENNARTZ, K. J.: Proliferationskinetik von Tumorzellen. In: Fortschritte der Krebsforschung (Ed.: C. G. SCHMIDT, O. WETTER). Stuttgart: Schattauer 1969.
19. LENNARTZ, K. J., MAURER, W., EDER, M.: Autoradiographische Untersuchung über die Dauer der DNS-Verdopplung und die Generationszeit bei Ascitestumoren (Maus) mit unterschiedlichen Chromosomen-Stammlinien und von verschiedener Abstammung. Z. Krebsforsch. 71, 267 (1968).
20. MITTERMAYER, C.: Der mitotische Cyclus und seine Beeinflussung durch Cytostatica. In: Fortschritte der Krebsforschung. (Eds C. G. SCHMIDT, O. WETTER). Stuttgart: Schattauer 1969.
21. PFEIFFER, S. E., TOLMACH, L. J.: Selecting synchronous populations of mammalian cells. Nature 213, 139 (1967).
22. PILGRIM, C., LENNARTZ, K. J., WEGENER, K., HOLLWEG, S., MAURER, W.: Autoradiographische Untersuchungen über tageszeitliche Schwankungen des H-3-Index und des Mitose-Index bei Zellarten der ausgewachsenen Maus, des Ratten-Fetus und bei Ascites-Tumorzellen. Z. Krebsforsch. 68, 138 (1965).
23. QUASTLER, H., SHERMAN, F. G.: Cell population kinetics in the intestinal epithelium of the mouse. Exp. Cell Res. 17, 420 (1959).
24. RAJEWSKY, M. F.: Synchronization in vivo: Kinetics of a malignant cell system following temporary inhibition of DNA synthesis with hydroxyurea. Exp. Cell Res. 60, 269 (1970).
25. RAJEWSKY, M. F.: Proliferative parameters of mammalian cell systems and their role in tumor growth and carcinogenesis. Z. Krebsforsch. 78, 12 (1972).
26. RAJEWSKY, M. F., HÜLSER, D. E., FABRICIUS, E.: Untersuchungen zur Synchronisation in vivo: Temporäre Inhibition der DNA Synthese durch Hydroxyharnstoff in normalen und malignen Säugerzellsystemen. Z. Krebsforsch. 76, 266 (1971).
27. SINCLAIR, W. K.: Methods and criteria of mammalian cell synchrony. In: Fortschritte der Krebsforschung. Normal and malignant cell growth (Eds R. J. M. FRY, M. L. GRIEM, W. H. KIRSTEN). Berlin, Heidelberg, New York: Springer 1969.
28. STUBBLEFIELD, E.: Synchronization methods for mammalian cell cultures. In: Methods of cell physiology, Vol. 3 (Ed. D. M. PRESCOTT). New York, London: Academic Press 1968.
29. WIMBER, D. E., QUASTLER, H.: A C-14- and H-3-thymidine double labeling technique in the study of cell proliferation in Tradescantia root tips. Exp. Cell Res. 30, 8 (1963).
30. ZEUTHEN, E. (Ed.): Synchrony in cell division and growth. New York: Wiley 1964.

Critical Survey of Experimental Data on *in vivo* Synchronization by Hydroxyurea

M. Tubiana, E. Frindel, and F. Vassort

The use of drugs capable of causing partial synchronization of malignant cells has been advocated in cancer chemotherapy. The purpose of this paper is to review some of the data on which such treatments might be based and to evaluate the practicality of cell synchronization in cancer therapy.

Many agents kill cells preferentially during certain phases of the cell cycle. Moreover, some of these agents can also temporarily block the progress of proliferating cells throughout the cell cycle. Selective killing and reversible block change the age distribution of the cell population and increase the proportion of cells in one of the phases of the cell cycle, thereby producing a cycling variation of the sensitivity of surviving cells to drugs or ionizing radiations. This cell reassortment has been called synchronization by some authorities.

The so-called synchronizing effect of ionizing radiation due to preferential killing (55, 16) and mitotic delay has been described in experiments in which mice received sublethal doses of total-body irradiation followed by second doses at various intervals (28). Synchronization has also been described for erythroblastic cells (44), hemopoietic stem cells (15), intestinal crypt cells (68, 19) epidermal cells (8, 69) and roots of vicia faba (21). It has been also observed in tumors (27, 52): solid mouse tumors were irradiated in vivo and cell survival assayed in vitro. After a conditioning dose a cyclic fluctuation in the radiosensitivity of surviving cells was observed for about 40 hours (52) and was consistent with that predicted for a synchronous cohort of surviving cells moving through the phases of the cell cycle, taking into account the cell-cycle data and the age response of these cells. Attempts have been made to build mathematical models based on these data, in order to increase cell death and optimize fractionation in radiotherapy (58, 70).

Many drugs have been reported to cause some cell synchrony in vivo e.g. cytosine arabinoside (20, 35), bleomycin (2), fluorouracil (31), vincristine (32) and hydroxyurea. We shall concentrate mainly on the experimental data obtained with this last drug.

In-vitro tests have shown that hydroxyurea (HU) kills the cells synthesizing DNA and causes a reversible block at the boundary between G1 and S (54). Experimental data suggest that a similar effect is achieved in vivo; for instance, partial cell synchronization has been reported in mouse skin (56), bone-marrow stem cells (4, 66) and differentiated cells (42, 43), duodenal crypt cells (9, 19), rat cartilage cells (30) hair matrix cells (40), and a few experimental tumors (49, 50, 20, 36, 41, 53, 45).

On the basis of these data, it has been suggested that the synchronizing effect of HU should be exploited in human cancer therapy. It was hoped that with the correct time interval between the conditioning dose of HU and the administration of a second therapeutic agent, the damaging effect on normal tissues could be minimized while the killing effect on malignant cells could be enhanced. This goal is of such importance that any information on which potential clinical application could be based ought to be critically evaluated.

A. METHODOLOGY

Various methods have been used to study the kinetics of cell proliferation after HU administration, such as labeling index, cytophotometry, and rate of DNA synthesis, evaluated by the incorporation of tritiated thymidine in DNA.

The changes in the time course of the labeling index after pulsed tritiated thymidine administration has been used in many experiments to assess cell reassortment (9, 10, 13, 35). Although this method provides useful information, the results it yields are by no means conclusive. The only cells which need to be considered in cancer therapy are those that can proliferate and give rise to viable progeny. Normal tissues and tumors are composed of differentiated cells which can only divide a few times, and of clonogenic cells. The proportion of clonogenic cells varies, but is often small. Moreover, after treatment with radiation or medication, the damaged cells may divide a few times but all their progeny will eventually die, and these doomed cells cannot be distinguished on morphological grounds from viable clonogenic cells.

Conventional cytophotometry on smears or imprints (6, 17) is similar to autoradiography, but automated cytophotometry with modern equipment (50) is open to more discussion, as the DNA content of all the cells is measured without taking their morphology into account. Cells of different types are pooled and the data obtained for a tumor, for example, reflects the state of all the cells located inside the tumor, whether malignant or belonging to connective tissue.

The same is true of data obtained by measurement of tritiated thymidine incorporation with liquid scintillation. Furthermore, with this technic the variation of DNA-specific activity corresponds not only to changes in the proliferative status of the cell population and in the rate of DNA synthesis, but also to changes in the pools of precursors (48). Comparisons between labeling index and DNA-specific activity have shown a good correlation in some experiments (9, 2, 35) and a wide discrepancy between the two sets of data in others (15, 53), indicating the possible unreliability of the ^{3}H-incorporation method (Fig. 1).

A reliable technic for the measurement of the number of surviving cells is cloning, either in vivo (24, 59) or in vitro (1). The proliferative status of the surviving clonogenic cells can be assayed by an in-vitro suicide technic (3) that has recently been adapted to the study of the kinetics of cell proliferation in an experimental tumor after administration of HU (53). Unfortunately, these technics are time consuming and elaborate, and they can be used only for a few normal tissues or experimental tumors. They have been used to follow the effect of administration of HU on bone-marrow stem cells (65, 66, 67) and on the EMT-6 tumor (53).

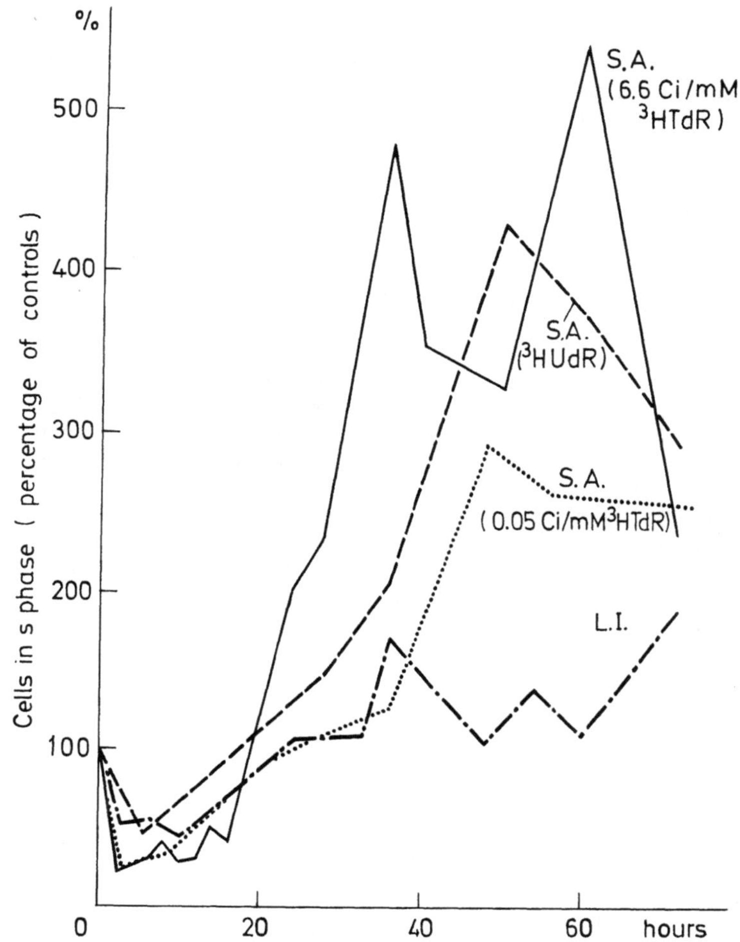

Fig. 1. Influence of irradiation with 250 rad (at time zero) on the synthesis of DNA in bone-marrow nucleated cells measured with various techniques:
- – – – – – labeling index (L. I.),
- ············ specific activity of DNA 1 hour after a single injection of 20 μCi of tritiated thymidine (^{3}HTdR), specific activity 0.05 Ci/mMol,
- ---------- tritiated deoxyuridine (^{3}HUdR), specific activity 2.8 Ci/mMol
- ———— tritiated thymidine (^{3}HTdR), specific activity 6.6 Ci/mMol (data from FRINDEL et al., 1966)

A simpler, but still reliable, method of studying the synchronizing effects is to follow the time course changes of cell or tissue radiosensitivity after administration of HU (40, 19, 36, 52, 45).

It is generally implicitly assumed that the few surviving viable clonogenic cells progress throughout the cell cycle synchronously with the large population of differentiated cells and of doomed cells. A few data support the assumption that doomed cells and viable cells have the same kinetic parameters during the first cell cycle (12, 23, 35), however other data show differences in their proliferative patterns in some tumors (53). Moreover, the cell cyle duration and proliferative status of clonogenic cells and more mature cells may differ widely. For instance, in normal mouse bone marrow, the multiponential stem cells may have a low growth fraction while the differentiated cells are actively dividing (65).

When methods based on tritiated-thymidine incorporation or DNA content are used, they should be checked, at least for a few time intervals, by a more elaborate procedure.

B. INFLUENCE OF HU CONCENTRATION ON THE DURATION OF THE BLOCK

The duration of the G1/S block depends upon the concentration of HU in the tissue. This is demonstrated by the data of VASSORT et al. on the percentage of bone-marrow stem cell in the S-phase after a single administration of various doses of HU (Fig. 2). The duration of the block varies from 2 to 5 hours for single doses of HU between 1 and 50 mg (Fig. 2). With cells on the epidermis a block of 1 to 4 hours was observed after doses ranging from 1 to 30 mg (22). However, with very high doses (20 to 60 mg) the influence of the dose on the duration of the block is small (9, 10). The duration of the first cell cycle of surviving bone marrow CFU also varies with different doses of HU (Figs. 3 and 4).

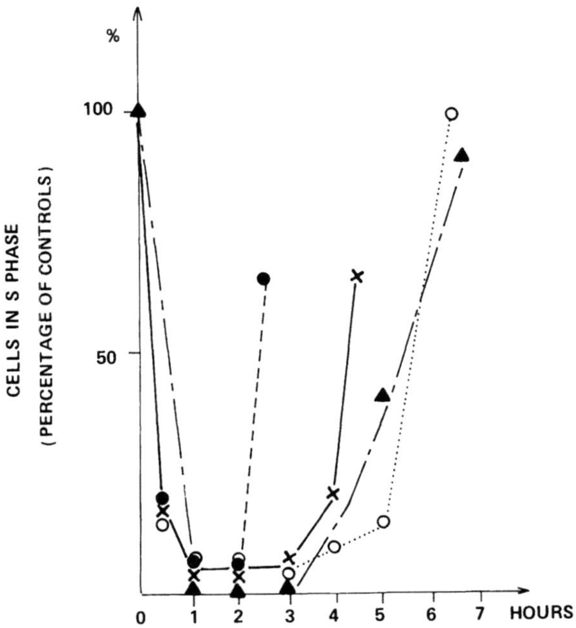

Fig. 2. Time course changes in the percentage of bone-marrow cells in S-phase after i.p. administration of various doses of hydroxyurea (HU): percentage of CFU in S-phase (measured by in-vitro suicide technic)
●-----------● after 1 mg HU per mouse.
x———————x after 10 mg HU.
o-----------o after 50 mg.
▲- - - - - - -▲ labeling index of nucleated bone marrow cells after 50mg HU (from F. VASSORT, unpublished data).

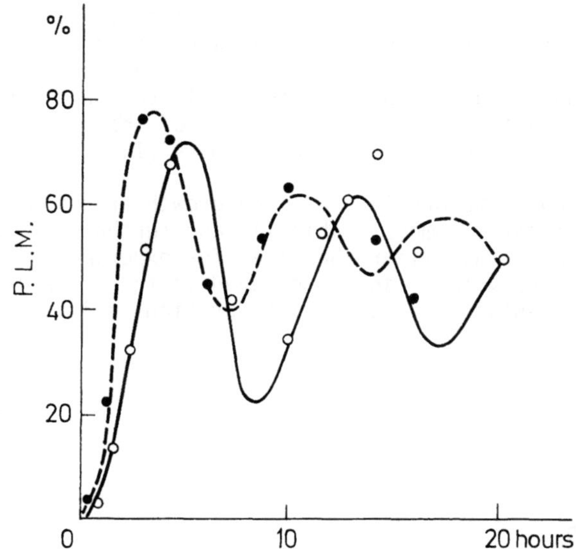

Fig. 3. Percentage of labeled mitoses in bone-marrow cells 46 hours after i.p. administration of 10 mg HU (●-----●), and in control mice (o——o) after HU the duration of the cell cycle is not significantly different (F. VASSORT)

HU concentration in a tissue or tumor is influenced by 3 factors: the amount of HU administered, the rate of HU disappearance, and the vascularization of the tissue. The disappearance rate of HU in plasma has been measured by RAJEWSKY; it can vary from species to species and values cannot be extrapolated from experimental animals to human beings.

The influence of vascularization on HU concentration in normal and malignant tissues has not been studied, but it is well known that tumors are not uniformly vascularized. This may introduce differences in HU concentrations between various zones of a tumor, in particular the central part and the periphery.

C. DEGREE OF SYNCHRONY AND PARAMETERS OF CELL KINETICS

The extent of synchrony that can be achieved in a cell population by administration of HU depends upon the distribution of the cell-cycle duration. When there is a wide range of cell-cycle duration the synchrony is less well achieved. It also depends upon the proliferative status of the population. When all the cells are engaged in a proliferative cycle, a high degree of synchrony can be achieved after a G1/S block of a few hours. Subsequently, desynchronization is caused by the differences among the surviving cells in the rate of progression through the cell cycle. The cyclic fluctuations in chemosensitivity or radiosensitivity of the cell population are progressively damped after a few cycles, and the time after which they will be damped is reduced with widening spread of cell-cycle duration.

In some tumors the cell cycle is longer at the center of the tumor than at the periphery (23). The timing of the synchronizing effect may be different in the two zones. After irradiation of the NCTC 2472 fibrosarcoma in the ascites form with 250 rad a marked difference was observed between the effects on the young, fast-growing 4-day tumors and those on the 12-day slow-growing tumors in which the cell cycle was longer (14). Division was longer in old tumors, and the recovery of the duration of the cell cycle was more rapid in young than in old tumors (14).

In human tumors (38, 61) the growth fraction is generally lower than in experimental tumors (Table 1), and furthermore, the distribution of cell-cycle time is much wider than that for experimental tumors (Fig. 5). The degree of synchrony that can be achieved is therefore inferior to that obtained in experimental tumors, and its duration is likely to be shorter.

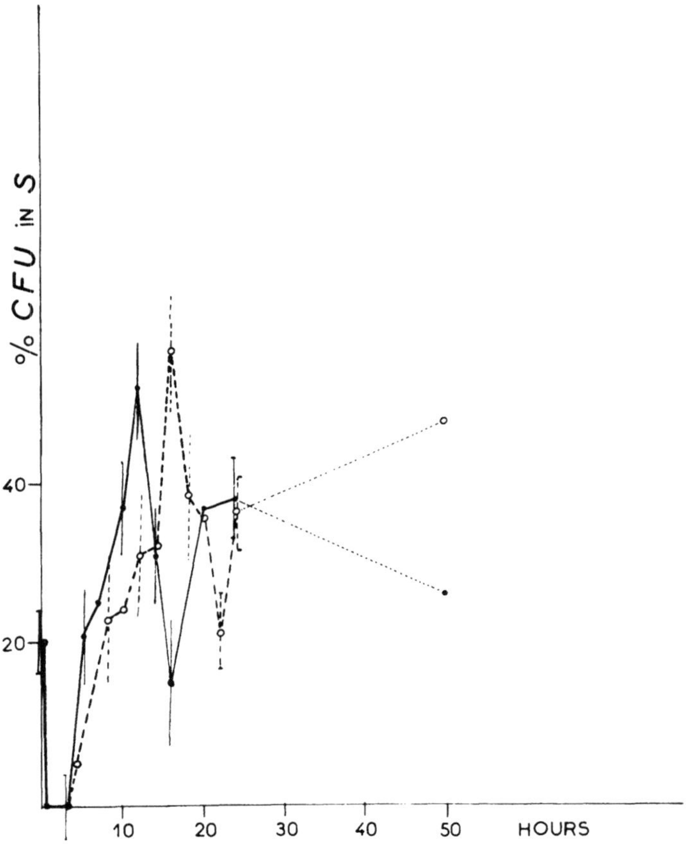

Fig. 4. Percentage of bone-marrow stem cells (CFU) in S-phase, measured by in vitro suicide technique after 2 doses of HU (——— 10 mg HU, ------- 50 mg HU). From F. VASSORT et al. (66)

A correlation has been observed between the histologic type of human tumor and the mean values for the parameters of cell kinetics (labeling index, doubling time, rate of cell loss) (Table 1). However, in some histologic types, the spread of the individual value of these parameters is wide (38) and an overlap is observed between the various histologic types (Table 2).

Table 1. Mean kinetic parameters of various histological types of human tumors[a]

Histological type	Doubling time (days)	Labeling index (%)	Growth fraction (1) (%)	Cell loss factor (2) (%)	Absolute cell loss per 10^9 cel. per day (3)	Daily cell renewal rate per cent per day (4)	Radiosensitivity (Mean tumor control dose in rad)	Chemosensitivity
Embryonal	27	30	90	93	$420 \cdot 10^6$	42	2500-3000	++
Tumors	(76)	(6)						
Malignant	29	29	90	94	$510 \cdot 10^6$	51	3500-4000	++
Lymphoma	(41)	(15)						
Mesenchymal	41	15	15	76	$55 \cdot 10^6$	5.5	8500	-
Sarcoma	(87)	(68)						
Squamous cell	58	8	25	89	$100 \cdot 10^6$	10	6000-7000	+
Carcinoma	(51)	(68)						
Adenocarcinoma	83	2	6	56	$11 \cdot 10^6$	1	6000-8000	±
	(134)	(121)						

[a] (See 38, 5)
The numbers in brackets indicate the number of patients for whom data were available

(1) Calculated from L.I, assuming $T_c/T_S = 3$.

(2) Calculation based on doubling time and labeling index, assuming $T_s = 15$ h and $\lambda = 0.7$

(3) Equal to the product: birth rate x cell loss factor.

(4) Equal to: absolute cell loss/number of cells.

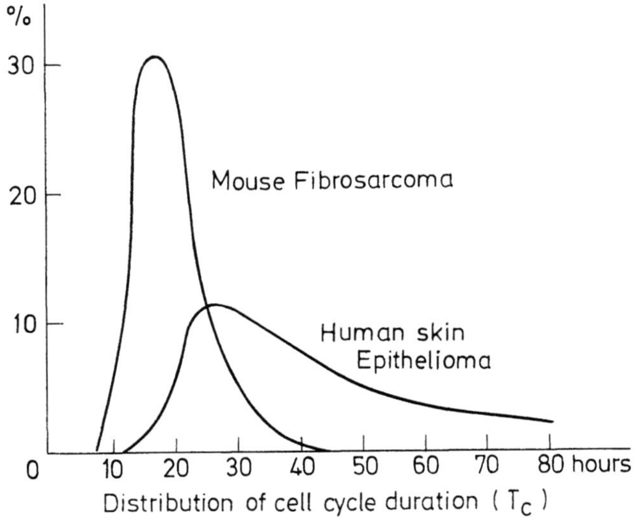

Fig. 5. Distribution of cell-cycle durations in a human epidermoid cancer of the skin and in the NCTC 2472 fibrosarcoma of the C_3H mouse. The spread of the cell cycle is much wider in the human tumor. (Data from FRINDEL et al. see 61

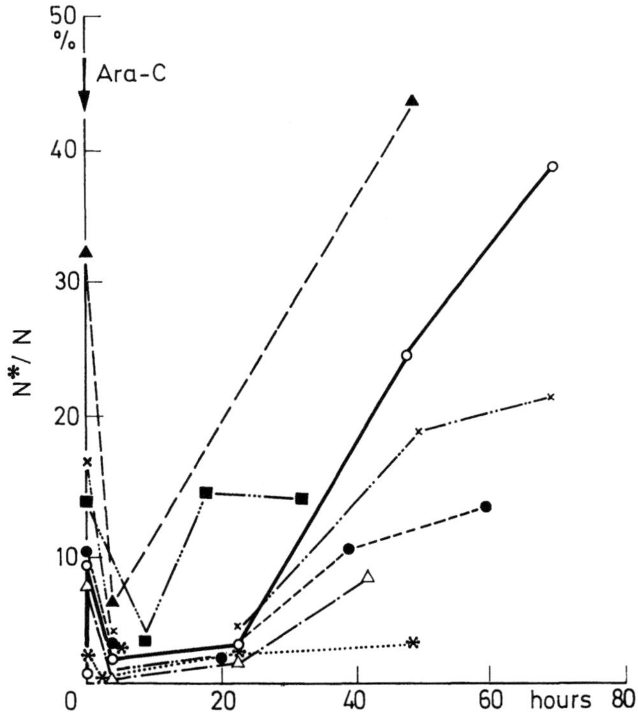

Fig. 6. Time course changes of the labeling index of bone-marrow leukemic cells in patients treated with cytosine arabinoside. ■—···—···—■ patient with acute myeloblastic leukemia treated by ERNST et al. (13) with 2 mg/kg of cytosine arabinoside. The other patients had acute lymphoblastic leukemia and were treated by LAMPKIN et al. (35), receiving 5 mg/kg cytosine arabinoside

Table 2. (from ref. 5, 38)

	Labeling Index	L.I. 97.5/L.I. 2.5	Doubling time	D.T. 97.5/D.T. 2.5
Embryonal Tumors	30.0	8	27.0 days	60
Hematosarcomas	29.2	11	28.9 days	60
Squamous Cell Carcinomas	8.3	23	58.0 days	60
Mesenchymal Sarcomas	4.1	142	41.4 days	60
Adenocarcinomas	2.1	275	82.7 days	60

The ratio of the lower and the higher values of the 95% confidence interval is an indicator of the spread of the individual values. For the labeling index, the spread is wide for all the histological groups but is larger in the groups with the slower growth rates. For the doubling times, the spread is similar in all histological groups.

Tumors of the same histologic type can therefore react differently to HU. Fig. 6 compares some of the human data obtained in patients with acute leukemia (13, 35). Although there is a general trend, the time courses of the labeling index vary notably among patients.

D. RECRUITMENT

Damage to a normal tissue triggers a homeostatic mechanism (34) and recruitment of previously quiescent cells into the proliferative pool (65).

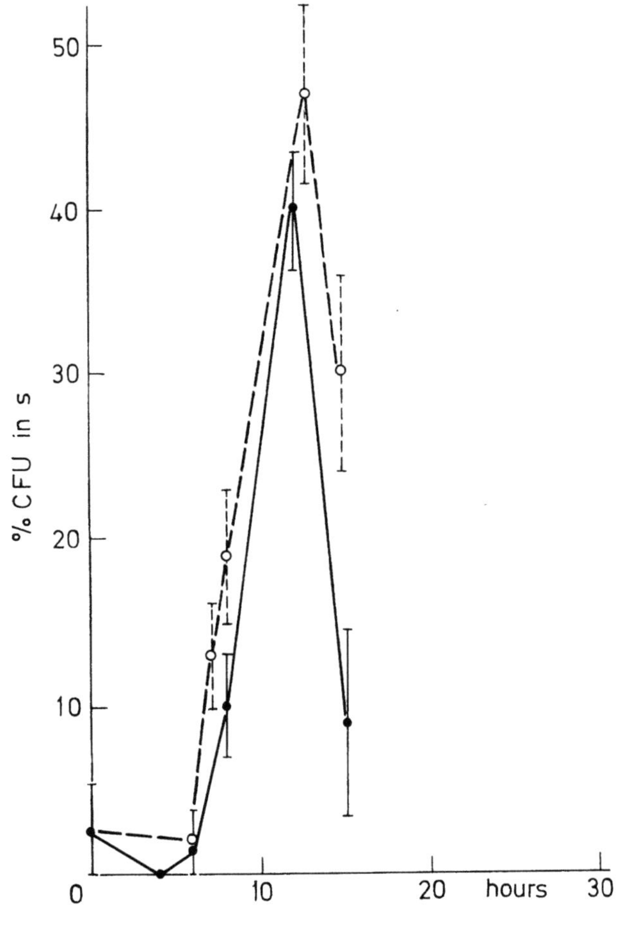

Fig. 7. Time course changes of the proportion of bone-marrow stem cells (CFU) in S-phase after administration at time zero of 1 mCi radioactive thymidine (———) or of 10 mg HU (------) to $C_{57}Bl$/mice. In these mice only 5% of the CFU are in S-phase before treatment. The recruitment of quiescent stem cells into proliferation starts 6 to 8 hours after treatment. (Data from VASSORT et al. 65 and 66)

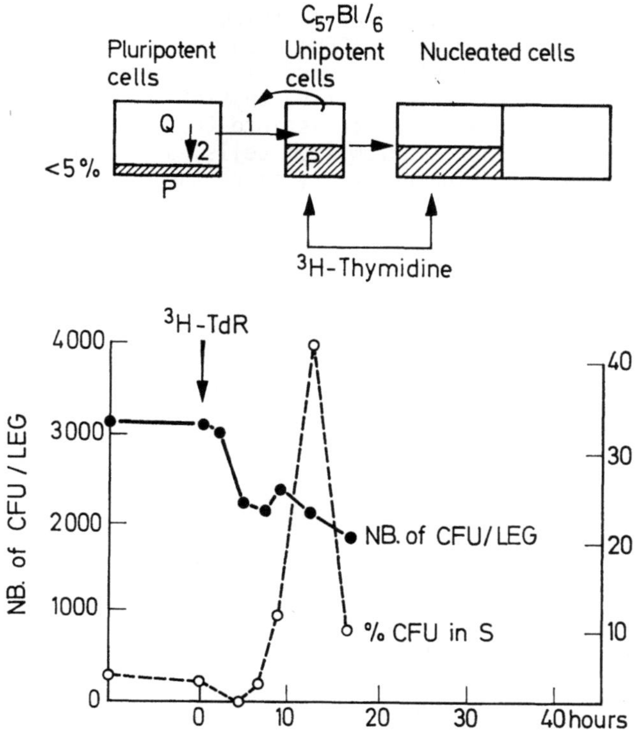

Fig. 8. Time course changes of the number of bone-marrow stem cells (CFU) per leg (●———●) and of the proportion of stem cells in S-phase (o----o) after administration of 1 mCi radioactive thymidine to C_{57}Bl mice. The direct effect of tritiated thymidine on pluripotential stem cells (CFU) is negligible since most of these cells are quiescent. Unipotential stem cells and nucleated cells are proliferating, and about 40% - 50% of these cells are in S-phase. Radioactive thymidine kills cells in S-phase, and the damage caused to these cell compartments triggers the differentiation of pluripotential stem cells. The depletion of the pluripotential cell compartment triggers the entry of quiescent stem cells into cell cycle. (Data from VASSORT et al., 66)

For hemopoietic tissues it is important to appreciate that drugs do not only have a synchronizing effect, but also are able to cause recruitment. The entry of bone-marrow stem cells into the proliferative compartment can be detected 8 to 10 hours after the administration of HU to mice. The number of stem cells is measured by means of the spleen colony technic (59) and the proportion of stem cells in S-phase is measured with an in-vitro suicide technic (3), i.e. incubation in vitro with radioactive thymidine before injection into sublethally irradiated recipient mice. In a strain of mice in which practically all the stem cells are quiescent, the proportion of stem cells in S-phase remains very low for the first few hours after drug administration and suddenly rises at about the 8th hour (Fig. 7). The peak is reached 12 hours after administration of HU; at this time 45% of colony-forming units (CFU) are in S-phase (66, 67). The same effect is observed after in-vivo injection of radioactive thymidine (67), which has a selective effect on cells in S-phase and no toxic effect for cells which are not synthesizing DNA (Fig. 8). This demonstrates that the damage caused to bone-marrow cells in the compartment of cells in the process of maturation and proliferation triggers recruitment of previously quiescent multipotential stem cells (CFU) into the proliferative pool (67). In strains of mice in which about one third of the stem cells are in cycle, an equivalent amount of HU or radioactive thymidine causes the entry of about half the previously quiescent stem cells into the cycle after a similar time interval (65). Thus, for bone-marrow stem cells, synchronization and recruitment cannot be considered independently since they occur concurrently (65, 67).

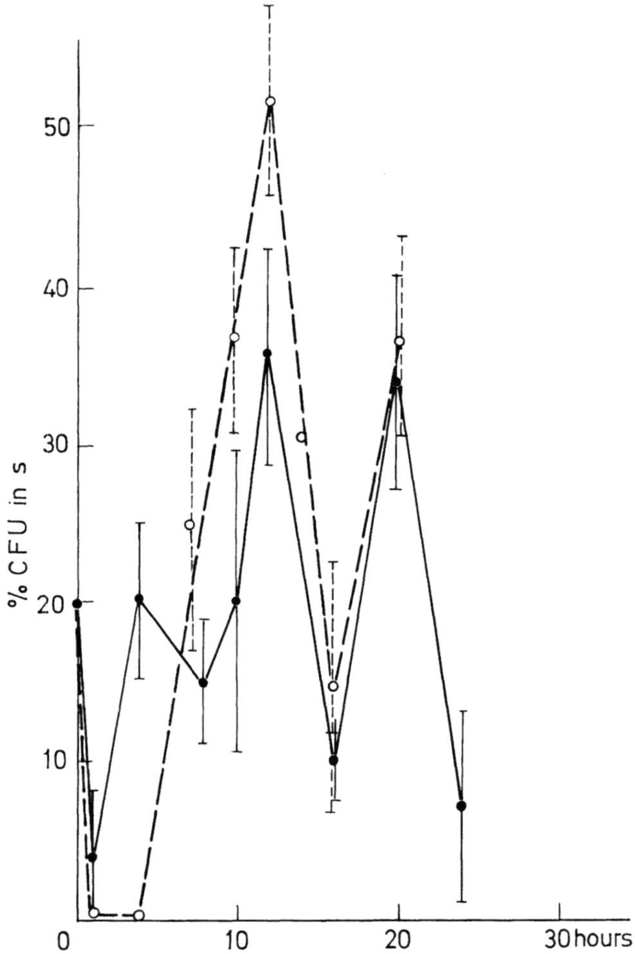

Fig. 9. Percentage of CFU in S-phase in C_3H mice after administration of 1 mCi of tritiated thymidine (●——●) and of 10 mg of HU (o ------- o). (Data from VASSORT et al. 66)

Recruitment of bone-marrow stem cells has also been observed after X-ray irradiation (7) or the administration of many drugs (64). Recruitment has also been described in many normal tissues (34). The lapse of time between administration of the drug or X-ray irradiation and the onset of regeneration varies in different tissues, but it is generally a few days (2-3 days in the intestine and 5-8 days in the skin); it is shorter for bone marrow (6-8 h) (67).

Recruitment has been reported in experimental tumors after X-ray irradiation (39, 1, 23) and after chemotherapy (57). However, in these cases the lapse of time between administration of the drug and the recruitment seems to be of the order of 4 to 8 days.

Little work on human tumors has yet been reported. Some authors (51, 63, 37) have found an acceleration of the rate of growth after irradiation in pulmonary and skin metastases. Others (18, 35, 13) have demonstrated recruitment of quiescent leukemic cells in patients after chemotherapy.

It should be stressed that the tissue sensitization to cycle-specific agents that is caused by recruitment is more pronounced in bone-marrow than in other normal or malignant tissues during the first few days.

E. TIMING

The last, and perhaps most important, point that must be dealt with is the scheduling. It would be desirable to determine the time interval between two administrations of a drug that will afford the optimum protection for normal critical tissue while increasing the kill of tumor cells.

In clinical chemotherapy with HU the untoward effects are primarily hematologic and gastrointestinal toxicity. Fortunately, data on the hematologic and gastrointestinal effects are available. Figs. 10 and 11 summarize information reported for mice in various papers after two ranges of single doses of HU.

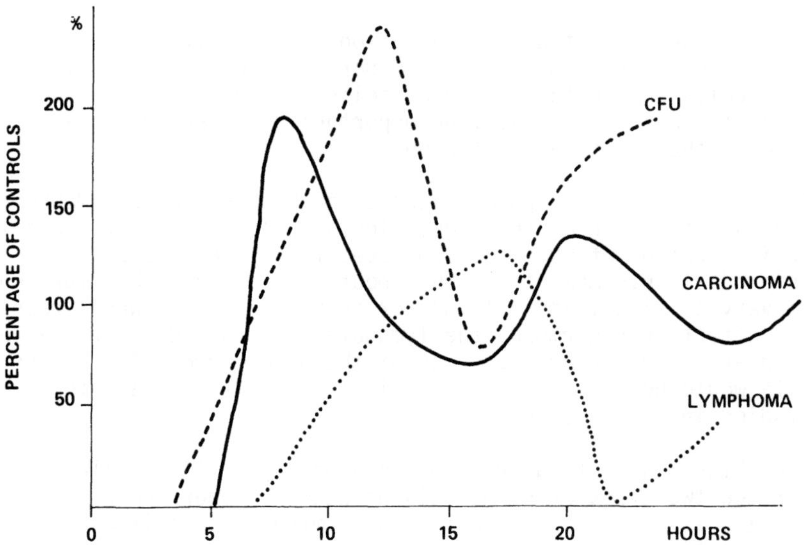

Fig. 10. Time course changes of proportion of cells in S-phase after administration at time zero of 0.5 mg/g of HU for bone-marrow stem cells (-----) in mice (CFU) (from VASSORT et al., 65) and (———) carcinoma in rat (from RAJEWSKY et al., 49); and after 0.5 mg/mouse of HU (.......) for lymphoma in mice (from MADOC-JONES et al., 36)

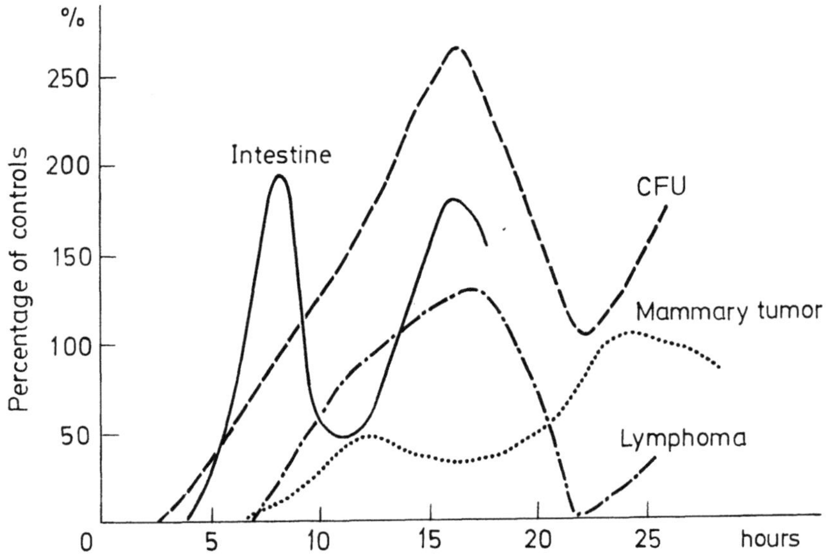

Fig. 11. Time course changes of proportion of cells in S-phase after administration at time zero of 50 mg HU per mouse (------) bone marrow stem cells in S-phase (from VASSORT et al., 65); after administration of 60 mg HU per mouse (———) labeling index of epithelial cells of intestine; (......) DNA specific activity of mammary tumor (from DETHLEFSEN et al., 9, 10); and after administration of 0.5 mg/mouse of HU (— - — - —) lymphoma (from MADOC-JONES et al., 36)

Fig. 10 indicates that the variations in the time course of the relative number of cells in S-phase after HU perturbation are very similar in bone-marrow stem cells and in the malignant cells of the carcinoma studied by RAJEWSKY (49). There is practically no opportunity for achieving a differential effect between these 2 types of tissue.

The timing in the lymphoma, studied by MADOC-JONES and MAURO (36), is different, and the peak of the proportion of cells in S is reached 16 hours after administration of HU. If a drug specifically active on cells in S were administered at this moment the therapeutic ratio would be improved, but the timing is very critical, and a longer or shorter interval would result in a detrimental effect. Furthermore, the lymphoma was studied after smaller doses of HU than are used during the study of the bone marrow. The interpretation of the data would be easier if the critical normal tissue and the tumor had been studied in the same animals.

When high doses of Hu are administered (Fig. 11), similar results are obtained. For the two types of normal tissue and the tumors considered, the optimum interval, if any, is difficult to determine, and if it were known, it would be very critical.

The discussion stresses that even when all the necessary kinetic data are available, the procedure has the potential capacity for being appreciably more effective than conventional therapy in only a few situations. However, the extreme importance of the goal merits further work to assess what improvement might be achieved in experimental tumor therapy.

Relevant clinical data are extremely difficult to collect. As already discussed, human tumors of the same histologic type may vary widely from a kinetic point of view (38, 61). For instance, when single doses of cytosine arabinoside were administered, an increase of the labeling index was observed between 25 and 96 hours afterwards in 7 patients with acute lymphoblastic leukemia, while 2 patients showed no apparent response (35).

Solid tumors are much more difficult to study, since an investigation of this type requires multiple biopsies whose interpretation is complicated by the possible heterogeneity of the tumor. Furthermore, investigations for each type of drug and each dose used would be necessary. The amount of work required to evaluate the feasibility alone of synchronization in the clinic is impressive.

Thus the choice of interval between the two drug administrations should be based on the characteristics of the critical normal tissue, which may vary less in response from patient to patient than do neoplastic tissues.

While research of this nature is carried out, other avenues for progress deserve consideration. In particular, the differences in timing of recruitment in normal tissues and in tumors may provide opportunities for optimization of a differential effect. As previously discussed, acceleration of cell proliferation is observed after chemotherapy or irradiation in normal tissues and in tumors. The homeostatic mechanism is very efficient in normal hemopoietic stem cells. The lapse of time between drug administration and the start of cell regeneration is of the order of hours, and the number of stem cells and their proliferation rate return to normal in about one week. In experimental tumors the recruitment of G_0-cells starts about 4 days after drug administration (57) or irradiation (I) and the proliferative fraction returns to its initial value in about two weeks when the tumor is back to its pretreatment volume. Recovery of the critical normal tissues thus seems to be complete before the end of tumor repopulation.

Knowledge of these time factors for human bone marrow and for human tumors would provide a basis for intermittent chemotherapy. The few data available for human metastases in lung (37) or skin (51) suggest that the phase of accelerated growth rate has a duration of a few weeks or one month and is longer than the recovery time of bone marrow and of the other critical normal tissues. Cycle-dependent drugs presumably have a more specific effect on tumor cells initially during the first few hours after irradiation or drug administration, i.e. before the recruitment of normal bone-marrow stem cells, and again later, after the completion of regeneration in normal critical tissues. A time interval between doses of the drugs equal to the recovery time of hemopoietic tissues would therefore appear adequate.

In tumors with a low growth fraction, radiotherapy or proliferative independent drugs should be used at the beginning of the treatment in order to produce cell depletion among the quiescent or slowly dividing cells and subsequently to speed up proliferation and to trigger resting cells into division. For these tumors, the time interval between courses of chemotherapy can be lengthened without risk since the rate of tumor growth is slow.

In conclusion, despite the encouraging clinical results reported in some papers (2, 32, 35, 46, 47), further experimental work and clinical investigation on the cell kinetics of perturbed normal critical tissues and tumors are badly needed. Even a crude analysis requires a voluminous amount of data that is not presently available.

REFERENCES

1. BARENDSEN, G. W., BROERSE, J. J.: Experimental radiotherapy of a rat rhabdomyosarcoma with 15 MeV neutrons and 300kV X-rays. I- Effects of single exposure. Europ. J. Cancer 5, 373 (1969).
2. BARRANCO, S. C., LUCE, L. K., ROMSDAHL, M. M., HUMPHREY, R. M.: Bleomycin as a possible synchronizing agent for human tumor cells in vivo. Cancer Res. 33, 882 (1973).
3. BECKER, A. J., MCCULLOCH, E. A., SIMINOVITCH, L., TILL, J. E.: The effects of differing demands for blood cell production of DNA synthesis by hemopoietic colony forming cells of mice. Blood, 26, 296 (1965).
4. CHAFFEY, J. T., HELLMAN, S.: Differing responses to radiation of murine bone-marrow stem cells in relation to the cell cycle. Cancer Res. 31, 1613 (1971).
5. CHARBIT, A., MALAISE, E., TUBIANA, M.: Relation between the pathological nature and the growth rate of human tumours. Europ. J. Cancer 7, 307 (1971).
6. COOPER, E. H., PECKHAM, M., MILLARD, R. E., HAMLIN, I. M. E., GERARD-MARCHANT, R.: Cell proliferation in human malignant lymphomas. Analysis of labeling index and DNA content in cell populations obtained by biopsy. Europ. J. Cancer 4, 287 (1968).
7. CROIZAT, H., FRINDEL, E., TUBIANA, M.: Proliferative activity of the stem cells in the bone marrow of mice after single and multiple irradiations (total or partial body exposure). Int. J. Radiat. Biol. 18, 347 (1970).
8. DENEKAMP, J., BALL, M., FOWLER, J. F.: Recovery and repopulation in mouse skin as a function of time after X-irradiation. Radiat. Res. 37, 361 (1969).
9. DETHLEFSEN, L. A., RILEY, R. M.: Hydroxyurea affects in the C3H mouse. I - Duodenal crypt cell kinetics. Cell Tiss. Kinet. 6, 3 (1973).
10. DETHLEFSEN, L. A., RILEY, R. M.: II - Mammary tumor cell kinetics. Cell Tiss. Kinet. 6, 173 (1973).
11. EGAMI, N.: Kinetics of recovery from injury after whole body X-irradiation of the fish Oryzias latipes at different temperatures. Radiat. Res. 37, 192 (1969).
12. ELKIND, M. M., HAN, A., VOLZ, K. W.: Radiation response of mammalian cells grown in culture. IV - Dose dependance delay and post-irradiation growth of surviving and nonsurviving chinese Hamster cell. J. nat. Cancer Inst. 30, 705 (1963).
13. ERNST, P., FAILLE, A., KILLMAN, S. A.: Perturbation of cell cycle of human leukemic myeloblast in vivo by cytosine arabinoside. Scand. J. Haematol. 10, 209 (1973).
14. FRINDEL, E., VASSORT, F., TUBIANA, M.: Effects of irradiation on the cell cycle of an experimental ascites tumor of the mouse. Inter. J. Radiat. Biol. 17, 329 (1970).
15. FRINDEL, E., CHARRUYER, R., TUBIANA, M., KAPLAN, H. S., ALPEN, E. L.: Radiation effects on DNA synthesis and cell division in the bone marrow of the mouse. Int. J. Radiat. Biol. 11, 345 (1966).
16. FRINDEL, E., TUBIANA, M.: Radiobiology and the cell cycle. In: The cell cycle and cancer, p. 389. New York: Marcel Dekker 1971.
17. FRINDEL, E., VALLERON, A. J., VASSORT, F., TUBIANA, M.: Proliferation kinetics of an experimental ascites tumor of the mouse. Cell Tiss. Kinet. 2, 51 (1969).
18. GABUTTI, J. V., PILERT, A., TAROCCO. R. P., GAVOSTO, F., COOPER, E. H.: Proliferative potential of out of cycle leukemia cells. Nature 224, 375 (1969).

19. GILLETTE, E. L., WITHERS, H. R., TANNOCK, I. F.: The age sensitivity of Epithelial cells of mouse small intestine. Radiology 96, 639 (1970).
20. GIBSON, M. H. L., BERTALANFFY, F. D.: In vivo synchrony of solid B16 melanoma by cytosine arabinoside, an inhibitor of DNA synthesis. J. nat. Cancer Inst. 49, 1007 (1972).
21. HALL, E. J., MARTIN-BROWN, J., CANAVAGH, J.: Radiosensitivity and the oxygen effect measured at different plases of the mitotic cycle using synchronously dividing cells of the root meristen of Vicia Faba. Radiat. Res. 35, 622 (1968).
22. HENNINGS, H., DEVICK, F.: Comparison of cytotoxicity of hydroxyurea in normal and rapidly proliferating epidermis and small intestine in mice. Cancer Res. 31, 277 (1971).
23. HERMENS, A. F.: Variations in the cell kinetics and the growth rate in an experimental tumour during natural growth and after irradiation. The Netherlands:Radiobiological Institute TNO 1973).
24. HEWITT, H. B., WILSON, C. W.: A survival curve for mammalian leukemia cells irradiated in vivo. Brit. J. Cancer 13, 69 (1959).
25. HURWITZ, C., TOLMACH, J. L.: Time lapse cinemicrographic studies of X-irradiated HeLa C_3 cells. I - Cell progression and cell desintegration. Biophys. J. 9, 607 (1969).
26. HYODO-TAGUCHI, Y.: Effect of X-irradiation on DNA synthesis and cell proliferation in the intestinal epithelial cells of goldfish at different temperatures with special references to recovery process.
27. KALLMANN, R. F., BLEEHEN, N. M.: Post-irradiation cyclic radiosensitivity changes in tumors and normal tissues. In: Proceedings of a symposium on dose rate in mammalian radiation biology, April 29 - May 1, Oak Ridge, Tenn., 1968, USAEC Conf. 680410
28. KALLMANN, R. F., SILINI, G., TAYLOR, H. M.: Recuperation from lethal injury by whole-body irradiation. II - Kinetic aspects in radiosensitive BALB/e mice, and cyclic fine structure during the four days after conditioning irradiation. Radiat. Res. 29, 362 (1966).
29. KALLMANN, R. F., SILINI, G.: Recuperation from lethal injury by whole-body irradiation. I- Kinetic aspects and the relationship with conditioning dose in C_{57}Bl mice. Radiat. Res. 22, 622 (1964).
30. KEMBER, N. F.: Hydroxyurea and the differentiation of growth cartilage cells in the rat. Cell Tiss. Kinet. 5, 199 (1972).
31. KISSEL, P., DUPREZ, A., BESSOT, M.: Essais de synchronisation in vivo de la synthèse de l'ADN de cellules malignes humaines par le 5-fluorouracile. Etude autohistoradiographique. C. R. Acad. Sci. (Paris) 262, 2558 (1966).
32. KLEIN, H. O.: Synchronization of tumor cell proliferation and the timing of cytostatic drugs. Europ. J. clin. biol. Res. 17, 835 (1972).
33. LAMERTON, L. F.: Donnés sur les relations entre la chimiosensibilité et la cinétique de prolifération cellulaire des tumeurs et des tissus sains. Bull. Cancer 60, 105 (1973).
34. LAMERTON, L. F.: Cell proliferation and the differential response of normal and malignant tissues. Brit. J. Radiol. 45, 161 (1972).
35. LAMPKIN, B. C., NAGAO, T., MAUER, A. M.: Synchronization and recruitment in acute leukemia. J. clin. Invest. 50, 2204 (1971).
36. MADOC-JONES, H., MAURO, F.: Age responses to X-rays, Vinca Alkaloids and hydroxyurea of murine lymphoma cells synchronized in vivo. J. nat. Cancer Inst. 45, 1131 (1970).
37. MALAISE, E., CHARBIT, A., CHAVAUDRA, N., COMBES, P. F., DOUCHEZ, J., TUBIANA, M.: Changes in volume of irradiated human metastases. Brit. J. Cancer 26, 43 (1972).

38. MALAISE, E., CHAVAUDRA, N., TUBIANA, M.: The relationship between growth rate, labeling index and histological type tumours. Europ. J. Cancer 9, 305 (1973).
39. MALAISE, E., TUBIANA, M.: Croissance des cellules d'un fibrosarcoma expérimental irradié chez la souris C3H. C. R. Acad. Sci. (Paris) 270 D, 539 (1966).
40. MALKINSON, F. D., GRIEM, M. L., MARIANOVIC, R.: Effects of hydroxyurea and radiation on hair matrix cells. Cell Tiss. Kinet. 6, 395 (1973).
41. MAURO, F., MADOC-JONES, H.: Age Response to X-radiation of murine lymphoma cells synchronized in vivo. Proc. nat. Acad. Sci. 63, 686 (1969).
42. NAJEAN, Y.: Action de la chimiothérapie sur la cinétique cellulaire. I - Evolution, en fonction du temps, de la prolifération erythroblastique. Influence de cette donnée pour le choix de l'espacement des drogues dans un traitement sequentiel. Nouv. Rev. franc. hématol. 11, 185 (1971).
43. NAJEAN, Y., FAILLE, A.: Action de la chimiothérapie sur la cinétique cellulaire. II - Leucémies murine de Rauscher et de Moloney. Nouv. Rev. franc. hématol. 13, 51 (1973).
44. ODARTCHENKO, N., COTTIER, H., FEINENDEGEN, L. E., BOND, P. V.: Mitotic delay in more mature erythroblasts of the dog, induced in vivo by sublethal doses of X-rays. Radiation Res. 21, 413 (1964).
45. PIVER, M. S., HOWES, A. E., SUIT, H. D., MARSHALL, N.: Effect of hydroxyurea on the radiation responses of C3H mammary tumors. Cancer 29, 407 (1972).
46. POUILLART, P., SCHWARZENBERG, M., MATHÉ, G., SCHNEIDER, M., JASMIN, C., HAYAT, M., WEINER, R., de VASSAL, F., AMIEL, J. L., BEYER, H. P., FAJ-BISOWICK, S.: Essai clinique de combinations chimiothérapiques basée sur la notion de synchronisation cellulaire. Administration première d'un antimitotique suivie de l'application de produits cycle ou phase dépendants. Nouv. Presse méd. 1, 1757 (1972).
47. POUILLART, P., MATHE, G., SCHWARZENBERG, L.: Essai de recrutement cellulaire par synchronisation partielle pour l'établissement d'une combinaison chimothérapique. Bull. Cancer 60, 187 (1973).
48. QUASTLER, H.: Effects of irradiation on synthesis and loss of DNA. Actions chimiques et biologiques et radiations 6, 149 (1963).
49. RAJEWSKY, M. F., HULSER, D. F., FABRICIUS, E.: Untersuchungen zur synchronisation in vivo: Temporäre inhibition der DNA-synthese durch hydroxyharnstoff im normalen und malignen Säugerzellsystem. Z. Krebsforsch. 76, 266 (1971).
50. RAJEWSKY, M. F.: Cinétique de prolifération des populations cellulaires et traitement des cancers. Regroupement dans le cycle cellulaire de cellules en prolifération par les drogues. Bull. Cancer 60, 143 (1973)
51. RAMBERT, P., MALAISE, E., LAUGIER, A., SCHLIENGER, M., TUBIANA, M.: Données sur la vitesse de croissance des tumeurs humaines. Bull. Cancer 55, 323 (1968).
52. ROCKWELL, S., KALLMANN, R. F.: Cyclic radiation induced variations in cellular radiosensitivity in a mouse mammary tumor. Radiat. Res. 57, 132 (1974).
53. ROCKWELL, S., FRINDEL, E., TUBIANA, M.: Cell survival and cell proliferation in EMT6 tumors treated with single doses of X Rays or Hydroxyurea. Cell, Tiss. Kin. (in press).
54. SINCLAIR, W. K.: Hydroxyurea effects on chinese Hamster cells grown in culture. Cancer Res. 27, 297 (1967).
55. SINCLAIR, W. K.: Cell cycle dependence of the lethal radiation response in mammalian cells. Current Topics in Radiation Research 7, 264 (1972).
56. SINGER, R. M., GELFANT, S.: Continuous inhibition of DNA synthesis in mouse ear epidermis using hydroxyurea. Exp. Cell Res. 73, 270 (1972).
57. SKIPPER, H. E.: Kinetic behavior versus response to chemotherapy. Nat. Cancer Inst. Monographs. 34, 2 (1971).

58. STEWARD, P. G., HAHN, G. H.: The application of age response function to the optimiaztion of treatment schedules. Cell. Tiss. Kinet. 4, 279 (1971).
59. TILL, J. E., MCCULLOCH, E. A.: A direct measurement of the radiation sensibility of normal mouse bone-marrow cells. Radiat. Res. 14, 213 (1961).
60: TUBIANA, M.: The kinetics of tumour cell proliferation and radiotherapy. Brit. J. Radiol. 44, 325 (1971).
61. TUBIANA, M., MALAISE, E. P.: Cinêtique de prolifêration cellulaire des tumeurs et traitement des cancers. Pathologie Biologie. 21, 647 (1973).
62. UENO, Y.: Cellular kinetics in the mouse hemopoietic system after exposure to ionizing radiation. Int. J. Radiat. Biol. 14, 307 (1968).
63. VAN PEPERZEEL, H. A.: Effects of single doses of radiation on lung metastase in man and experimental animals. Europ. J. Cancer 8, 665 (1972).
64. VAN PUTTEN, L. M.: Recrutement, une arme à double tranchant dans la chimiothêrapie du cancer. Bull. Cancer 60, 131 (1973).
65. VASSORT, F., FRINDEL, E., TUBIANA, M.: Cinêtique cellulaire des cellules souches hêmatopoietiques et chimiothêrapie. Bull. Cancer 60, 163 (1973).
66. VASSORT, F., FRINDEL, E., TUBIANA, M.: Effects of hydroxyurea on the kinetics of colony forming units of bone marrow in the mouse. Cell Tiss. Kinet. 4, 423 (1971).
67. VASSORT, F., WINTERHOLER, M., FRINDEL, E., TUBIANA, M.: Kinetics parameters of bone-marrow stem cells using in vivo suicide by tritiated thymidine or by hydroxyurea. Blood 41, 789 (1973).
68. WITHERS, H. R., ELKIND, M. M.: Radiosensitivity and fractionation response of crypt cell mouse jejunum. Radiat. Res. 41, 450 (1969).
69. WITHERS, H. R.: Recovery and repopulation in vivo by mouse skin epithelial cells during fractionated irradiation. Radiat. Res. 32, 227 (1967).
70. YOUNG, J. M., FOWLER, J. F.: The effect of X-ray induced synchrony on two dose cell survival experiments. Cell Tiss. Kinet. 2, 95 (1969).

Cell Synchronization in Solid Tumors

J. Schumann, F. Ehring, and W. Göhde

1. INTRODUCTION

Problems of cell synchronization are of importance in the treatment of malignant tumors because the sensitivity of the cells to cytostatics and irradiation can alter considerably during the course of the cell-division cycle (2, 22, 14, 21). For this type of sensitivity change to be exploited for treatment, however, would require that the cells in solid tumors could also be synchronized.

Most experiments on synchronization in tumor cells have so far been limited to cell cultures and suspended cell populations (e.g. ascites tumors). During the logarithmic phase of growth, such systems consist almost exclusively of proliferating cells, and their growth fraction consequently amounts to nearly 100%. Conditions are different in solid tumors. In these cases only part of the tumor takes part in the proliferation, depending on the vascularization. In the main, it is the external layer of the tumor that contains the proliferating cells. These form the P-pool. Under this there is frequently a layer of cells which are capable of dividing, but are in the resting stage, forming the Q-pool. These cells are also called the G_0-phase cells. In addition, the center of the tumor may still contain cells incapable of division and necroses (15, 16, 23).

A number of authors have now shown that cells in solid human tumors can also be partially synchronized by cytostatics with a cell-kinetic action (10, 11, 4, 13). On the basis of this discovery, various therapy models were developed and introduced into clinical practice. Fluorouracil (FU), hydroxyurea and vincristine are some of the substances that were used as synchronizing agents. In spite of the encouraging clinical results with some of these therapy models, important problems of phase-specific treatment of solid tumors are still unsolved and must be borne in mind.

In attempts to subject solid tumors to synchronization treatment, the fact that at first only the growth fraction of the tumor is affected must be taken into consideration. But it is possible that during, and because of, the chemotherapy recruitment, i.e. further colonization of the tumor with proliferating cells, occurs. Cells may thus migrate from the Q-pool to the P-pool. If this should occur during treatment, these cells may also be affected by phase-specific agents, but if it does not occur until the end of the treatment, a further course may be necessary (12, 17), which gives rise to a further complication; the kinetics of the proliferation of the tumor cells can also change during the treatment (9). A maximal synchronizing effect produced by substances with a cell-kinetic action is consequently only observed after treatment periods that do not correspond to normal cell-cycle periods (1, 3, 20). A rapid method of determination is therefore necessary to check whether a cell-synchronizing treatment has been successful.

Our attempts to improve the experimental basis for irradiation and chemotherapy after partial synchronization of the tumor cells were carried out with the aid of a more modern technique for cell-kinetic analysis, i.e. pulse cytophotometry. This procedure allows a rapid check for changes in the relative composition of collectives of cells in different phases of the cell cycle. In this way, the extent and duration of the cell-kinetic action of the drug can be quickly recognized and consequently the correct time for the application of the second step of the treatment can be determined more accurately.

2. MATERIAL AND METHODS

Our experiments were carried out with the cytostatics FU and bleomycin in hamster sarcoma HS-6, in solid Ehrlich carcinoma in the mouse and Ehrlich ascites tumor cells (EAT) in vivo. The cell-kinetic effect of the agents was determined with the aid of a pulse cytophotometer (ICP 11, PHYWE AG, Göttingen). This method makes the distribution of the quantities of DNA of the tumor cells available only one hour after a biopsy, which gives direct information on the relative composition of the sample of cells in the different phases of the cell cycle. The cell-kinetic effect on human tumors was also checked with the pulse cytophotometer after a sample had been taken during the course of treatment.

The reader is referred to other publications for details of the pulse cytophotometry technique (8, 20, 5-7).

For the survival experiment, adult NMRI mice with EAT cells in the logarithmic phase of growth (on day 5 after inoculation) were inoculated intraperitoneally with 100 mg bleomycin per kg bodyweight. One group of the mice were irradiated with 2000 R (200 kv, 0.5 mm Cu filter) immediately after and the second group 48 hours after the administration of bleomycin; 49 hours after treatment with bleomycin, the EAT cells of both groups were inoculated into 14-day old mice and the death rate was determined.

3. RESULTS

The DNA-distribution patterns determined by pulse cytophotometry in the tumor-cell populations examined are shown in histograms. In these histograms, the first peak always represents the cells which showed a 2c DNA content at the time of taking the sample; both G_1 and G_0-phase cells can be involved. The second peak, at 4c, shows the measure of cells with double DNA content, the (G_2+M7)-phase cells. In between, cells with DNA values between 2c and 4c -- i.e. S-phase cells -- were observed.

In solid Ehrlich carcinoma in the mouse, cells were arrested at the beginning of the S-phase after a 12-hour treatment with FU (Fig. 1). Eight hours after

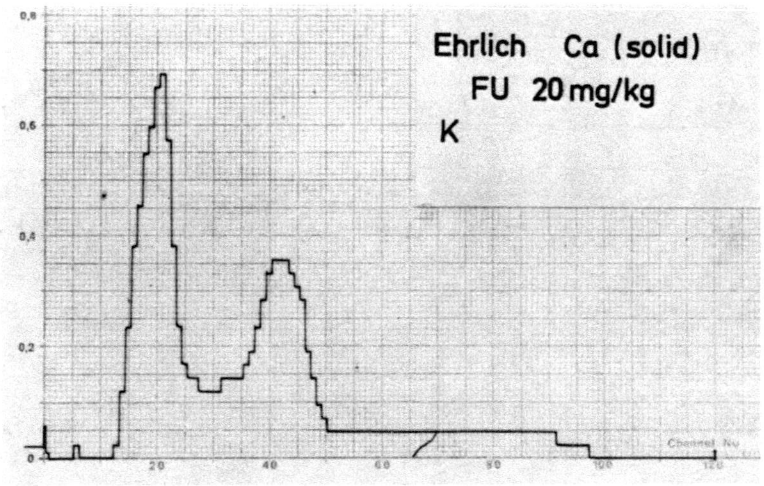

Fig. 1 a

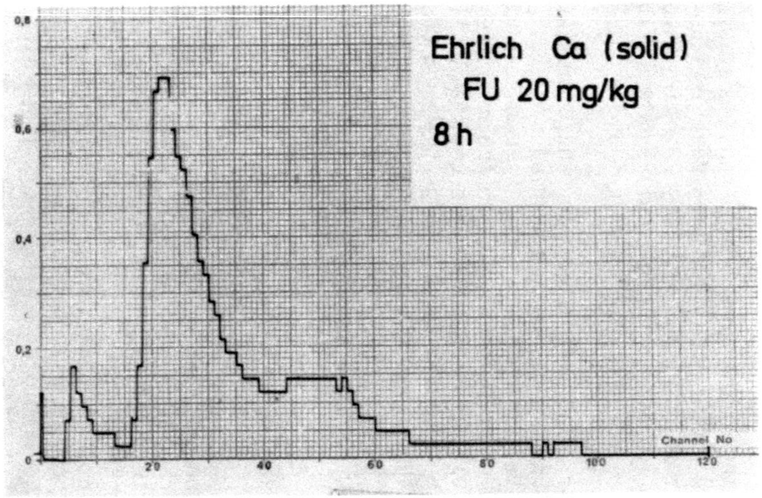

Fig. 1 b

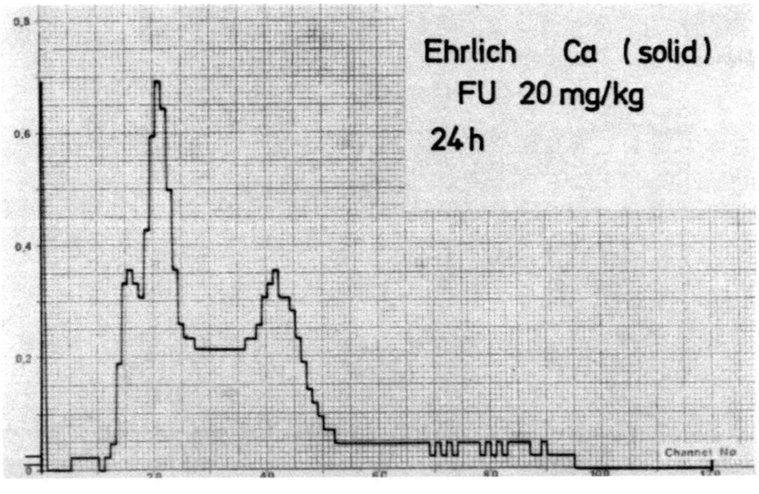

Fig. 1 c

Fig. 1 a - c. Distribution of amounts of DNA in solid Ehrlich, (a) untreated tumor, (b) tumor 8 h after 12 h infusion with FU, (c) tumor 24 h after 12 h infusion with FU

the end of the treatment with FU, the (G_2+M) portion of the population was still below the control level, a large proportion of the cells being still in the early S-phase. The DNA histogram showed a higher proportion of (G_2+M) only 24 hours after the end of the treatment, when a higher proportion of S-phase cells was recorded than in the controls. The duration of the S-phase, which is about 10 to 12 hours in untreated Ehrlich carcinoma cells, was approximately doubled in this test. The same results were also obtained in hamster sarcoma HS-6 (19).

In patients who had been treated for 12 hours with FU by intravenous drip, pulse cytophotometry revealed that a substantial increase in the (G_2+M) fraction could only be achieved in a few cases, and in these cases, a higher proportion of (G_2+M) was only demonstrable 10 to 14 hours after discontinuation of the FU infusion (24).

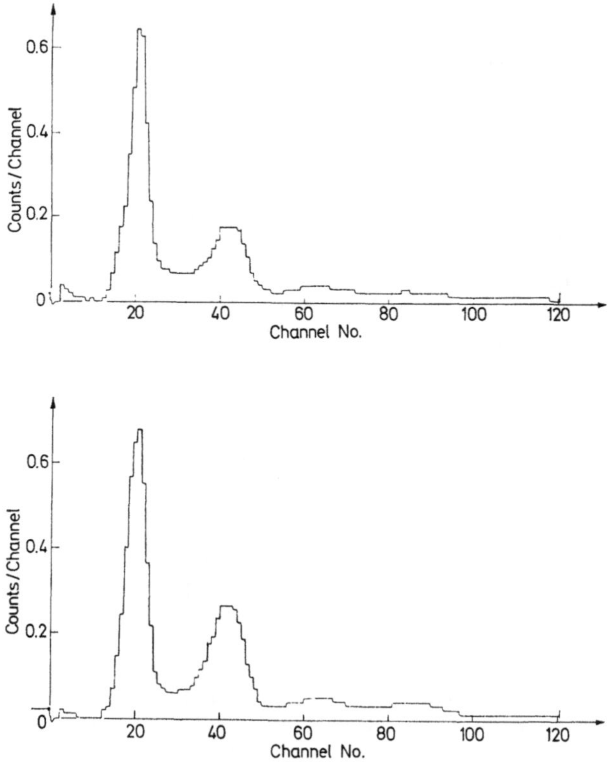

Fig. 2. Distribution of amounts of DNA in solid Ehrlich carcinoma above: untreated tumor (G_2+M); proportion = 23%, below: tumor 30 hours after beginning of treatment with bleomycin (G_2+M); proportion = 32%

It has already been shown that, in doses between 50 and 250 mg/kg body weight, bleomycin produces a distinct arrest of EAT cells in vivo, and in vitro in the (G_2+M)-phase and at the end of the S-phase (7, 18). Fig. 2 shows the corresponding results obtained in the solid Ehrlich carcinoma in the mouse. After two single applications, each of 20 mg/kg body weight, given 24 hours apart, the DNA histogram of the Ehrlich carcinoma cells was obtained (Fig. 2, below). The increase in (G_2+M)-phase cells amounted to about 45% compared with the controls (Fig. 2, above).

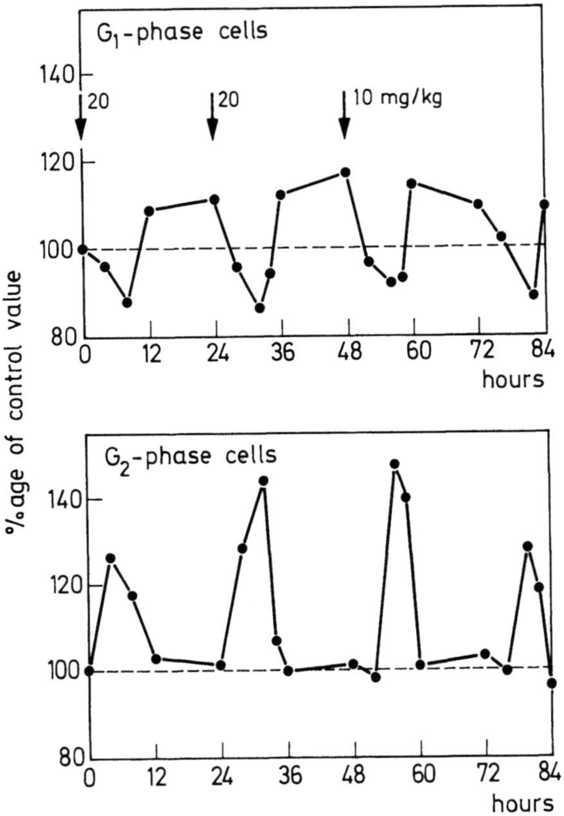

Fig. 3. Changing of relative proportions of G_1- and (G_2+M)-phase cells in solid Ehrlich carcinoma during bleomycin treatment

Fig. 3 shows that this effect on the proliferation of solid Ehrlich carcinoma cells was reproducible with repeated subcutaneous administration of bleomycin. The mice were treated with bleomycin at the times indicated in Fig. 3 (arrows) The times samples were taken from the tumors for pulse cytophotometry are shown on the abscissa (dots). It can be seen from this illustration that the maximum values for the arrest of cells in the (G_2+M)-phase is always attained 4 to 8 hours after the injection of bleomycin. The bleomycin-induced blocking of tumor cells at the end of the cell cycle is only of short duration. Fig. 3 also shows that bleomycin produces partial synchronization of the tumor cells; this effect is still visible even after bleomycin has been discontinued (72 to 84 h on the abscissa).

Our investigations were carried out with the intention of sensitizing the tumor cells to irradiation by means of a cell-synchronizing pretreatment. From a large number of investigations (22, 2, 21) it can be deduced that in mammalian cells sensitivity to irradiation is greatest at the end of the cell

cycle. Synchronizing or arresting as many cells as possible in a cell collective in the (G_2+M)-phase must consequently lead to an improvement in the therapeutic effect of irradiation. This question was examined in a preliminary survival experiment. Mice with EAT cells in the logarithmic phase were treated with bleomycin as described above. One group of mice were subjected to whole-body irradiation immediately after the intraperitoneal injection of bleomycin. Fig. 4 (top) shows the cell-kinetic state of the EAT cells at the time of irradiation. The second group of animals were not irradiated until 48 hours after the administration of bleomycin. The composition of the EAT cells at the time of irradiation is shown in Fig. 4 (below). The proportion of (G_2+M)-phase cells in the total population was increased to six times the level of the controls in this group.

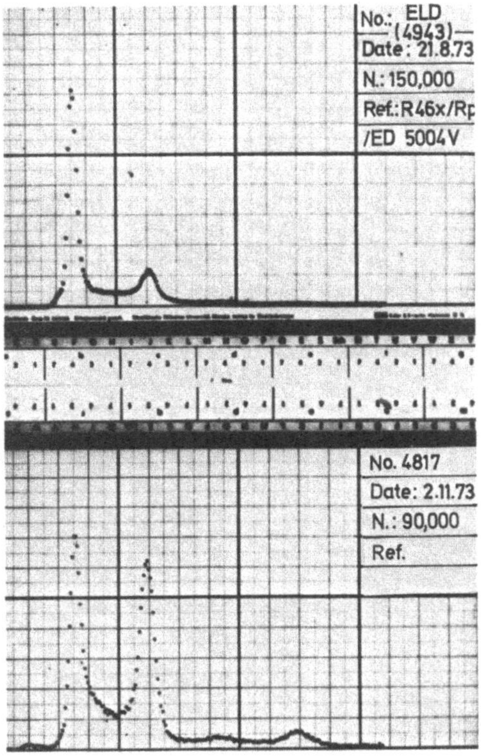

Fig. 4. DNA histogram of EAT cells above: before treatment, below: 48 hours after application of bleomycin (125 mg/kg b.w. i.p.)

Forty-eight hours after administration of bleomycin, the EAT cells of both groups were inoculated into 14-day old mice. Fig. 5 shows the death rate among these mice. Mice inoculated with EAT cells after irradiation causing partial synchronization survived about 8 days on average, while those with EAT cells not subjected to irradiation causing partial synchronization only survived for about 5 days.

Measurements with the pulse cytophotometer in tumor biopsies from patients treated with bleomycin confirm our experimental results (Fig. 6), although

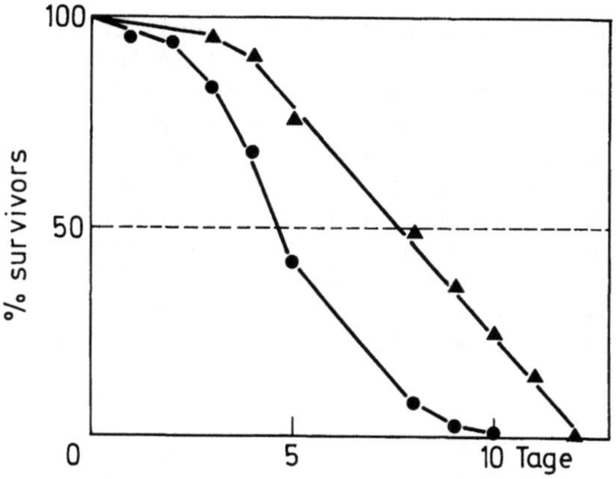

Fig. 5. Death rate of 14-day old mice inoculated with EAT cells in logarithmic phase of growth, ■ simultaneous application of bleomycin (125 mg/kg b.w.) and irradiation (2000 R), ▲ Irradiation (2000 R) 48 h after application of bleomycin (125 mg/kg b.w.)

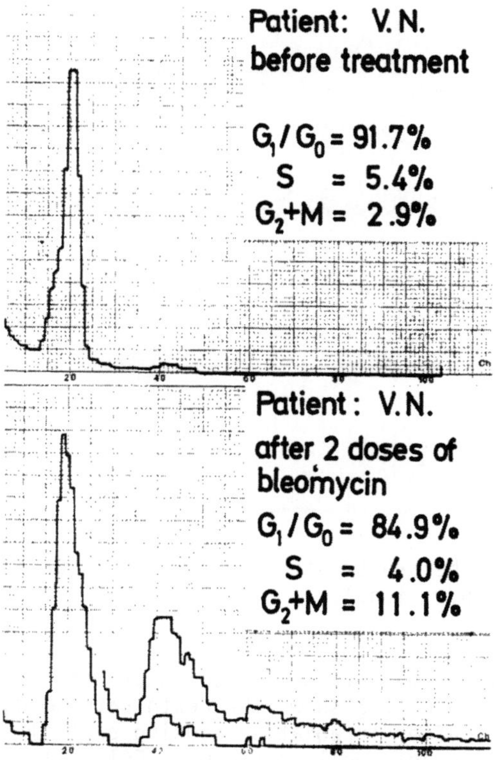

Fig. 6. Distribution of amounts of DNA in human squamous epithelial carcinoma, above: untreated tumor, (G_2+M); proportion = 3%, below: tumor 30 h after beginning treatment with bleomycin (2 x 15 mg); (G_2+M) proportion = 11%

the extent of the synchronizability of the tumor cells is less in such cases, because of the smaller proportion of proliferating cells. The initial clinical observations after irradiation of partially synchronized tumor cells are encouraging to some extent, but no definite conclusion can be drawn from them as yet.

4. DISCUSSION

The results show that partial synchronization of cells in solid tumors -- even in humans -- is possible to an extent which can be exploited for combination therapy with some prospect of success. In contradistinction to other treatment models, an attempt was made to arrest the cells in that phase of the cell cycle in which the second step of the treatment can take place directly. When chemotherapy and irradiation are combined, which can only be done in regionally confined tumors, arrest of the cells in the radio-sensitive phase before irradiation can be recommended if healthy proliferating tissue can be largely spared during irradiation by suitable limitation of the field. In the case of tumors that have metastasized, chemotherapy is recommended after cell synchronization. The reader is referred to the descriptions of other models elsewhere in this volume.

Individual supervision of the effect of cytostatics on cell kinetics and individual determination of proliferation parameters should not, however, be dispensed with during the testing and application of synchronization therapy. The findings on the state of cell kinetics of a treated tumor should be obtained as soon as possible, to allow calculation of the most favorable time to introduce the second step of the treatment safely. The automatic cytophotometers which work with cell suspensions offer the best means of obtaining this information currently available.

Acknowledgements

These investigations were supported by the Arbeitsgemeinschaft für Krebsbekämpfung (Anti-Cancer Campaign) in Nordrhein-Westfalen.

We should like to thank Fräulein R. Upmann and Fräulein J. Spiess for their conscientious assistance.

REFERENCES

1. BROWN, A. L., BERRY, R. J.: Effects of X-irradiation on the cell population kinetics in a model tumor and normal tissue system: implications for the treatment of human malignancies. Brit. J. Radiol. 42, 372 (1969).
2. DEWEY, W. C., HUMPHREY, R. M.: Relative radiosensitivity of different phases in the life cycle of L-P 59 mouse fibroblasts and ascites tumour cells. Radiat. Res. 16, 503 (1962).
3. FEINENDEGEN, L. E.: Zelluläre Aspekte der Strahlensensibilisierung. Strahlentherapie 143, 257 (1972).

4. GANZER, U., NITZE, H. R.: Mitoseindexbestimmungen an in vivo synchronisiertem menschlichen Tumorgewebe. Arch. klin. exp. Ohr- Hals- u. Kehlk.-Heilk. 194, 388 (1969).
5. GÖHDE, W.: Automation in der quantitativen Zytologie mit dem Impulscytophotometer. Mitteilungsdienst der Ges. z. Bekämpfung der Krebskrankheiten, Nordrhein-Westfalen e. V. 6, 255 (1972).
6. GÖHDE, W.: Zellzyklusanalysen mit dem Impulscytophotometer. Thesis, Med. Fak. Münster 1973.
7. GÖHDE, W.: Impulscytophotometrietest der Zytostatikawirkung, In: Aktuelle Probleme der Therapie maligner Tumoren (Ed. G. WÜST), p. 241. Stuttgart: Thieme 1973.
8. GÖHDE, W., DITTRICH, W.: Impulsfluorometrie - ein neuartiges Durchflußverfahren zur ultraschnellen Mengenbestimmung von Zellinhaltsstoffen. Acta histochem. Vol. 10, Suppl., 429 (1971).
9. GREMMEL, H., QUÄCK, J.: Zum Problem der Synchronisation von Tumorzellen bei kombinierter Zytostatika- und Strahlenbehandlung. Strahlentherapie 144, 35 (1972).
10. KISSEL, P., DUPREZ, A., BESSOT, M.: Essais de synchronisation in vivo de la synthèse de l'ADN de cellules malignes humaines par le 5-fluorouracile. Étude autohistoradiographique. C. R. Ser. D 262, 24: 2558 (1966).
11. KLEIN, H. O., GROSS, R., LENNARTZ, K. J.: Untersuchungen zur Proliferationskinetik und Synchronisation menschlicher Tumorzellen. Ihre Bedeutung für die zytostatische Therapie. Verh. dtsch. Ges. inn. Med. 77, 738 (1971).
12. LAMPKIN, B. C., NAGAO, T., MAUER, A. M.: Synchronization and recruitment in acute leukemia. J. clin. Invest. 50, 2204 (1971).
13. LENNARTZ, K. J., KLEIN, H. O., FEAUX DE LA CROIX, W., KLEIN, P. J.: Vergleichende in vivo- und in vitro-Untersuchung der Zellkinetik experimenteller Tumoren und die Bestimmung des Generationszyklus von Tumorzellen des Menschen in vitro. Verh. dtsch. Ges. Path. 55, 591 (1971).
14. MADOC-JONES, H., MAURO, F.: Age responses to X-rays, vinca alkaloids, and hydroxyurea of murine lymphoma cells synchronized in vivo. J. nat. Cancer Inst. 45, 1131 (1970).
15. MENDELSOHN, M. L.: Autoradiographic analysis of cell proliferation in spontaneous breast cancer of C3H mouse. III. The growth fraction. J. nat. Cancer Inst. 28, 1015 (1962).
16. MENDELSOHN, M. L.: Cell cycle kinetics and mitotically linked chemotherapy. Cancer Res. 29, 2390 (1969).
17. RAJEWSKY, M. F.: Proliferative parameters of mammalian cell systems and their role in tumor growth and carcinogenesis. Krebsforsch. 78, 12 (1972).
18. SCHUMANN, J.: Die Wirkung von Bleomycin auf die DNS von Tumorzellen in vivo und in vitro. In: Aktuelle Probleme der Therapie maligner Tumoren (Ed. G. WÜST). Stuttgart: Thieme 1973.
19. SCHUMANN, J., HATTORI, S.: Impulscytophotometrie der DNS bei soliden Tumoren unter Cytostatikaanwendung in vivo und in vitro. Vortrag: Symposium, Impulscytophotometrie; Heidelberg 1973.
20. SCHUMANN, J., EHRING, F., GÖHDE, W., DITTRICH, W.: Impulscytophotometrie der DNS in Hauttumoren. Arch. klin. exp. Derm. 239, 377 (1971).
21. SINCLAIR, W.: Cell cycle dependence of the lethal radiation response in mammalian cells. Current Topics in Radiat. Res. Quarterly 7, 264 (1972).
22. TERASIMA, T., TOLMACH, L. J.: Variation in several responses of HeLa cells to X-irradiation during the division cycle. Biophys. J. 3, 11 (1963).
23. TUBIANA, M.: The kinetics of tumor cell proliferation and radiotherapy. Brit. J. Radiol. 44, 325 (1971).
24. WANNENMACHER, M., GLUPE, J., ESSER, E., SCHUMANN, J.: Klinische Erfahrung mit der Strahlenbehandlung inoperabler maligner Tumoren nach Teilsynchronisation. Strahlentherapie (in press).

Experimental and Clinical Results of Chemotherapy after Partial Synchronization of Cell Proliferation*

H. O. KLEIN and R. GROSS

The planning of cytostatic treatment of malignant diseases should be based on precise knowledge of the mechanism of action and the pharmacokinetics of cytostatic drugs as well as of the proliferation kinetics of tumor cells. These conclusions are drawn from the investigations of SKIPPER and his co-workers (14).

In recent years numerous reports have been published showing that several cytostatic drugs attack specifically cell metabolism and kill proliferating normal and neoplastic cells in certain cycle phases. Others, however, display their cytocidal effects only in a certain phase, after damaging the metabolism in previous phases. The results were mainly obtained with partially synchronized cells in culture. They vary according to the cell lines, the drug concentration, and duration of exposure to the drug used. The serum half-life of these drugs is short and varies between 3 minutes for cytosine arabinoside and about 5 hours for hydroxyurea (9).

From the aspect of the proliferation behavior of malignant cell systems, the crucial points for therapy are wide deviations in the single cell-cycle times from the mean generation time of the proliferating cell compartment, and in particular, varying fractions of nonproliferating cells within a tumor.

But besides these kinetic data the mode of proliferation, i.e. asynchronous or synchronous growth, also seems to be of importance. In general, according to DUBLIN (2) and to our own (7) investigations, human tumor cells proliferate asynchronously.

Theoretically, these facts, i.e. asynchronous growth, varying fractions of nonproliferating tumor cells, and wide deviations of the single cell-cycle times from the mean generation time, are real obstacles to effective cytostatic treatment with drugs whose action is phase-specific. Provided that there is no primary resistance to the cytostatic agent, asynchronously proliferating malignant cells could be killed by a certain phase-specific drug only if, by the time of drug application they are in the sensitive cycle phase or will reach it while the cytotoxic blood level is still high. Thus a cytostatic drug being slowly eliminated from the blood is most effective on those asynchronously proliferating cells whose cycle time is equal to or shorter than the serum half-life of the drug.

---

*Supported by Deutsche Forschungsgemeinschaft

To make chemotherapy of tumors more effective it seemed it would be useful to accumulate asynchronously proliferating cells in the cycle phases most sensitive to certain cytostatic drugs. This means changing the asynchronous to synchronized proliferation. Synchronization of cell proliferation has long been performed in vitro. The criteria of cell synchrony have been well described (1).

In 1969, our group began to investigate the combination of partial synchronization of tumor-cell proliferation and the cell phase-specific application of a cytostatic drug. Some of these data have already been published (4-8). We used low doses of the spindle poison vincristine as inductor of synchronization and cyclophosphamide, which displays its cytocidal effects mainly during the S- and G2-phases, as an example of a cytostatic drug.

The degree of synchrony is dependent upon 1) the extent of deviation from the mean generation time, 2) the velocity of cell progression into the stage where the inductor displays its transitory effect, 3) the size of the growth fraction, and 4) the serum half-life of the inductor. Rapid desynchronization is due to a wide spread of single cell-cycle times (1).

Cytostatic treatment after induction of partial synchronization was studied in rapidly proliferating diploid and tetraploid Ehrlich-Ascites tumors at day 5 after tumor inoculation (log-phase growth). The proliferation data and the proof of synchronization are described by LENNARTZ and KLEIN elsewhere in this volume.

This section will show some experimental data collected in these animal tumors and relating to the therapeutic effect of cyclophosphamide after partial synchronization, and also the results of a pilot study in some human tumors.

A. ANIMAL EXPERIMENTS

The possibility of inducing partial synchronization of cell proliferation in vivo and knowledge of the cell-cycle and DNA-synthesis time of these Ehrlich-Ascites tumors (dipl. EAT and tetrapl. ELT) were used for cytostatic treatment with cyclophosphamide. DNA synthesis in both partially synchronized tumor cell populations began at the 35th hour for the EAT and the 26th hour for ELT after application of vincristine (LENNARTZ and KLEIN, this volume). The upper half of Fig. 1 shows the percentage of necrobiotic EAT cells in untreated animals and at various times after a single injection of vincristine (0.028 μg/g) or cyclophosphamide (0.1 mg/g) and also after cyclophosphamide (0.1 mg/g) during the DNA synthesis of partially synchronized EAT cells and after simultaneous application of vincristine (0.028 μg/g) and cyclophosphamide (0.1 mg/g). Necrobiotic tumor cells were determined by means of the supravital dye lissamine green (1% solution). The main conclusion drawn from this experiment is that cyclophosphamide is most effective when given during DNA synthesis in the partially synchronized EAT cells. There is a statistically significant increase in the necrobiotic index over a period of 24 hours. Vincristine applied alone in a dose which induces partial synchronization has no increased cytocidal effect compared to the spontaneous necrobiotic index in untreated animals.

Similar results were observed in tetraploid Ehrlich-Ascites tumor cells (ELT), as is shown in the lower half of Fig. 1. The highest number of necrobiotic cells was caused by cyclophosphamide applied during DNA synthesis in the partially synchronized cells.

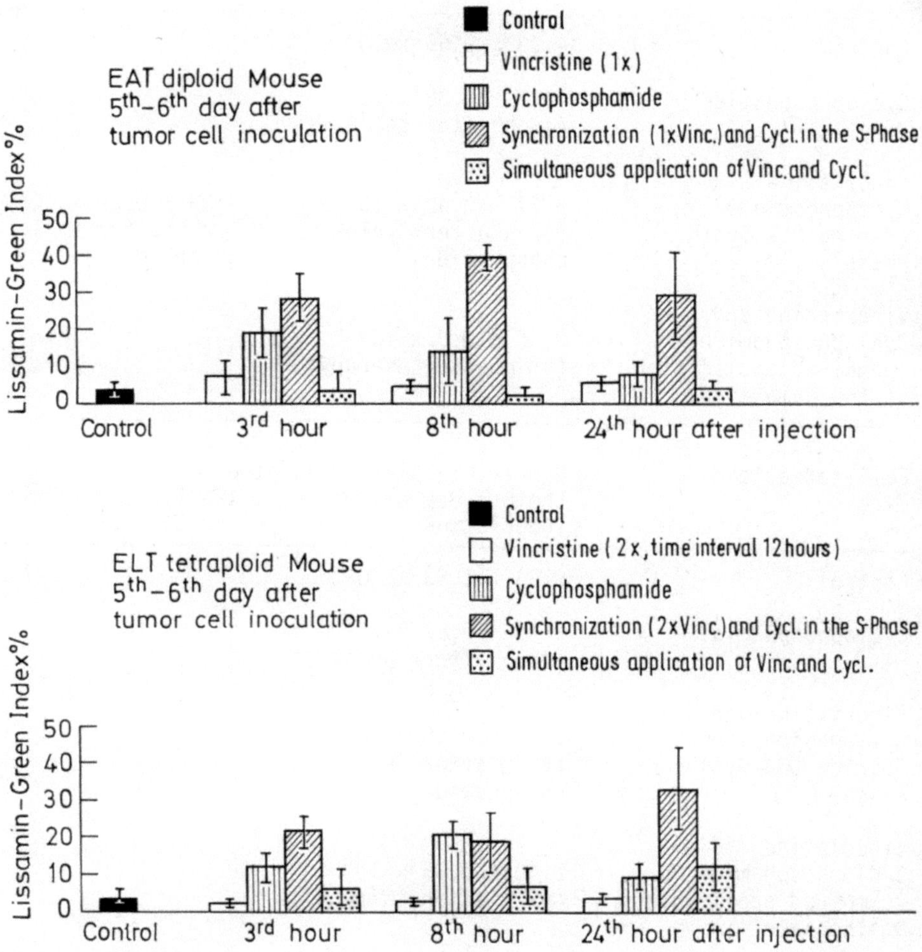

Fig. 1. Percentage of necrobiotic diploid (EAT) and tetraploid (ELT) Ehrlich-Ascites-Tumor cells in mice as a function of time after different cytostatic treatments. Confidential limits of the average values for p=5%. As supravital dye served Lissamine-Green. Intraperitoneal inoculation of 15-17x10^6 tumor cells

These results were also supported by cell counting (Fig. 2). Cyclophosphamide given during the S-phase of the synchronized cells (EAT and ELT) reduces the number of tumor cells in the abdominal cavity by a factor of almost two compared with the untreated controls and mice that have received cyclophosphamide alone. Simultaneous application of both vincristine and cyclophosphamide does not have any significant effect.

The survival rate of tumor bearing (EAT, ELT) animals is also better (by a factor of approximately two at the 50% level) when cyclophosphamide is given again during DNA synthesis in the partially synchronized cells.

EAT (diploid) Mice	Number of Tumor Cells at the 8th day after inoculation	the 9th day after inoculation
Control	$4.29 \pm 0.55 \times 10^8$	
Cyclophosphamide	$4.21 \pm 0.36 \times 10^8$ (48 h after therapy)	
Vincristine and Cyclophosphamide (during DNA Synth. Phase)	$2.77 \pm 0.49 \times 10^8$ (48 h after Cyclophosphamide)	$3.09 \pm 0.22 \times 10^8$ (72 h after Cyclophosphamide)
Vincristine and Cyclophosphamide (combined application at the same time)	$3.56 \pm 0.5 \times 10^8$ (48 h after therapy)	

ELT (tetraploid) Mice	Number of Tumor Cells at the 8th day after inoculation	the 9th day after inoculation
Control	$5.93 \pm 1.53 \times 10^8$	
Cyclophosphamide	$2.78 \pm 0.57 \times 10^8$ (48 h after therapy)	
Vincristine and Cyclophosphamide (during DNA Synth. Phase)	$1.31 \pm 0.98 \times 10^8$ (48 h after Cyclophosphamide)	
Vincristine and Cyclophosphamide (combined application at the same time)	$2.40 \pm 0.05 \times 10^8$ (48 h after therapy)	

Fig. 2. The influence of different cytostatic treatments on the number of diploid (EAT) and tetraploid (ELT) Ehrlich-Ascites-tumor cells in mice at the 8th and 9th (EAT) and 8th (ELT) day after intraperitoneal tumor-cell inoculation. Average values and standard deviations

Results similar to those in the ascitic tumors were observed in a diploid Ehrlich tumor growing subcutaneously (Fig. 3). The growth fraction of this solid tumor was in the range of 50%. As the figure shows, the best treatment is again the application of cyclophosphamide during the S-phase of the partially synchronized tumor cells. During four courses of treatment the tumor volume decreased to nearly unmeasurable values. However, after cessation of therapy, tumor growth recommences. From a theoretical point of view, this therapeutic result can only be explained by the assumption that after the individual courses of treatment, which followed one another at time intervals of 10 days, cells of the very large nonproliferating compartment were triggered into cycle and were consequently affected by the next cytostatic attack. Experiments are already under way to test this hypothesis.

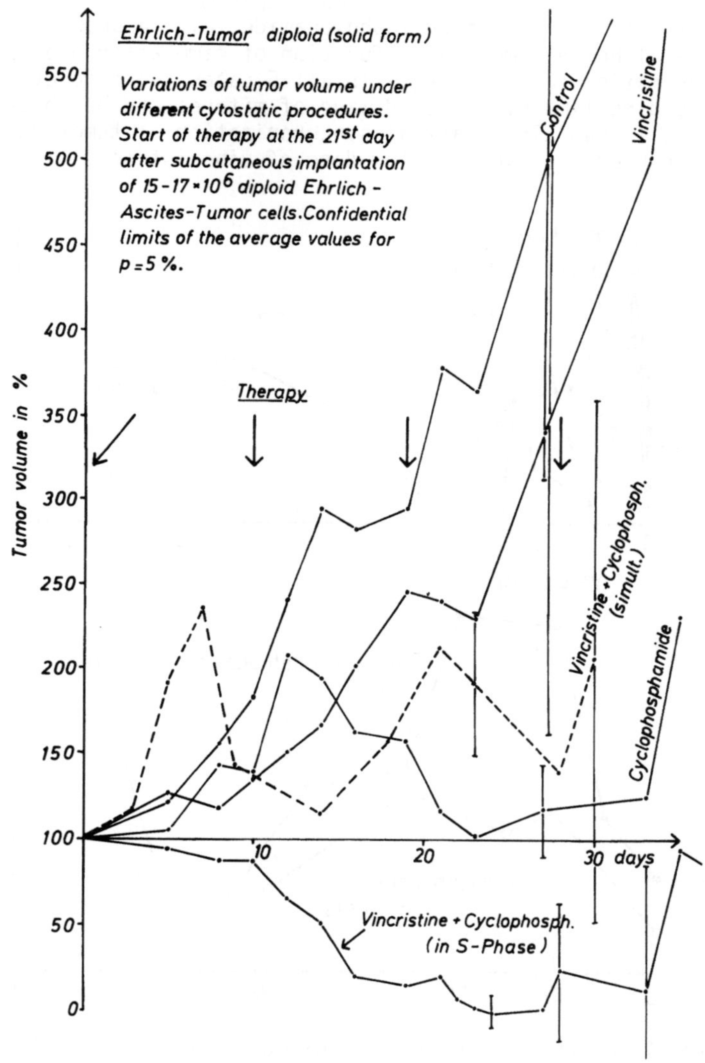

Fig. 3

These animal experiments show that pharmacological induction of partial synchronization of tumor cell proliferation can be exploited for therapy with cyclophosphamide. The therapeutic result is most marked after therapy during the S-phase of the synchronized cells. Recent findings (15) are consistent with our own; these authors showed (a) that partial synchronization can also be induced in L 1210 leukemia cells by vincristine, and (b) that this phenomenon can be exploited in an effective therapy with cytosine arabinoside during DNA synthesis of the synchronized cells.

B. INVESTIGATIONS IN HUMAN TUMORS

It was the aim of our investigation to test whether partial synchronization of cell proliferation in human tumors could be pharmacologically induced and whether, in analogy to the animal experiments, it might also make it possible to treat tumors with cyclophosphamide. Fig. 4 shows the mitotic curves of several human tumors as a function of time after one or two injections of vincristine (0.025 mg/kg). In all 5 cases two complete mitotic waves or the ascending limb of a second wave of mitoses can be observed. That indicates that, in man also, partial synchronization of tumor cell proliferation can be induced *in vivo* by a low dose of vincristine.

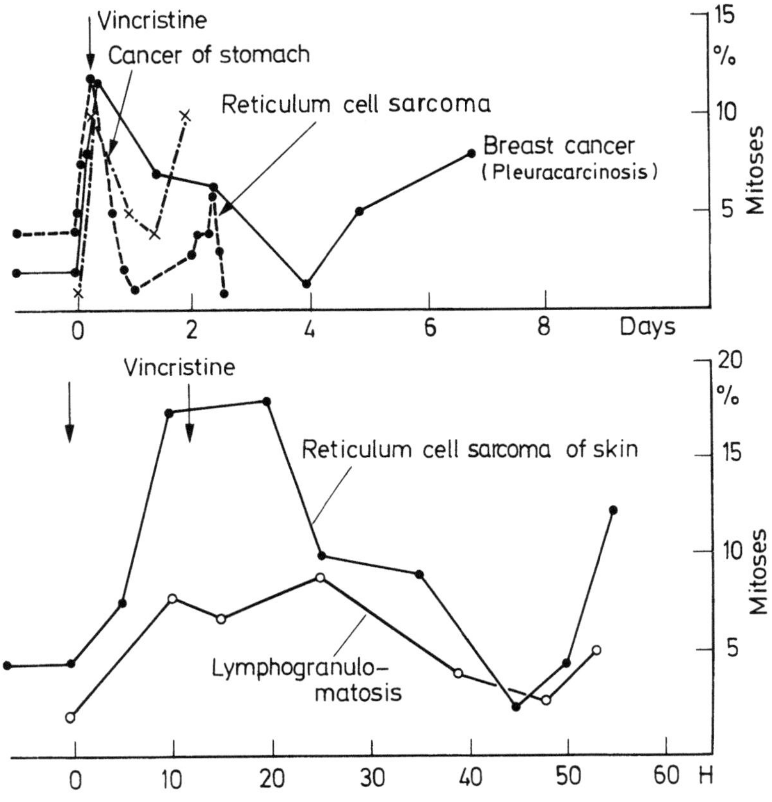

Fig. 4. Percentage of mitoses of malignant cells in human reticulum-cell sarcoma, breast cancer, cancer of stomach, and lymphogranulomatosis, as a function of time after one or two injections of vincristine

The essential prerequisite for phase-specific cytostatic treatment after partial synchronization is knowledge of the mean generation time and the duration of its subphases. In human tumors this is the crucial point. We tried to obtain approximate information on cell kinetics by means of an *in-vitro* method applying the double-labeling technique with H^3- and C^{14}-thymidine. Freshly explanted tumor tissue prepared as cell suspension and tissue pieces, and also bone-marrow aspirates are incubated for two hours in autologous plasma at

2.2 atm of oxygen and + 37°C. During the first hour, plasma contains 1 μC C^{14}-TdR/ml. At the end of the first hour cells are centrifuged, labeled plasma is removed, and after washing the cells are incubated again in fresh plasma containing 10 μC H^3-TdR/ml. At the end of the second hour, smears, histological sections, and autoradiograms are prepared. Staining is performed with Giemsa, H.-E., and PAS. The labeling index and the duration of the S-phase are measured directly. The minimal length of G_2 is determined according to the first appearance of labeled mitoses. The mean cell-cycle time is calculated from the labeling index and the duration of S, and corrected for log-phase growth. The mean duration of mitoses is calculated from the mitotic index and the mean cell-cycle time. Further technical details and results in several tumor types and methodological investigations are published elsewhere (3, 9, 12).

We are now also able to determine the approximate size of the growth fraction in vitro. We use two methods, one of which is a modification of the stathmokinetic method of ASTALDI. We combine the application of a spindle poison with that of H^3-TdR. Instead of colchicine we apply vincristine. For three hours the fraction of labeled mitoses/unlabeled mitoses is determined as a function of time. This curve allows us to calculate the flux of cells in mitosis. Under steady-state conditions this flux is constant throughout the cell cycle. Therefore, this value and the duration of S determined by the double-labeling technique are recorded in order to facilitate calculation of the real labeling index and the cell-cycle time for cells in the proliferating compartment. Furthermore, the quotient of the labeling index observed and the real labeling index calculated by means of the stathmokinetic method represents the fraction of cells in the proliferating compartment (growth fraction).

The size of the growth fraction can also be determined by means of the double-labeling technique. We measure the flux of cells in and out of the S-phase and calculate the real labeling index and the real cell-cycle time, as well as the size of the growth fraction in the way mentioned above.

Both methods work very well, as methodological in-vivo and in-vitro investigations in several animal tumors have shown. Preliminary results and further technical details will be published elsewhere (KLEIN et al., in preparation).

The values for the mean cell-cycle time yielded by the double-labeling technique can now be corrected according to the real size of the growth fraction. It is true that the value of these in-vitro data determined in a small specimen may be limited where the proliferation kinetics of cells in the whole tumor and its metastases are concerned. As mentioned above, the presence of numerous subclones of cells having different kinetic behavior within a tumor can lead to wide deviations from the mean generation time. The same is true for varying fractions of nonproliferating cells in different areas of a tumor. In general, however, zones of proliferation are mainly in the marginal areas of a tumor. For our studies we took specimens from this region, Our in-vitro data for cells of lymphoreticular tumors are consistent with those published in the literature (7, 9).

On the basis of these in-vitro data of proliferation kinetics we established a therapy scheme for the administration of cyclophosphamide during the S-phase of partially synchronized human tumor cells. For technical reasons, it was not possible to investigate every patient treated in this pilot trial completely with regard to synchronization or proliferation kinetics, and the following assumptions were made: 1) human tumor cells proliferate asynchronously, 2) in man partial synchronization of tumor-cell proliferation can be induced pharmacologically with vincristine, 3) a higher degree of synchronization can be obtained with two injections of vincristine , 4) the generation time of human tumor cells is lengthened by vincristine by a factor of 1.5.

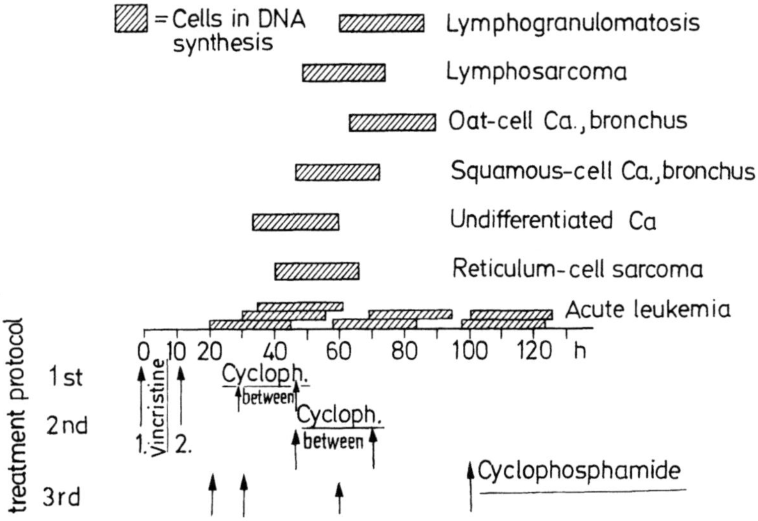

Fig. 5. Cytostatic treatment regime with high doses of cyclophosphamide given during DNA-synthesis phase of partially synchronized human tumor cells. Estimation of frequency of tumor cells synthesizing DNA as a function of time after two injections of vincristine according to in-vitro data on cell kinetics

In Fig. 5, the hatched boxes show the position of DNA-synthesizing cells after vincristine. This position was calculated from the duration of the mitotic block (about 10 hours) and the mean duration of G_1 lengthened by a factor of 1.5. According to this scheme, three treatment protocols can be deduced: 1) in patients with undifferentiated carcinoma, squamous-cell carcinoma of the bronchus, reticulum-cell sarcoma, and lymphosarcoma, cyclophosphamide was usually administered between 30 and 48 hours after the first injection of vincristine, 2) for patients with Hodgkin's disease and oat-cell carcinoma of the bronchus between 48 and 72 hours after the first injection of vincristine, 3) for patients with acute leukemia, because of the wide range of cell-cycle times, therapy was scheduled according to the individual values.

Our therapeutic results are as follows: Out of 67 cases - all previously treated with either X-rays or chemotherapy - 40 (about 59%) experienced transitory complete remission, and 20 (about 29%) partial remission; in 7 cases (about 12%) there was no response. The best results were obtained in lymphoreticular tumors. About 80% of patients with advanced disease (stages III and IV) experienced complete remission. These and the other results can be seen in the Table.

Other workers who have exploited synchronization have obtained similar therapeutic results in human solid tumors (13) and in acute leukemia of children and adults (10, 11, 16).

Table. Results of high-dose therapy with cyclophosphamide in rapidly growing human tumors after partial synchronization of the tumor cells

	Number of patients	Remission complete	Remission partial	Remission none
Acute leukemia	7	4	2	1
Reticulum cell sarcoma (advanced)	14	9	3	2
Lymphogranulomatosis	III B 9	9	-	-
	IV 10	1	7	2
Lymphosarcoma (advanced)	15	12	3	-
Bronchus Ca. (advanced)	7	1	5	1
Undifferentiated carcinoma (unknown primary tumor)	2	1	-	1
Undifferentiated adenoca of the stomach, skin metastases	1	1	-	-
Undifferentiated carcinoma of the tonsil; lung metastases	1	1	-	-
Malignant testicular teratoma, multiple lung metastases	1	1	-	-
Total	67	40 (ca.59%)	20 (ca.29%)	7 (ca.12%)

These favorable results led to the inception of a randomized trial with the MOPP scheme of DeVita and "synchronization therapy" in patients with advanced Hodgkin's disease, lymphosarcoma, and reticulum-cell sarcoma. The main goals of the trial are to compare 1) the remission rate, 2) the duration of maintained remission, 3) the percentage of severe side effects. The number of cases is still too small to allow firm conclusions. But as a preliminary result we can state that so far the remission rate is similar in the two groups. Should this be confirmed later, it would mean that therapy with a single drug given during a certain cycle phase of cells that are partially synchronized is as effective as a four-drug combination therapy given in the presence of asynchronously proliferating cells - at least in these tumors.

REFERENCES

1. CAMERON, J. L., PADILLA, G. M. (Eds): Cell synchrony. New York, London: Academic Press 1966.
2. DUBLIN, W. B.: Northw. Med. 43, 232 (1944).
3. KLEIN, H. O., LENNARTZ, K. J., EDER, M., GROSS, R.: Histochemie 21, 369 (1970).
4. KLEIN, H. O., LENNARTZ, K. J., HABICHT, W., EDER, M., GROSS, R.: Klin. Wschr. 48, 1001 (1970).
5. KLEIN, K. O., LENNARTZ, K. J., GROSS, R.: III. Internat. Congr. Lymphol., Brussels 1970, Abstr. Vol. , p. 10.
6. KLEIN, H. O., GROSS, R., LENNARTZ, K. J.: Verh. dtsch. Ges. inn. Med. 77, 738 (1971).
7. KLEIN, H. O., LENNARTZ, K. J., GROSS, R., EDER, M., FISCHER, R.: Dtsch. med. Wschr. 97, 1273 (1972).
8. KLEIN, H. O., LENNARTZ, K. J., TEICHMÜLLER, W., GROSS, R.: Proc. VII. Internat. Congr. Chemother. 2, 431 (1972).
9. KLEIN, H. O., LENNARTZ, K. J.: Sem. Hematol. 11, 203 (1974).
10. LAMPKIN, B. C., NAGAO, T., MAUER, A. M.: Nature 222, 1274 (1969).
11. LAMPKIN, B. C., NAGAO, T., MAUER, A. M.: XIII Internat. Congr. Hematol., Munich 1970, Abstr. Vol., p. 226.
12. LENNARTZ, K. J., KLEIN, H. O., FEAUX DE LA CROIX, W., KLEIN, P. J.: Verh. dtsch. Ges. Path. 55, 591 (1971).
13. POUILLART, P., SCHWARZENBERG, L., MATHÉ, G., SCHNEIDER, M., JASMIN, C., HAYAT, M., WEINER, R., DEVASSAI, F., AMIEL, J. L., BEYER, H. P., FAJ-BISOWIC, S., Nouv. Presse méd. 1, 1757 (1972).
14. SKIPPER, H. E.: The cell cycle and chemotherapy of cancer. In: The cell cycle and cancer (Ed. R. BASERGA), p. 355. New York: Marcel Dekker 19/1.
15. VADLAMUDI, S., GOLDIN, A.: Cancer Chemother. Rep. 55, 547 (1971).
16. VINCENT, P. C., CROSSEN, P., BUDDENDIECK, M., MELLOR, J., GUNZ, F. W.: XIII Internat. Congr. Hematol., Munich 1970, Abstr. Vol. 226.

Problems in the Treatment of Slow-Growing Tumors*

L. M. van Putten

The various aspects of the kinetics of slow-growing tumors in man are important in relation to the possibility of synchronization. Volume growth of many human tumors is slow compared to the tumors that grow so rapidly in small rodents. Three factors can be involved in this slow growth, and most often a combination of these factors is present. One is the prolongation of cell-cycle time, the second is the increasing fraction of cells that are not in cycle and which are not participating in the proliferation (Q-cells), and the third factor in some tumors is a significant degree of cell death. Cell death can be caused by different mechanisms; in some cells it may be due to an inherent deficiency which is incompatible with life, or it may be related to the structural environment of the tumor cells. The latter is probably the more frequent cause, and this cell death seems to be based on crowding and poor nutrition of the cells and is a direct or indirect consequence of overproduction of cells.

For our understanding of the importance of tumor growth rate it is necessary to introduce quantitative analysis of the cell destruction with and without synchronization: it is possible to make a model for a fast-growing tumor in which 10 - 20% of the cells are passing simultaneously through the sensitive phase and could be killed by a drug without synchronization, whereas with ideal synchronization 90% or more of the cells could pass through the sensitive phase simultaneously and be killed. Thus the ratio of cell destruction after synchronization to that before would be 5 : 10. Some animal models presented in this volume are based on long-transplanted tumors which could be synchronized very easily. On the basis of very extensive data on the cell kinetics, synchronization was effective, but the destruction after the same dose of the drug used was usually increased by a factor of about two. In the clinical situation we should not expect to obtain a very much higher level of effectiveness than in the experimental situation, since 1) our information on the cell cycle of each individual tumor is less complete and 2) the different clones of a primary tumor vary more widely in cell-kinetic parameters than is usually the case in transplanted tumors in mice. In our quantitative analysis even for fast-growing human tumors a gain factor of two is thus optimistic. But the effect in slow-growing tumors is still slighter, as shown by a quantitative estimate of the effects of cell synchronization: Fig. 1 presents a comparison of the effects which synchronization could have on tumors with different cell-kinetic parameters. The two columns on the left represent the composition of a tumor which has a high growth fraction (i.e. the majority

*Some of the studies reported here were carried out in the program of the EORTC Screening and Pharmacology Group.

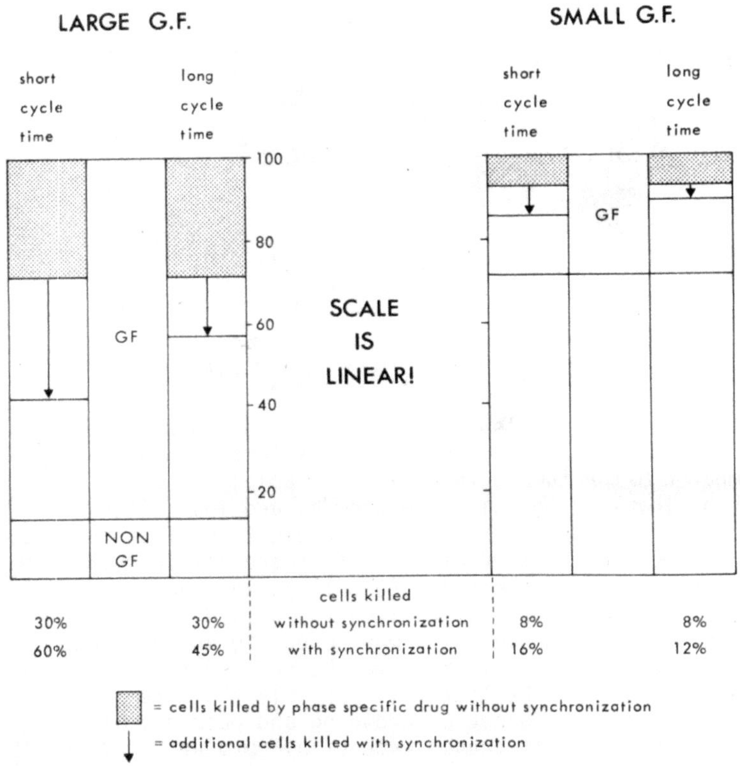

Fig. 1. Graphic representation of the effect of phase-specific cell destruction after synchronization of the proliferating cells in tumors with different proliferation parameters. The length of the downward arrow is an indication of the extra fraction of cells killed as a consequence of synchronization. P = proliferating cells, Q = quiescent cells. Columns I and II: tumors with a large growth fraction. Columns III and IV: tumors with a small growth fraction. Tumors in columns II and IV are characterized by a long cell-cycle time which is responsible for less complete synchronization

of the cells are in the cell cycle and therefore amenable to synchronization). The columns on the right represent tumors in which the growth fraction is much lower. But there are other differences; within each of these groups tumors vary in the length of the cell cycle. In this context a "long" cell cycle is one that is long in comparison to the duration of the synchronizing action. If cells are synchronized by being held up at a certain phase of the cycle, and if they are held there for two days, whereas the duration of the cell cycle is 5 days, for example, 40% of the cells will be collected at the holding point and synchronization will not be complete. There is presumably an upper limit to the time cells can be held for, which implies that the efficiency of cell synchronization is lower in tumors with a very long cell cycle. This is reflected in the second and fourth columns of Fig. 1; the destruction of the cycling cells when synchronization is achieved is not increased by 100% over the level without synchronization, but only by 50%. The numbers of cells killed are presented quantitatively as fractions of the totals with and without synchronization at the foot of each column. The figures range from 30% without and 60% with synchronization for a fast-growing tumor in which all cells have a short cell cycle and in which there is a large growth fraction, to 8% without and 12% with synchronization for the slowest-growing tumor.

This analysis has taken no account of the factor of cell death. Cell death is generally due to factors inherent in the structure of the tumor. This cell death can take place only if the number of cells increases beyond a certain figure. Destruction of cells by drugs may imply that the same number of cells is prevented from dying spontaneously due to crowding, and therefore this has the effect of decreasing the efficacy of any kind of therapy.

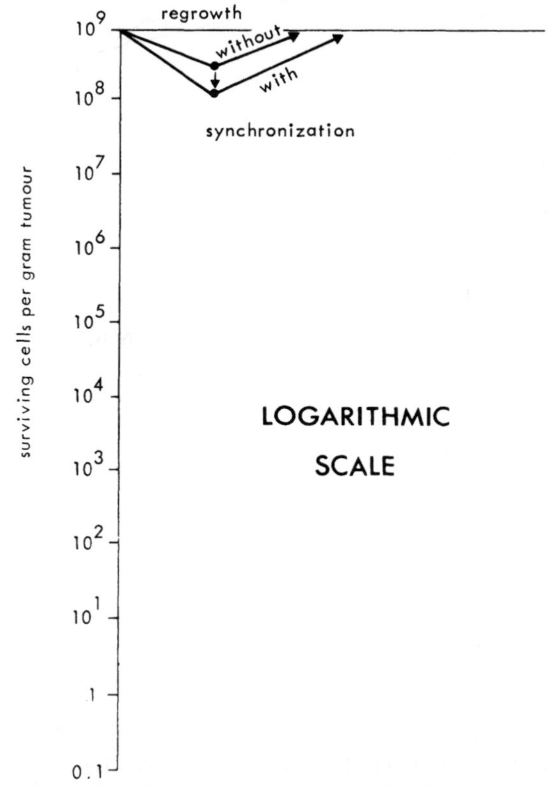

Fig. 2. The cell kill with and without synchronization, plotted in relation to the total number of tumor cells to be eliminated. Treatment with phase-specific agents in a single dose will almost never reduce cell survival by more than one decade. By synchronization, cell killing is increased from 30% to 60% in the fast-growing tumor. This implies a delay of about one doubling time in growth; for the most rapidly growing human tumors this is a few days. If the drugs kill only cells in cycle no major effect can be expected

In one series of treatment the percentage of tumor cells killed, ranged from 8 to 60. The object of treatment is the decrease in size or elimination of a tumor, and Fig. 2 shows how far short of this the effect falls, even in the best situation where the number of cells killed is doubled by synchronized treatment from 30 to 60%. This obviously does not result in cure of the disease. This is the situation in which the tumor grows rapidly, there is a short cell cycle and a short tumor-doubling time. It implies that the number of tumor cells will be approximately halved, which will be compensated by regrowth in one doubling time. Since this is short, it will cause only a brief decrease in tumor volume or the disease may remain stationary, since it may not be possible to measure the decrease during this period, which is probably of the order of a few days. Therefore the effect of treatment either with or without synchronization is not very significant.

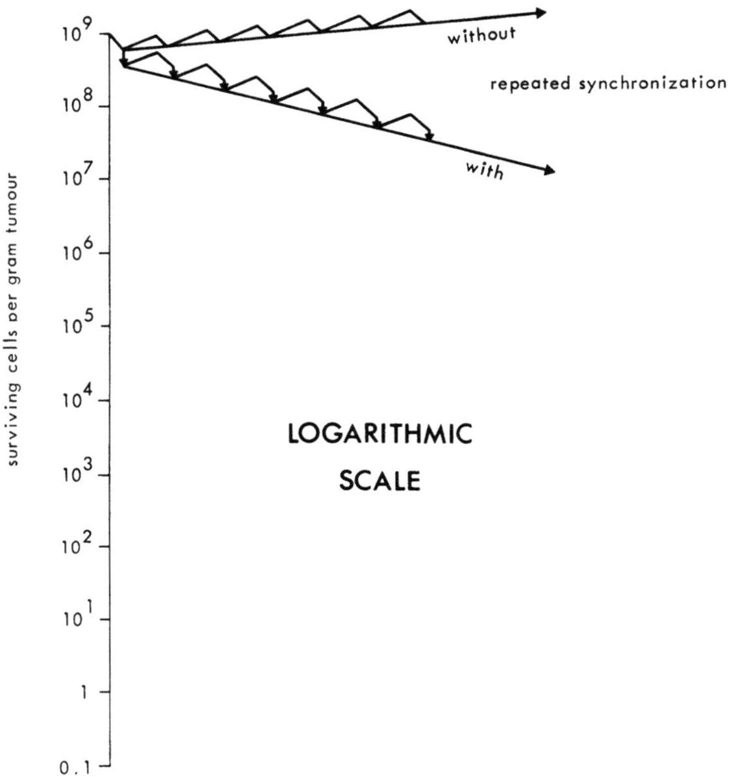

Fig. 3. Repeated synchronization followed by a phase-specific drug may be much more effective than a single exposure. Treatment without synchronization may permit a continuous increase in the number of tumor cells but when synchronization doubles the cell kill for each treatment there is a progressive decrease in surviving tumor cells

The alternative is illustrated in Fig. 3, and consists of repeated administration of drugs and repeated application of the whole schedule of synchronization. With this treatment it is possible that repeated administration over a long period may produce a prolonged remission of malignant disease. This graph also shows the effect in fast-growing tumors; for the slow-growing tumors the effects are obviously much slighter than a 30% increase in cell destruction; the effect is very much weaker initially, but the phenomenon of recruitment is observed; every time the treatment is repeated, additional cells enter the cycle and the tumor grows faster. As a result of this, two things will change in relation to the time scale depicted here; the down strokes on each treatment will be deeper, since the treatment will be more effective, but in addition the upstrokes will be steeper, since in each time interval between treatments there will be more repopulation. But, as on the whole the tumor will become more similar to the fast-growing tumor discussed earlier, it seems likely that with more treatment, the efficacy may actually improve and become similar to that depicted here. Thus repeated synchronization would in theory be preferable. The feasibility of this, i.e. the question as to whether there may be a synchronization scheme that disturbs the normal tissues so little that it can be used repeatedly seems an important point for further study. However, it may not be necessary.

Practicing physicians are very happy with the clinical results of synchronization schedules. Yet my analysis has just shown that we cannot expect major effects from a single synchronization treatment. There are two possible reasons for this:

1. My conclusions are based on false premises and synchronization is highly effective, even in a single application;
2. The good results would also be seen without synchronization and other factors are involved.

For obvious reasons it is the second possibility that I would like to discuss in more detail. It seems especially relevant to the group of the slow-growing tumors, which may contain the majority of the tumors treated in man. This category may also include most of the tumors that have been exposed to synchronization, with the exception of childhood leukemia. The fact that most of these tumors have many cells which are not in cycle makes it of the greatest interest to see what a drug which has multiple actions would do. Most alkylating agents are not only effective on the cycling cells, but also on cells which are out of cycle and do not belong to the growth fraction. These cells are usually killed with less efficiency but still to a significant extent (2, 14, 7). The use of alkylating agents as phase-specific drugs after synchronization will be associated with an effect on resting cells. The effect on resting cells can be weaker by a factor of two (expressed on the basis of dose). This effect is not negligible, and a glance at Fig. 1 shows that even half the effectiveness in killing noncycling cells with a drug of this kind will have an effect on the slow-growing tumors which could by far exceed the effect of killing the much smaller synchronized population. Of course we do not know whether the data collected on the effects of alkylating agents on hemopoietic stem cells are also valid for cells in solid tumors, but this possibility must be considered. This implies that before the success obtained with synchronization treatment can be convincingly shown to be really due to the synchronization and not to the use of particular drug combinations, controlled trials in which similar drugs are used with and without synchronization must be run.

There are two reasons for some distrust of the clinical importance of the data collected on phase specificity of cytostatic drugs: the curves observed for the dose-effect relationship in the killing of hemopoietic stem cells show a plateau, usually at doses much higher than the equivalent of the usual clinical dose (e.g. Fig. 5, upper part). If the dose that reduces cell survival to the plateau region is so high that it is never given to a patient, the plateau is less important and the rationale of the difference between phase-specific drugs and cycle-specific drugs is lost for clinical use under certain conditions.

In addition, there is reason to doubt whether findings which are valid for the resting cells in the mouse hemopoietic system are equally valid for tumor cells. The vinca alkaloids are clearly cell cycle phase-specific agents when applied to hemopoietic stem cells (2, 14, 7) or to HeLa cells and Chinese hamster cells in tissue culture (6). Yet other authors (5) have found that vincristine affects noncycling immunocompetent cells when these are exposed before they start to proliferate upon stimulation with phytohemagglutinin, and STRYCKMANS that vincristine can kill noncycling leukemic cells (1971).

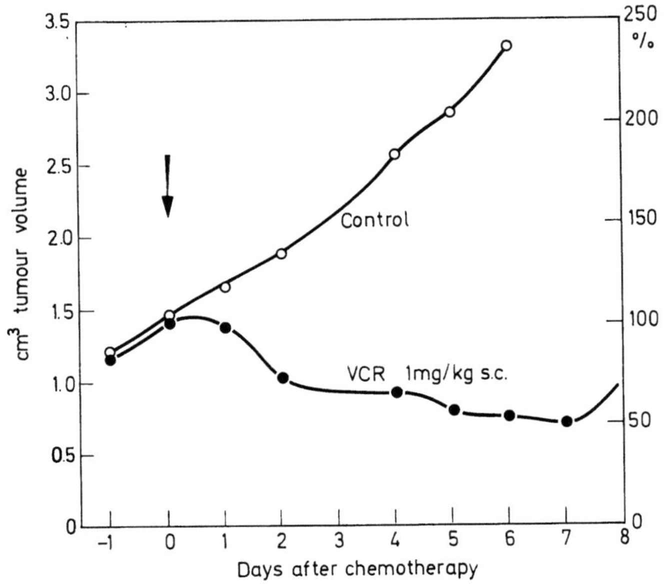

Fig. 4. Tumor volume measurements of subcutaneous rabdomyosarcoma implants in WAG/Rij rats. C = control rats; VCR = rats treated on day 0 with a single subcutaneous injection of 1 mg vincristine/kg body weight. Tumor volume decreases to about 50% on day 7. This indicates that cell survival must have been less than 50%. Yet the growth fraction in rabdomyosarcomas of this size is about 0.30 (3, 4). This indicates that vincristine must also have killed quiescent cells

Recently we observed marked volume reduction in a slow-growing solid tumor in rat after exposure to vinca alkaloids. In a first experiment we used a midlethal dose of vinblastine and noted a decrease of more than 80% in tumor volume, although the growth fraction of the large tumors of the type used is about 30% (4, 3). We considered the possibility that this might be an indirect effect due to the toxicity of the midlethal drug dose. In another study a single dose of 1 mg/kg vincristine was given, which also caused a protracted volume decrease to about 50% of this tumor in rats not ill from toxicity (Fig. 4). Two other possible explanations for the loss of noncycling cells in this tumor were ruled out. The first was loss by immune reactions; no tumor cell loss is observed in immunized rats (9, 12). The other explanation was based on an hypothetical lack of proliferation potential of noncycling cells, which has now also been ruled out (1). The inevitable conclusion seems to be that the vinca alkaloids also kill noncycling cells. Studies are in progress to obtain more quantitative determinations of the actual cell survival in tumors of this type in order to verify these conclusions, which have so far been drawn only on the basis of tumor-volume reduction. Nevertheless, it seems likely that our expression "phase-specific drugs" may be incomplete; it could be that the vinca alkaloids are phase-specific for certain tissues only or for certain cell types only.

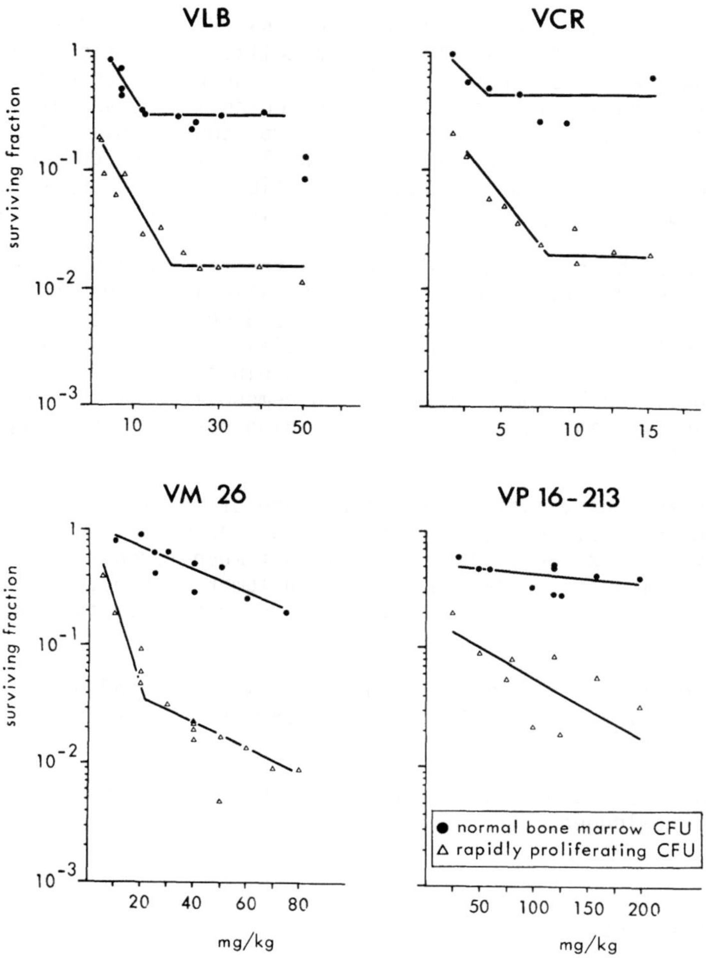

Fig. 5. Cell-survival curves for mouse spleen colony forming hemopoietic stem cells after exposure in vivo to spindle poisons. In each graph the upper curve and closed circles represent the survival of resting stem cells; lower curves and open triangles the survival of rapidly proliferating stem cells (7)

This possibility is consistent with the dose-effect curves of other spindle poisons, as is illustrated in Fig. 5. The curves for vincristine and vinblastine clearly show a plateau indicating that the resting cells are resistant. The curve for VM26[a] does not show a true plateau, showing that the resting subpopulation is not completely resistant to this drug; there is increased cell destruction with higher doses, although the latter part of the curve is not as steep as the initial component, which probably reflects destruction of part of the rapidly proliferating subpopulation. For VP 16-213[b] there is no plateau in the curve and no resistant subpopulation can be identified.

---

[a] 4'-demethyl epipodophyllotoxin-thenylidene glucoside

[b] 4'-demethyl epipodophyllotoxin-ethylidene glucoside

Evidence has been published (10) that VP 16-213 differs from the other spindle poisons in its fixed binding to cells. Drug action cannot be modified by washing the cells exposed in vitro. In contrast, suspensions exposed to vincristine and vinblastine show increased cell survival after the drugs have been washed out. A mechanism of this type could explain the toxicity of VP 16-213 for cells out of cycle, and it would also open up the possibility of a differential response of cell populations to these spindle poisons if the drug binding were partially reversible in some cell types but not in others.

These observations indicate that the terminology we use in distinguishing phase-specific from non-phase-specific agents may be rather loose, and at least for the spindle poisons should be reserved for certain drug-cell combinations in which phase specificity can be demonstrated, whereas this might not be true of other drug-cell combinations. The fact that these agents may specifically spare some resting hemopoietic stem cells is an advantage which may explain the good results of high doses of these agents used as introduction drugs.

These considerations show that some of the schedules described in the papers in this volume may be effective for reasons which have nothing to do with synchronization. It is evident that much further work must be done, both in experimental systems and in human tumor therapy, before we can fully understand the mechanisms responsible for effective therapy with cytostatic drugs.

The studies reported in this paper were carried out in collaboration with Mrs. J. DE RUITER, Mrs. L. KRAM and Mrs. M. PIJPERS.

Gifts of samples of VM 26 and VP 16-213 from Sandoz, Basle are gratefully acknowledged.

REFERENCES

1. BARENDSEN, G. W., ROELSE, H., HERMENS, A. F., MADHUIZEN, H. T., VAN PEPERZEEL, H. A., RUTGERS, D. H.: Clonogenic capacity of proliferating and nonproliferating cells of a transplantable ratrhabdomyosarcoma. J. nat. Cancer Inst. 51, 1521 (1953).
2. BRUCE, W. R., MEEKER, B. E., VALERIOTE, F. A.: Comparison of the Sensitivity of Normal Hematopoietic and Transplanted Lymphoma Colony-Forming Cells to Chemotherapeutic Agents administered in Vivo. J. nat. Cancer Inst. 37, 233 (1966).
3. HERMENS, A. F.: Variations in the cell kinetics and the growth rate in an experimental tumour during natural growth and after irradiation, Thesis. Rijswijk:Radiobiological Institute TNO 1973.
4. HERMENS, A. F., BARENDSEN, G. W.: Changes of Cell Proliferation Characteristics in a Rat Rhabdomyosarcoma Before and After X-Irradiation. Europ. J. Cancer 5, 173 (1969).
5. MCWILLIAMS, N. B., MAUER, A. M., LAMPKIN, B. C.: Dose dependent vincristine effects. Clin. Res. 19, 494 (1971).
6. MAURO, F., MADOC-JONES, H.: Age Response of Cultured Mammalian Cells to Cytotoxic Drugs. Cancer Res. 30, 1397 (1970).

7. PUTTEN, L. M. van, KRAM-IDSENGA, L. K. J.: Cell-Cycle Specificity and Therapeutic Effectiveness of Cytostatic Agents. Cancer Chemother. Reports 56, 691 (1972).
8. PUTTEN, L. M., van, LELIEVELD, P., KRAM-IDSENGA, L. K. J.: Abhängigkeit der Wirksamkeit Phasen-spezifischer Zytostatika vom Zellzyklus; Interpretation von Dosis-Wirkungskurven. In: Aktuelle Probleme der Therapie maligner Tumoren. Ed. by: G. W. WÜST, pp.197-208. Stuttgart: Georg Thieme 1973.
9. REINHOLD, H. S.: Evaluation of the Radiosensitivity of Cells of a Transplantable Rhabdomyosarcoma in the Rat. Europ. J. Cancer 2, 33 (1966).
10. STÄHELIN, H.: Reversibility of the cytostatic effect of the podophyllotoxin derivative VP 16-213. Abstract no. 150 in: Abstracts Volume B, 8th Intern. Congress of Chemotherapy, Athens (1973).
11. STRYCKMANS, P.: Kinetic Aspects of Leukemia Therapy. In: Cancer Chemotherapy, Ed. F. ELKERBOUT, P. THOMAS and A. ZWAVELING, p. 7. The Leiden University Press 1971.
12. TANNOCK, I. F.: Personal Communication 1971.
13. VALERIOTE, F., BRUCE, R. W.: Comparison of the Sensitivity of Hematopoietic Colony-forming Cells in different Proliferative States to Vinblastine. J. nat. Cancer Inst. 38, 393 (1967).
14. VALERIOTE, F. A., TOLEN, S. J.: Survival of Hematopoietic and Lymphoma Colony forming Cells In Vivo following the Administration of a Variety of Alkylating Agents. Cancer Research 32, 470 (1972).

Summary

R. Gross

Both normal and neoplastic cells can be divided into cells in proliferation, cells leaving the cycle on dying, and cells in the G_0-phase which can be stimulated to renewed proliferative activity. A cell population is determined mainly by the following factors: The length of the cycle (ranging from 1.5 months for human epidermis, to 15 - 18 hours for neutrophilic precursor cells), the fraction of dying cells, and that of G_0-cells. DNA and histones alternate in synthesis until DNA and histones are replicated and finally the cell divides. When WJ-38 human diploid fibroblasts in culture were used in tests, it was shown that the increase in chromatin template activity observed 1 hour after stimulation was not inhibited by actinomycin D, for example, whereas cycloheximide, an inhibitor of protein synthesis, was efficient in this respect. A nonhistone protein fraction with a middle weight of about 40,000 was distinctly increased 30 min after stimulation. There is an obvious difference between the nonhistone proteins of normal cells and those activated by certain viruses, e.g. SV 40.

In his study on proliferative parameters relevant to cancer-chemotherapy, M. RAJEWSKY (Tübingen) distinguished a P-compartment of proliferating cells from a Q-compartment with or without the capacity for re-entry of the cycle. Cytocidal effects may be connected with a higher sensitivity of dividing cells in general, and with a more or less phase-dependent specificity. However, for many agents the critical molecular interaction is still unknown. In addition, the phase specificity depends on the actual concentration of the drug at cell level. Furthermore, the phase of maximum sensitivity may be different from that in which arrest is observed. With the methods available it seems impossible to recognize small subpopulations of dividing cells against a background of large groups of nondividing cells. The majority of the nondividing cells have a G_1-DNA content, while a smaller fraction contain G_2+M-DNA. Only a small proportion of cells seem to be actually "clonogenic," i.e. to give rise to new cell clones, whereas other cells remain in a state of only potential clonogenic capacity.

The conditions of synchronization were described by A. CAPUTO (Rome) in terms of DNA synthesis and its control by different metabolites and enzymes, especially by transscriptase. Emphasis was laid on the problem of "cell-repair," which he differentiates from _de-novo_ synthesis.

Observations on synchronization by K. J. LENNARTZ and H. O. KLEIN (Cologne) started with _in-vitro_ models of diploid and tetraploid Ehrlich ascites tumors, a solid form and a solid mammary carcinoma. The asynchronous proliferating tumors were partially synchronized by one or two low doses of vincristine

(0.025 μg/g body weight). Cycle parameters were estimated by single and double labeling with ^3H or ^{14}C-thymidine respectively and also by means of Feulgen cytophotometry. The viability of cells was tested by staining with lissamin green. The authors demonstrated that the cells of all the tumors mentioned could be partially synchronized. However, the data revealed that only a moderate degree of synchronization was obtained, or that synchrony was lost again rather rapidly in further development. Vincristine prolonged the generation time by a factor of 1.5 - 3.0.

M. TUBIANA (Villejuif) started from very simple models and calculations and progresses through mouse experiments (determination of colony-forming units) to discuss the chances and limits of growth synchronization. Bone-marrow cells were killed in the S-phase by means of hydroxyurea, and remarkable recruitment was observed as little as 8 - 10 hours later. In addition, the cycle is changed by blocking maneuvers. Thus, it seems very difficult or even impossible to distinguish the interfering phenomena of synchronization and recruitment. In general terms, counteraction of neoplastic growth is efficient if 10^9 or more tumor cells are lethally damaged in relation to 10^4 or less bone-marrow cells.

Further examinations into the conditions of partial synchronization were performed with the aid of impulse cytophotometry. This method was found particularly well suited for quick determination of proportions in different cycle phases, as shown by J. SCHUMANN and his co-workers (Münster). Values of about 2 c correspond with the G_0 or G_1-phases, and values of 4 c with the G_2-phase, whereas the values for cells in the S-phase vary between these two limits. Bleomycin arrests cell division in the (G_2+M)-phase. This effect can be increased by repeated application. The result is effective partial synchronization, since the increase in the values for G_2 were also observed in subsequent cycles.

In the report by H. O. KLEIN and R. GROSS (Cologne) on experimental and clinical results of chemotherapy with partial synchronization, the standard schedule consisted of in-vitro predeterminations of the growth fraction, of the period of generation, and of different cycle phases in human neoplastic tissue samples taken by aspiration, biopsy or surgery. After a given time the application of 2 low doses of vincristine (usually 0.03 mg/kg body weight) was followed by one single dose of 30 - 60 mg/kg cyclophosphamide. The preliminary results with 69 patients were encouraging. The method proved at least as efficient as those yielding the best published results obtained by authors using polychemotherapy without adaptation to cell kinetics. A co-operative study involving several oncologic centers and comparing "blind" chemotherapy against partial synchronization is in progress.

In slow-growing tumors, the growth fraction of cells is reduced and/or the cell cycle is prolonged while the death rate of cells increases. After mentioning the difficulties encountered even with fast-growing tumors, L. M. van PUTTEN (Rijswijk) demonstrated that for slow-growing tumors the chances of chemotherapy are far worse. In fact, the majority of human tumors are slow-growing, and include various types which have been exposed to partial synchronization within the first series of his experiments.

Papers and an extensive discussion reproduced in this volume have promoted the understanding of cell kinetics as a basis for partial synchronization in tumor chemotherapy. They have also, however, shown up the remaining difficulties and the large gaps in general knowledge. More appropriate methods are required in particular for research on human neoplasias. The initial clinical experiences reported and demonstrated by several groups seem, nevertheless, to mark some advance on conventional polychemotherapy.

Subject Index

Recent Results in Cancer Research

Sponsored by the Swiss League against Cancer. Editor in Chief: P. Rentchnick, Genève

1 Schindler, R.: Die tierische Zelle in Zellkultur. Geb. DM 22,—, US $ 9.50
2 Neuroblastomas — Biochemical Studies. Edited by C. Bohuon (Symposium). Cloth DM 22,—; US $ 9.50
3 Hueper, W. C.: Occupational and Environmental Cancers of the Respiratory System. Cloth DM 45,—, US $ 19.40
4 Goldman, L.: Laser Cancer Research. Cloth DM 22,—; US $ 9.50
5 Metcalf, D.: The Thymus. Its Role in Immune Responses, Leukaemia Development and Carcinogenesis. Cloth DM 32,—; US $ 13.80
6 Malignant Transformation by Viruses. Edited by W. H. Kirsten (Symposium). Cloth DM 43,—; US $ 18.50
7 Moertel, Ch. G.: Multiple Primary Malignant Neoplasms. Their Incidence and Significance. Cloth DM 25,—; US $ 10.80
8 New Trends in the Treatment of Cancer. Edited by L. Manuila, S. Moles, and P. Rentchnick. Cloth DM 43,—; US $ 18.50
9 Lindenmann, J., and P. A. Klein: Immunological Aspects of Viral Oncolysis. Cloth DM 25,—; US $ 10.80
10 Nelson, R. S.: Radioactive Phosphorus in the Diagnosis of Gastrointestinal Cancer. Cloth DM 21,—; US $ 9.10
11 Freeman, R. G., and J. M. Knox: Treatment of Skin Cancer. Cloth DM 21,—; US $ 9.10
12 Lynch, H. T.: Hereditary Factors in Carcinoma. Cloth DM 32,—; US $ 13.80
13 Tumours in Children. Edited by H. B. Marsden and J. K. Steward. Cloth DM 96,—; US $ 41.30
14 Odartchenko, N.: Production Cellulaire Erythropoïétique. Relié DM 38,—; US $ 16.40
15 Sokoloff, B.: Carcinoid and Serotonin.
16 Jacobs, M. L.: Malignant Lymphomas Cloth DM 32,—; US $ 13.80 and Their Management. Cloth DM 25,—; US $ 10.80
17 Normal and Malignant Cell Growth. Edited by R. J. M. Fry, M. L. Griem, and W. H. Kirsten (Symposium). Cloth DM 70,—; US $ 30.10
18 Anglesio, E.: The Treatment of Hodgkin's Disease. Cloth DM 30,—; US $ 12.90
19 Bannasch, P.: The Cytoplasm of Hepatocytes during Carcinogenesis. Electron- and Lightmicroscopical Investigations of the Nitrosomorpholine-intoxicated Rat Liver. Cloth DM 40,—; US $ 17.20
20 Rubidomycin. A new Agent against Cancer. Edited by J. Bernard, R. Paul, M. Boiron, C. Jacquillat, and R. Maral. Cloth DM 59,—; US $ 25.40
21 Scientific Basis of Cancer Chemotherapy. Edited by G. Mathé (Symposium). Cloth DM 34,—; US $ 14.70
22 Koldovský, P.: Tumor Specific Transplantation Antigen. Cloth DM 30,—; US $ 12.90
23 Fuchs, W. A., J. W. Davidson, and H. W. Fischer: Lymphography in Cancer. With contributions by G. Jantet and H. Rösler. Cloth DM 93,—; US $ 40.00
24 Hayward, J.: Hormones and Human Breast Cancer. An Account of 15 Years Study. Cloth DM 42,—; US $ 18.10
25 Roy-Burman, P.: Analogues of Nucleic Acid Components. Mechanisms of Action. Cloth DM 34,—; US $ 14.70
26 Tumors of the Liver. Edited by G. T. Pack and A. H. Islami. Cloth DM 68,—; US $ 29.30
27 Szymendera, J.: Bone Mineral Metabolism in Cancer. Cloth DM 40,—; US $ 17.20
28 Meek, E. S.: Antitumour and Antiviral Substances of Natural Origin. Cloth DM 20,—; US $ 8.60
29 Aseptic Environments and Cancer Treatment. Edited by G. Mathé (Symposium). Cloth DM 30,—; US $ 12.90
30 Advances in the Treatment of Acute (Blastic) Leukemias. Edited by G. Mathé (Symposium). Cloth DM 46,—; US $ 19.80
31 Denoix, P.: Treatment of Malignant Breast Tumors. Indications and Results. Cloth DM 58,—; US $ 25.00

32 NELSON, R. S.: Endoscopy in Gastric Cancer. Cloth DM 58,—; US $ 25.00
33 Experimental and Clinical Effects of L-Asparaginase. Edited by E. GRUNDMANN and H. F. OETTGEN (Symposium). Cloth DM 71,—; US $ 30.60
34 Chemistry and Biological Actions of 4-Nitroquinolin 1-Oxide. Edited by H. ENDO, T. ONO, and T. SUGIMURA. Cloth DM 40,—; US $ 17.20
35 PENN, I.: Malignant Tumors in Organ Transplant Recipients. Cloth DM 30,—; US $ 12.90
36 Current Concepts in the Management of Lymphoma and Leukemia. Edited by J. E. ULTMANN, M. L. GRIEM, W. H. KIRSTEN, and R. W. WISSLER (Symposium). Cloth DM 53,—; US $ 22.80
37 CHIAPPA, S., R. MUSUMECI, and C. USLENGHI: Endolymphatic Radiotherapy in Malignant Lymphomas. With contributions by G. BONADONNA, B. DAMASCELLI, G. FAVA, F. PIZZETTI, U. VERONESI. Cloth DM 53,—; US $ 22.80
38 KOLLER, P. C.: The Role om Chromosomes in Cancer Biology. Cloth DM 53,—; US $ 22.80
39 Current Problems in the Epidemiology of Cancer and Lymphomas. Edited by E. GRUNDMANN and H. TULINIUS (Symposium). Cloth DM 64,—; US $ 27.60
40 LANGLEY, F. A., A. C. CROMPTON: Epithelial Abnormalities of the Cervix Uteri. Cloth DM 64,—; US $ 27.60
41 Tumours in a Tropical Country. A Survey of Uganda (1964—1968). Edited by A. C. TEMPLETON. Cloth DM 79,—; US $ 34.00
42 Breast Cancer: A Challenging Problem. Edited by M. L. GRIEM, E. V. JENSEN, J. E. ULTMANN, and R. W. WISSLER (Symposium). Cloth DM 53,—; US $ 22.80
43 Nomenclature, Methodology and Results of Clinical Trials in Acute Leukemias. Edited by G. MATHÉ, P. POUILLART, and L. SCHWARZENBERG (Symposium). Cloth DM 64,—; US $ 27.60
44 Special Topics in Carcinogenesis. Edited by E. GRUNDMANN (Symposium). Cloth DM 58,—; US $ 25.00
45 KOLDOVSKÝ, P.: Carcinoembryonic Antigens. Cloth DM 38,—; US $ 16.40
46 Diagnosis and Therapy of Malignant Lymphoma. Edited by K. MUSSHOFF (Symposium). Cloth DM 62,—; US $ 26.70
47 Investigation and Stimulation of Immunity in Cancer Patients. Edited by G. MATHÉ and R. WEINER (Symposium). Cloth DM 96,—; US $ 41.30
48 Platinum Coordination Complexes in Cancer Chemotherapy. Edited by T. A. CONNORS and J. J. ROBERTS (Symposium). Cloth DM 68,—; US $ 29.30
49 Complications of Cancer Chemotherapy. Edited by G. MATHÉ and R. K. OLDHAM (Symposium). Cloth DM 58,—; US $ 25.00
50 Cancer Registry. Edited by E. GRUNDMANN and E. PEDERSEN (Symposium). Cloth DM 48,—; US $ 20.70
51 Gliomas. Current Concepts in Biology, Diagnosis and Therapy. Edited by J. HEKMATPANAH (Symposium). Cloth DM 54,—; US $ 23.30
52 The Ambivalence of Cytostatic Therapy. Edited by E. GRUNDMANN and R. GROSS (Symposium). Cloth 58,—; US $ 25.00

Special Supplement: Biology of Amphibian Tumors. Edited by M. MIZELL. Cloth DM 106,—; US $ 45.60

Prices are subject to change without notice

MIX
Papier aus verantwortungsvollen Quellen
Paper from responsible sources
FSC® C105338

If you have any concerns about our products,
you can contact us on
ProductSafety@springernature.com

In case Publisher is established outside the EU,
the EU authorized representative is:
Springer Nature Customer Service Center GmbH
Europaplatz 3, 69115 Heidelberg, Germany

Printed by Libri Plureos GmbH
in Hamburg, Germany